HEALTHCARE REFORM, QUALITY AND SAFETY

Healthcare Reform, Quality and Safety

Perspectives, Participants, Partnerships and Prospects in 30 Countries

Edited by

JEFFREY BRAITHWAITE
Macquarie University, Australia

YUKIHIRO MATSUYAMA
Canon Institute for Global Studies, Japan

RUSSELL MANNION
University of Birmingham, UK

&

JULIE JOHNSON
Northwestern University, USA

ASHGATE

Published by
Ashgate Publishing Limited
Wey Court East
Union Road
Farnham
Surrey, GU9 7PT
England

Ashgate Publishing Company
110 Cherry Street
Suite 3-1
Burlington, VT 05401-3818
USA

www.ashgate.com

British Library Cataloguing in Publication Data
A catalogue record for this book is available from the British Library

The Library of Congress has cataloged the printed edition as follows:
Healthcare reform, quality and safety : perspectives, participants, partnerships, and prospects in 30 countries / [edited] by Jeffrey Braithwaite, Yukihiro Matsuyama, Russell Mannion, and Julie Johnson.
    p. ; cm.
Includes bibliographical references and index.
ISBN 978-1-4724-5140-8 (hardback) -- ISBN 978-1-4724-5141-5 (ebook)
-- ISBN 978-1-4724-5142-2 (epub)
 I. Braithwaite, Jeffrey, 1954- , editor. II. Matsuyama, Yukihiro, 1953- , editor. III. Mannion, Russell, editor. IV. Johnson, Julie K., editor.
 [DNLM: 1. Health Care Reform. 2. Internationality. 3. Patient Safety. 4. Quality of Health Care. 5. Safety Management. WA 525]
 RA413.5.U5
 362.1'0425--dc23
                                                                                2014038604

ISBN: 978-1-4724-5140-8 (HBK)
      978-1-4724-5141-5 (EBK)
      978-1-4724-5142-2 (EPUB)

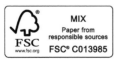

Printed in the United Kingdom by Henry Ling Limited, at the Dorset Press, Dorchester, DT1 1HD

Contents

List of Figures

List of Tables

List of Contributors

William Adu-Krow BSc, MB, ChB, MPH, DrPH is presently the Pan American Health Organization/World Health Organization (PAHO/WHO) representative of Guyana. He was previously the WHO country representative for Papua New Guinea between September 2010 and January 2014. He also serves on a pro bono basis as an Adjunct Professor at the Center for Population and Family Health of the Mailman School of Public Health at Columbia University, New York. He has worked in Ghana, New York, Washington DC, New Jersey, Solomon Islands, and Papua New Guinea. His main work has focused on violence against women and the impact of social determinants on global health architecture.

Ahmed Al-Mandhari MD, DTM&H, MRCGP (Int), PhD is a graduate of the College of Medicine & Health Sciences at Sultan Qaboos University, Oman and holds a Diploma in Tropical Medicine and Hygiene, PhD in Health Care Quality Management (2002), University of Liverpool, and a MRCGP (International). He was previously Head of Quality Management Department, Deputy Director General for Clinical Affairs, then Director General of the Sultan Qaboos University Hospital, and has acted as a WHO consultant on patient safety.

Hugo Arce MD, MPH, PhD is a physician. He was President and CEO of the Technical Institute for Accreditation of Healthcare Organizations 1994–2010 and President of the Argentine Society for Quality in Health Care. He is now Director of the Department of Public Health at the University Institute of Health Sciences, Barceló Foundation, Buenos Aires. He is the author of "The Territory of Health Decisions," "The Quality in the Health Territory," "The Health System: where it comes from and where it goes," as well as more than 150 articles and papers on health policy, hospital management, and quality in healthcare.

Arlene S Bierman MD, MSc, Dr is inaugural holder of the Ontario Women's Health Council (OWHC) Chair in Women's Health and Professor of Health Policy, Evaluation, and Management, Public Health, Nursing, and Medicine at the University of Toronto; and Senior Scientist in the Li Ka Shing Knowledge Institute at St. Michael's Hospital. She was a 2012–2013 Atlantic Philanthropies Health and Aging Policy Fellow/American Political Science Foundation Congressional Fellow. Her research examines service delivery and finance models on access, quality, and health outcomes among older adults, with a focus on socioeconomically disadvantaged populations.

Brette Blakely BA (summa cum laude), MA, PhD completed her undergraduate degree at Wellesley College in the US before migrating to Australia where she undertook her Masters degree in Bioethics. Subsequently she completed her PhD in Neuroscience at the Florey Institute for Neuroscience and Mental Health, University of Melbourne. Currently she is a Post Doctoral Research Fellow at the Australian Institute of Health Innovation, Macquarie University, Australia, working on projects related to patient safety and health reform. She has wide-ranging interests and expertise in health and medical challenges in differing settings.

Jeffrey Braithwaite BA, MIR (Hons), MBA, DipLR, PhD, FAIM, FCHSM, FFPH RCP (UK) is Foundation Director, Australian Institute of Health Innovation and Professor of Health Systems Research, Macquarie University, Australia. His research examines the changing nature of health systems, attracting funding of more than AU\$59 million. He has published extensively (more than 500 total publications) and he has presented at international and national conferences on more than 500 occasions, including over 60 keynote addresses. His co-edited books include *Resilient Health Care*, 2013 and *Culture and Climate in Health Care Organisations*, 2010.

Americo Cicchetti Laurea, Economia, PhD, Management is Professor of Management at the Catholic University, Faculty of Economics, Rome. He is Director of the Graduate School of Health Economics and Management at the Catholic University of Sacred Heart and a Member of the Price & Reimbursement Committee of the Italian National Drug Agency (AIFA). His research interests cover organizational design and human resource management in healthcare and the application of health technology assessment approaches for hospital management.

Silvia Coretti MSc, PhD, is a post doctoral researcher at the Catholic University of the Sacred Heart, Faculty of Economics, Rome (Italy). Her research interests include the economic evaluation of healthcare programs within the health technology assessment framework, with a particular focus on the issues concerning preference-based outcome measures.

Jacqueline Cumming BA, MA (1st class Hons), Economics, Dip Health Econ, PhD, Public Policy is Director of the Health Services Research Centre (HSRC), School of Government, Victoria University of Wellington, New Zealand. She has extensive public policy experience, having worked for New Zealand government organizations, including the Ministry of Health, prior to joining the HSRC. Her research interests are in priority setting, access to health services, primary healthcare and health systems reform, quality of care, and evaluation. She currently leads projects exploring the performance of the health system and key health services in New Zealand. She is currently president of the Health Services Research Association of Australia and New Zealand.

Ellen Catharina Tveter Deilkås Registered Specialist Internal Medicine, MD, PhD is a consultant in internal medicine with 20 years of clinical experience. She holds a PhD in patient safety culture and is a senior scientist at the Centre for Health Services Research at Akershus University Hospital. She conducts research on quality and patient safety improvement, and works part time with stroke rehabilitation. She holds a 20 percent position as a senior advisor for the Norwegian Knowledge Centre for Health Services, specifically responsible for national measurement of medical injury and patient safety culture. The measurements are part of the government's patient safety program.

Stephen Duckett BEc, MHA, PhD, DBA, DSc, DipEd(Tert), DipLegStud, FASSA FAICD is Director of the Health Program at Grattan Institute. He has a reputation for creativity, evidence-based innovation, and reform in areas ranging from the introduction of activity-based funding for hospitals, to new systems of accountability for the safety of hospital care. An economist, he is a Fellow of the Academy of the Social Sciences in Australia. He has extreme experience in health financing, health economics, and health policy.

Ezequiel García Elorrio MD, MSc, MBA, PhD is at the University of Buenos Aires. He specialized in Internal Medicine, Center for Medical Education and Clinical Investigation, and has an MA in Epidemiology, Harvard School of Public Health. Founder and board member of the Institute for Clinical Effectiveness and Health Policy (IECS) in Buenos Aires; Head of the Department of Health Care Quality and Patient Safety; Associate Professor of Public Health in the Faculty of Medicine CEMIC; Professor at the School of Public Health at UBA; and board member of the Master of Clinical Effectiveness at UBA. His primary interest is healthcare quality. He is currently funded by WHO, United States Agency for International Development/ Program for Appropriate Technology in Health (USAID/PATH), the Mapfre Foundation, and the Fogarty Center of the United States.

Carsten Engel MD is Deputy Chief Executive, Danish Institute for Quality and Accreditation in Healthcare (IKAS) and previously a specialist in anesthesiology. Since 2010 he has been a member of ISQua's Accreditation Council and an ISQua surveyor. He has contributed to the development and management of the Danish Healthcare Accreditation Program and is engaged in ensuring that IKAS draws upon and supports research in accreditation. He has an interest in healthcare as a complex system and the mechanisms by which accreditation can achieve an effect on the performance of healthcare providers.

Jesper Eriksen MSc, Political Science, is Special Advisor, Quality & Safety, the Danish Cancer Society. He holds a Master of Political Science degree and takes special interest in the interaction between the economic and political organization of the healthcare system and the quality of the healthcare efforts. He works with data-driven quality improvement in cancer treatment and is interested in monitoring progress from organizational, clinical, and user perspectives.

Hong Fung MBBS (HK), MHP (NSW), FRCS (Edin), FHKAM (Surg), FCSHK, FHKAM (Community Medicine), FHKCCM, FFPH (UK), FRACMA is currently Honorary Professor at the JC School of Public Health & Primary Care, the Chinese University of Hong Kong. He is also the President of the Hong Kong College of Community Medicine. His academic interest is in medical leadership and health system performance. Professor Fung was the Cluster Chief Executive of the New Territories East Cluster at the Hong Kong Hospital Authority in 2002–2013, responsible for the delivery of hospital care for a population of 1.3 million. He is acknowledged for his expertise in hospital planning and health informatics.

Tristan D Gloede Dipl.-Ges.-Ök. is currently a research associate at the Institute for Medical Sociology, Health Services Research and Rehabilitation Science, and is a graduate health economist from the University of Cologne, Germany. He is currently a doctoral candidate at the Faculty of Management, Economics, and Social Sciences at the University of Cologne. His research interests are organizational determinants of quality and efficiency of care, health economic evaluation, and outcomes research.

Adelia Quadros Farias Gomes MD, MBA, MSc has expertise in public health with an emphasis on hospital management. He was previously coordinator of the Outpatient Department of federal hospitals in Rio de Janeiro between 1998 and 2004. He is a Visiting Professor of the Master Course in Evaluation of Cesgranrio Foundation (discipline: Health Evaluation). Since 2001 he has been a consultant to the Brazilian Consortium for Accreditation of Health Systems and Services, in the Joint Commission International accreditation process. He also coordinates the Quality and Safety Committee of the federal hospitals in Rio de Janeiro.

Octavio Gómes-Dantés MD, MPH is senior researcher at the Center for Health Systems Research of the National Institute of Public Health of Mexico. His areas of academic expertise are health policy and global health. He holds a medical degree from the Autonomous Metropolitan University (Mexico) and two master degrees, one in Public Health and the other one in Health Policy and Planning, both from the Harvard School of Public Health (US).

Victor Grabois MD, MPH, MSc studied undergraduate Medicine at the Federal University of Rio de Janeiro and holds an MSc in Social Medicine. Since 2010 he has been a PhD student in Public Health at the ENSP/Fiocruz. Currently he is the General Coordinator of the National Qualification Course in Management of SUS, in the form of distance education and acts as coordinator (Fiocruz) of the process of developing educational modules and evaluative research under the Program for the Enhancement of Primary Care. He is also coordinator for the Executive Collaborating Centre for Quality of Care and Patient Safety.

Girdhar J Gyani BE, ME, PhD is currently the Director General, Association of Healthcare Providers (India). Prior to this he was Secretary General, Quality Council of India (2003–2012), a peak national body responsible for establishing and operating national accreditation structures and promoting quality in all walks of life. Dr Gyani was founding CEO of the National Accreditation Board for Hospitals and Healthcare Providers (NABH) and is currently an Honorary Member of Board. Dr Gyani served on the board of ISQua from 2009–2013.

Antje Hammer Dipl.-Soz is a state-examined nurse and graduate sociologist from the University of Bamberg, Germany. Her studies focus on quantitative and qualitative methods in empirical social research. Since 2008 she has been a research associate at the Institute for Medical Sociology, Health Services Research and Rehabilitation Science at the University of Cologne. Dr Hammer's main research fields are hospital management, safety cultures, patient safety, and quality of healthcare.

Sophia Hermawan DDS, MPH/Epidemiologist is Director of Human Resources Development at the National Brain Center Hospital, which is one of the hospitals owned and directly supervised by the Ministry of Health of the Republic of Indonesia. She is interested in quality improvement and especially in hospital accreditation. Dr Hermawan has been involved in the National Longterm Planning program, which was launched to reach international standards for government hospital services.

Valentina Iacopino PhD is postdoctoral researcher at the Catholic University of the Sacred Heart, Faculty of Economics, Rome (Italy). Her research interests focus on the diffusion and adoption processes of health technologies and on policy issues and governance of innovations in a healthcare context.

Tor Ingebrigtsen MD, PhD is CEO of the University Hospital of North Norway. He graduated from the University of Tromsø—the Arctic University of Norway (UiT) in 1988, trained as a neurosurgeon in Tromsø and Oslo, and has a PhD in the management of mild head injuries (1998). He was head of neurosurgery at UNN (1998–2005) and medical director for the Regional Health Authorities of North Norway (2005–2007). He is Associate Professor of Neurosurgery at UiT, and visiting Professor at the Australian Institute of Health Innovation, Macquarie, Australia. His recent research focuses on lean improvements and the impact of leadership on health IT.

Julie Johnson MSPH, PhD (evaluative clinical sciences) is Professor at Northwestern University (US). Previously she was Associate Professor in the Faculty of Medicine and Deputy Director of the Centre for Clinical Governance Research at the University of New South Wales in Sydney Australia. Her career interests involve building a series of collaborative relationships to improve the quality and safety of healthcare through teaching, research, and clinical improvement. She uses qualitative methods to study processes of care with the ultimate goal of translating theory into practice while generating new knowledge about the best models for improvement.

Abdelrahman A Kamel MBBS, MSc (Cardiology), DTQM (AUC) is currently acting Head of Technical Medical Affairs Department, Executive Board of the Health Ministers' Council for Cooperation Council States. He is Healthcare Quality & Patient Safety advisor, in addition to other responsibilities including facilitator for many Gulf Committee and Programs mainly concerning quality and patient safety, risk management, evidence-based medicine, and noncommunicable diseases control and prevention. He is co-author of more than eight books and manuals.

Tawfik Khoja MBBS, DPHC, FRCGP, FFPH, FRCP (UK) is Director General, Executive Board of the Health Ministers' Council for Cooperation Council States. He is a fellow of the Royal College of General Practitioners (UK), also of the Faculty of Public Health and of the Royal College of Physician (UK). He has been Adjunct Professor in Health Systems and Quality at Oklahoma University and received the professorial degree from Imperial College London (UK). He is a WHO temporary advisor. He is author and co-author of more than 40 books and manuals, and has published more than 70 research and scientific articles in international scientific journals.

Janne Lehmann Knudsen MD, Specialist in Public Health Medicine/ Community Medicine, PhD, MHM, is Director of Quality, Danish Cancer Society and specialist in Public Health Medicine. Since 2010 she has been board member of ISQua. She is a member of national committees and chairs the Advisory Council of Danish Knowledge Center for User Involvement. She has held positions as healthcare researcher and healthcare planner and has been a leading surveyor at the Danish Institute of Quality and Accreditation and Associate Professor at the University of Copenhagen. She has published several scientific papers and among others published a textbook on regulating quality in Danish healthcare.

Grace Labadarios MBChB, DRCOG, MRCGP graduated from the University of Stellenbosch in 1992 and was a GP in the UK until her return to South Africa in 2011. She holds a Diploma of the Royal College of Obstetricians and Gynaecologists, a Certificate of the Joint Committee on Postgraduate Training for General Practice and became a Member of the Royal College of General Practitioners in 2010. She joined The Council for Health Service Accreditation of South Africa (COHSASA) in 2011 as the GP Accreditation Program Coordinator and is now responsible for all standards development activities. She is currently completing her MMed in Public Health at the University of Cape Town.

Marion Lindh MD, Quality and Patient Safety Advisor, is currently affiliated with the Stockholm County Council as a senior advisor in patient safety. She has a medical background, specializing in internal medicine and geriatrics. She has been head of department for geriatrics and primary care as well as divisional Chief Executive Officer at the Western Stockholm County Council and Huddinge University Hospital. During her career she also served as Chief Medical Officer. She has developed and managed continuous quality improvement programs focusing on patient safety, quality costing, lean production, and management systems. She is author of the book "Safe Care."

Russell Mannion BA (Hons), PG Dip Health Econ, PhD, FRSA holds the Chair in Health Systems at the University of Birmingham where he is currently Director of Research at the Health Services Management Centre. He also holds professorial positions at the University of New South Wales and the University of Oslo. He was previously Director of the Centre for Health and Public Services Management at the University of York. His research embraces health systems reform, clinical governance, healthcare quality, and patent safety. He has won international awards for his research including the Baxter European book award. He provides advice to various international governments and health bodies, including WHO and the Organisation for Economic Co-operation and Development (OECD).

Carol Marshall MB, ChB, DTM&H, MSc is the interim CEO of the Office of Health Standards Compliance, South Africa. She has worked extensively in Mozambique and South Africa and was the Africa Regional Director for the Micronutrient Initiative for a number of years. Since early 2008 she has been responsible for guiding the development and monitoring the implementation of quality programs in South Africa, including the development of national standards for health establishments, the establishment of a national Inspectorate and Complaints Centre and supporting the Parliamentary process that led to the promulgation of the National Health Amendment Act.

Yukihiro Matsuyama PhD is Research Director, the Canon Institute for Global Studies, Affiliate Professor, Chiba University of Commerce, and Visiting Professor, the Center for Clinical Governance Research, Faculty of Medicine, University of New South Wales, Australia. His research examines the sustainability of safety-net systems in Japan including healthcare, pension, pandemic crisis, and employment through international comparative analyses. He is Advisor to the healthcare working group of the regulatory reform council of the Abe administration and Member, the welfare corporation reform committee of Ministry of Health, Labor & Welfare. He has published many books including *Health Reform and Economic Growth* (2010), which greatly influenced government policies.

Walverly Morales MD, MPH is a Medical Surgeon and holds a Master in Public Health degree. He has experience in health management, evaluation, and processes innovation in healthcare and patient safety, and the design and implementation of public healthcare strategies focused on quality improvement in México and Costa Rica. He currently collaborates as leader responsible for the State program for quality for the Ministry of Health in Morelos, Mexico.

José Carvalho de Noronha MD, DPH, PhD is Senior Researcher at the Oswaldo Cruz Foundation of the Brazilian Federal Ministry of Health, where he coordinates the Strategic Foresight of Brazilian Healthcare System Initiative. He is also Consultant to the Collaborating Center for Quality of Care and Patient Safety, International Advisor to the Consortium for Brazilian Accreditation of Health Systems and Services, and Member of the Joint Commission International Accreditation Committee. He is a former member of the International Society for Quality in Healthcare Advisory Council and Board. He has published book chapters and articles on health policy, healthcare evaluation policies, and quality measures.

Sun Niuyun MS, Director, NIHA (CN) is the Director of the Healthcare Safety and Risk Management Center of National Institute of Hospital Administration of China. She holds a Master of Management with a focus on hospital administration. She has worked at hospitals and at the Chinese Medical Doctor Association. Previously, she was a nurse practitioner, hospital manager, and manager for physicians' training. Her research is focused on the following areas: patient safety and healthcare quality, assessment of medical risks and design of its warning system, assessment and management of hospitals' operational performance, and assessment and management of health insurance payments.

John Øvretveit BSc (Hons), MPhil, PhD, C.Psychol, MIHM is Director of Research and Professor of Health Care Innovation Implementation and Evaluation at the Medical Management Centre, Karolinska Institute, Stockholm. He has studied and led health services quality improvement and evaluation over 30 years in many western and developing countries. His work is based on the belief that right organization design and management is critical for effective healthcare. Much of his work uses different social science disciplines to explain and predict events and processes in healthcare and clinical practice. He was awarded the 2014 Avedis Donabedian international quality award for his work on quality economics.

Holger Pfaff studied social and administrative sciences at the Universities of Erlangen-Nuremberg and Constance. Since 1997, he has held the Medical Sociology professorship at the University of Cologne. He is Director of the Institute for Medical Sociology, Health Services Research, and Rehabilitation Science at the University of Cologne since 2009. This "bridge institute" is a joint institution of the Faculties of Human Sciences and Medicine. Since 2009, he has held the professorship in Quality Development and Evaluation in Rehabilitation.

Martin Powell BA (Hons), PhD is Professor of Health and Social Policy at the Health Services Management Centre, University of Birmingham, UK. He has published over 10 books and 80 articles in the areas of health and social policy. Recent research interests include privatization, accountability, and human resource management in health services.

Ånen Ringard BA, MSc (Political Science), PhD is a postdoctoral researcher at the Health Services Research Unit, Akershus University Hospital, Norway. He is currently seconded to the Ministry of Health and Care Services, where he is heading the secretariat for a Royal Commission on Priority Setting in Health Care. He is also employed as project manager in the Norwegian Knowledge Centre for the Health Services. He holds a degree in political sciences (Cand.polit.), and a PhD in Health Policy/Health Services Research, both from the University of Oslo. His research focuses on patient empowerment, hospital choice, priority setting, quality and safety, and health system analysis.

Enrique Ruelas MD, MPA, MHSc is a physician trained in public and health administration in Mexico and Canada. He was the Dean of the National School of Public Health of Mexico, Program Director of the WK Kellogg Foundation for Latin America, President and CEO of Qualimed, Vice Minister of Health of Mexico, and Secretary of the General Health Council of Mexico. He was responsible for the design and implementation of the first national strategy for quality improvement in healthcare in Mexico; chaired the Mexican Commission on Accreditation of Health Care Facilities; was President of the Mexican Society for Quality in Health Care; the Mexican Hospital Association; and ISQua, the International Society for Quality in Health Care, between 1993 and 1995. He is a Senior Fellow of the Institute for Healthcare Improvement, and President of the Latin American Society for Quality in Health Care, and the National Academy of Medicine of Mexico.

Magna Andreen Sachs MD, PhD is currently affiliated to the Medical Management Centre, Karolinska Institutet, as senior advisor/researcher, involved in patient safety and patient safety culture research. Her background is in medicine, specializing in anesthesia and intensive care. She has served as head of the Department of Anesthesia and Intensive care and also as Chief Medical Officer at Danderyd hospital in Stockholm. During her service at Danderyd hospital she managed continuous quality improvement work with an emphasis on patient safety and patient centeredness. Over the past ten years she has managed the Stockholm County Council support of quality improvement within healthcare.

Paulinus LN Sikosana MD, MPH, MBA, CIRM (UK) is Team Leader for Health Systems Strengthening and Health Care Financing in the Papua New Guinea (PNG) World Health Organization Country Office. He was Health Adviser to the Australian Government's PNG health program, Senior Planning Adviser to the Mozambique

Ministry of Health, Technical Health Advisor for the Essential Health Package and Sector Wide Approach in Malawi, and Permanent Secretary for Health in Zimbabwe. His work encompasses public health practice, strategic planning, monitoring and evaluation, reforms, aid effectiveness, and health systems in developing countries. He authored *Challenges in Reforming the Health Sector in Africa: Reforming Health Systems under Economic Siege — the Zimbabwean Experience* (2010).

Sodzi Sodzi-Tettey BSc, MBChB, MPH is a trained Improvement Advisor, Public Health Physician and Executive Director of Project Fives Alive!—a partnership between the Institute for Healthcare Improvement (US) and the National Catholic Health Service, working in collaboration with the Ghana Health Service to reduce mortality in children under five through Quality Improvement methods. He writes a weekly column for the *Daily Graphic* and is the immediate past Vice President of the Ghana Medical Association.

Giorgio Solimano MD is Professor and Head of the Global Health Program at the School of Public Health "Dr. Salvador Allende G.," University of Chile; Technical Secretary of the Latin American Alliance for Global Health; Chief Editor of the Revista Chilena de Salud Pública; and Senior Lecturer in Epidemiology at the Mailman School of Public Health, Columbia University. He is former Dean of the School of Public Health; President of the Latin American Association of Schools of Public Health; Professor of Public Health at the Mailman School of Public Health; and Representative of the President of Chile in the Council of the University of Chile. He has published 12 books and over 60 scientific papers and articles on global health and health and nutrition policies.

David R Steel OBE, MA, DPhil, FRCP Edin is Honorary Senior Research Fellow at the University of Aberdeen and chairs the Prioritisation Panel of the National Institute for Health Research Health Services and Delivery Research Program. He worked for 25 years in NHS management and was Chief Executive of NHS Quality Improvement Scotland from its creation in 2003 until 2009. He is author of the Scottish health systems review published in 2012 as part of the European Observatory's Health Systems in Transition series. In 2008 he was awarded an OBE for services to healthcare.

Andrew Thompson BSc (Hons), PhD has key research interests in the field of citizenship and public policy, particularly in relation to health services. This includes the politics of healthcare, public participation in healthcare, perception and satisfaction measurement, quality management, and multi-level governance. He also works on the social justice agenda in relation to widening participation in higher education. He is a member of the Participatory and Deliberative Democracy Group of the UK Political Studies Association, the European Political Science Association, and the European Consortium for Political Research. He is also a statistical adviser to national and international research teams.

Leonel Valdivia BEd, DipEd, MEd, PhD is co-Director and founder of the Global Health Program of the School of Public Health, Faculty of Medicine, University of Chile and part of the directing team of the School. He chaired the School's Department of Health Promotion and Education. He has enjoyed a successful career in international development cooperation in the United States of America, having worked for UNFPA, PAHO/WHO, IPPF, and USAID. He started his academic career as a Lecturer at the University of Edinburgh, and holds a PhD and MEd from the University of Manchester. Valdivia's research interests focus on the effects of economic globalization on health equity and social justice.

Stuart Whittaker MBChB, FFCM(CH) MMed, MD is founder and CEO of the Council for Health Service Accreditation of Southern Africa. He is a leader in the field of healthcare quality improvement and accreditation and is a member of the Board Advisory Committee, Expert Group, and an international surveyor for ISQua. He is a Visiting Professor at the School of Public Health and Medicine, University of Cape Town. He holds Board positions on both the South African healthcare regulatory body the Office of Health Standards Compliance and the Regional Centre for Quality in Health Care, which aims to advance the quality of healthcare in the East, Central, and Southern regions of Africa.

Eng Kiong Yeoh MBBS (HK), FRCP (Edin), FHKCP, FRCP (Lond), FRCP (Glasg), FRACP, FHKAM, FHKCCM, FFPH (UK), FRACMA is Professor of Public Health and the Director of the JC School of Public Health and Primary Care, the Chinese University of Hong Kong. His research is in health systems, services, and policy with an interest in applying systems thinking. He is the Chairman of the Asia Network for Capacity Building in Health Systems Strengthening of the World Bank Institute since 2009. In addition, he is the International Advisory Board member, National University of Singapore's Initiative to Improve Health in Asia, and the President of the International Hospital Federation. He was also the former Secretary for Health, Welfare and Food of the Government of Hong Kong Special Administrative Region, and Head of the Hong Kong Hospital Authority.

Eyal Zimlichman MD, MSc (MHCM) is an internal medicine physician, a healthcare executive, and a researcher focused on healthcare quality, patient safety, and information technology. Dr Zimlichman is currently Deputy Director and Chief Quality Officer at Sheba Medical Center, Israel's largest hospital. Prior to this, Dr Zimlichman was a researcher at Brigham and Women's Hospital and Harvard Medical School affiliated Center for Patient Safety Research and Practice in Boston. He has served on several expert panels commissioned by the US Department of Health and Human Services and the Ministry of Health in Israel, centering on quality measurement and use of information technology.

Acknowledgements

The editors would like to acknowledge some of the many people from around the world who helped make this book possible. We are indebted to multiple people and groups.

For committing themselves to this idea, and taking time out of their busy schedules to write, the authors from the countries represented in the book must be thanked first and foremost. The wisdom contained across the pages is theirs, and it is their skills in telling their countries' stories that make the book what it is. The International Society for Quality in Healthcare (ISQua) helped us bring together this global expertise. It facilitated our initial meeting in Edinburgh and thus helped create the platform for our collaboration.

The job of editing this book was made manageable through the considerable work undertaken by several people. In particular, Brette Blakely did a marvellous job in coordinating the manuscript, corresponding with the editorial staff and authors, and providing her substantial expertise. Gina Lamprell spent many hours diligently double checking each comma, table number, and reference and offered comments of substance to sharpen the text. Danielle Marks assisted with editorial and referencing activities, and Jenny Plumb supported early efforts in establishing the project. We credit turning 27 chapters of material written by 51 authors into a unified book to this talented group.

No book is possible without the faith, support and guidance of great publishers. Ashgate is of the very highest rank amongst publishing houses. Thank you, Guy Loft and the Ashgate team, for seeing value in this idea and providing the means to make it a reality.

Finally, our colleagues Professor Cliff Hughes and David Bates have been strong supporters of our work. They have paid us a great compliment, and graciously endorsed the book.

Foreword

David W Bates and Clifford F Hughes

The Oxford English Dictionary defines "reform" as: "to make or become better by the removal of faults or errors." In this global compendium world experts have come to focus on this definition, working to bring together the positive potential impacts of system change and the principles of quality and safety to patient care.

What is remarkable is the range and depth of individuals involved in authoring this book. The coordinating editors have assembled an extraordinary wealth of experience. Many of the authors are known to us personally and have impressed with their wisdom, insight, and willingness to share. All are renowned experts within their own national boundaries but have practiced, presented, and written on the world stage.

One of the intriguing features of the book is the variation in context (represented by the sheer number of countries and their unique demographics) and yet there is an amazing similarity of values, goals, and aspirations of those who plan to deliver care to patients. The enormous breadth and scope of this review will help the reader understand the ubiquitous nature of reform, and safety and quality, in jurisdictions of different size, experience, technology use, and investment levels.

This book is especially timely, as the echoes of the Global Financial Crisis continue to reverberate, causing Governments to evaluate the economic outputs of their investments. It addresses the safety and quality outputs of health systems and as such will become an essential reference point for healthcare policymakers, planners and workers—tackling the difficult question of whether recent efforts in reforms are yielding the necessary returns.

The sum total of this experience is a window into health reform strategies that countries are experimenting with, and the quality and safety initiatives they are implementing and testing. The book does not tell us precisely what to do next—no one can do that. But it does provide many case-study examples of how heath systems are struggling to advance—sometimes making progress, sometimes marking time, and even sometimes stepping back—but always striving to improve. That is perhaps the most useful lesson for us all.

David W Bates MD, MSc
President, International Society for Quality in Health Care (ISQua)
Professor of Medicine, Harvard Medical School, and Professor of Health Policy and Management, Harvard School of Public Health, Boston, USA
&
Clifford F Hughes MBBS, DSc
President Elect, International Society for Quality in Health Care (ISQua)
Clinical Professor—Surgery, University of Sydney and Chief Executive Officer, Clinical Excellence Commission, Sydney, Australia

Chapter 1

Introduction

Jeffrey Braithwaite, Yukihiro Matsuyama, Russell Mannion and
Julie Johnson

The Genesis of This Compendium

As academic researchers, we have collectively and individually been interested in health reform for many years. Health reform at its most basic involves making changes (which are hoped to result in improvements) in the performance, operations, structures, process, or outcomes of health systems. (Of course, a key part of reform is to decide what to keep and what to change. Some things may be working well and not need reforming.) Nevertheless, reform is usually construed as a set of high-level, macro-system considerations concentrating on change. We have also been interested over the years in efforts to enhance the quality of care and make things safer for patients. Healthcare quality is a multi-faceted concept which embraces a number of dimensions, including: safety, cost-effectiveness, access, responsiveness, patient centeredness, and equity. Patient safety is about the prevention of harm to patients. Quality and safety interventions are typically thought of as targeted initiatives at the mid- to lower-levels of health systems—a set of meso- or micro-system considerations.

However, as we each conducted and participated in research on our own health systems, we rarely saw health reform explicitly related to quality and safety. It wasn't clear to us how big-picture, national-level reforms stood in relation to measures to improve the quality of care and safety of patients.

So, guided by an initial idea from the first-listed editor to develop our understanding of these interactions, the editors met at various times over several years, in Sydney, Australia; Tokyo, Japan; Birmingham, England; and Hong Kong, People's Republic of China, to consider a key question: what is the relationship between large-scale health system reforms and quality of care and patient safety? We did not expect that there would be a simple answer. We doubted that health reform and quality and safety would have a definite, positive relationship, because we know that healthcare is delivered in a complex adaptive system, and that complex constructs are rarely associated in a linear relationship. We also hypothesized—speculated, really—that disentangling the effects of health systems reform at the national level on quality and safety delivered at the front lines of care, would not be easy. However, it is a sufficiently important topic—if only because, at least in principle, the two *should* be related in a coherent, well-functioning system. We agreed to allocate some serious intellectual resources to analyzing it.

The Involvement of 30 Health Systems

To give effect to our interest in how, or whether, health reforms affect the quality and safety of care delivered on-the-ground in health systems, we set off in search of a way to inquire into the phenomenon. The first-listed editor hit on the idea of a book of invited chapters from a variety of health systems on the topic, and persuaded the other editors to join in support. We invited representatives from multiple countries, and ended up with over 30 countries each to give a talk at the International Society for Quality in Health Care (ISQuA) annual meeting held in Edinburgh, Scotland, in October 2013. Each country made a presentation and most accepted our subsequent invitation to develop a chapter for the book. Over the next six months, each devoted some of their valuable time to explicating their answer to the question we had posed.

We recognized a unique and very special opportunity. By inviting a range of lower-, middle-, and higher-income countries to contribute a chapter, we were poised to address, head-on, a problem that most international books on health systems fail to solve: to ensure there is adequate representation of countries beyond those in the Organization for Economic Cooperation and Development (OECD). In this, the final version of the book, as can be seen, we were successful in this quest, and we have assembled chapters from each of the key regions of the world.

The book provides an in-depth analysis of 24 health systems, in addition to a regional perspective provided on the Gulf States written by colleagues in the Kingdom of Saudi Arabia, adding a further six countries. In total, 30 health systems, providing care to more than four billion people, over 60 percent of the world's population, living in over 51,762,891 square kilometers of the earth, are represented (Figure 1.1) (worldatlas n.d.).

What Do We Know About This Issue to Date?

There are various sources of information which enable policymakers, researchers, and other interested parties to appreciate how healthcare systems are structured or perform comparatively. These include data sources and studies from the Commonwealth Fund in the United States, academic studies published in journals such as *Health Policy*, *Health Policy and Planning*, *BMJ Quality & Safety*, and *International Journal for Quality in Health Care,* and from reports and health systems or country profiles from the OECD, World Health Organization (WHO), the United Nations (UN), and the International Labour Organization (ILO).

From these sources, a set of meta-level conclusions can be drawn. At their most basic, health systems consume a sizeable proportion of their countries' gross

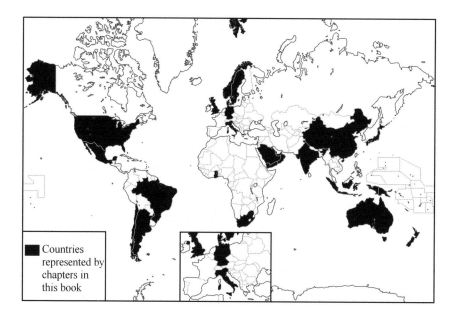

Figure 1.1   Representation of countries within the book

domestic product (GDP), and each face logistical challenges in delivering care equitably and efficiently across the populations they serve. Although healthcare must be targeted to localized and specific groups, equally it is always a national concern, too. Further, regardless of country, delivering healthcare to citizens is never merely an economic, financial, social, or logistical problem. It is also, inevitably, intensely political and ideological.

All health systems are accountable for spending budgetary allocations wisely and organizing care to meet needs. They are structured across sectors—acute, primary, secondary, tertiary, aged care, and community-based services. Every health system has a mix of publicly-funded and privately-provided services, although the particular balance of service provision across the public and private spheres differs greatly by country.

A key concern of health systems is to get the policy and legislative settings right, and there are always multiple measures in train in every country to improve, tweak or revamp the system. This is health reform—adjusting policy, legislative requirements, structures, responsibilities, funding mechanisms, and the like. There are also strenuous efforts, often funded as projects, programs, and initiatives, to improve things at the organizational level. These take the form of measures such as mandating hand hygiene behaviors, introducing root cause analysis training, specifying the use of checklists in theatres, training staff to be better at detecting deteriorating patients, and standardizing approaches to shift handovers. Additional efforts are in play at the clinical coalface—where individual providers and care-giving teams work to make sense of national mandates and organizational policies, while trying to provide the best possible care to their patients.

How the Chapters and Book are Structured

We gave the leading authors of each chapter a template to serve as a guide, specifying key issues and more detailed points we hoped they would address. Many of the invited authors involved co-authors in their countries, and occasionally beyond, to work with them and provide additional input into their chapter. Most but not all chapter-writers found this template useful, with some preferring to write under their own, purpose-designed headings and subheadings. This was fine with us, as we did not want to be excessively prescriptive, preferring instead to see authors express their answer to the question we had set them in their own way. However, as you read each contribution, you will find that even when the headings differ from chapter to chapter, similar points seem to be touched on, recurrently, throughout the book.

We partitioned the book into five sections. These map to five key geographical regions. This may seem in hindsight a natural, even inevitable division, but the book could have been structured differently. We discussed this as we edited the chapters, thinking about whether readers might prefer to see chapters grouped alphabetically, or by income (with sections on lower-, medium-, and higher-income countries), or similarly financed (more privately-oriented systems like America's and Japan's clustered together, contrasted with more predominantly tax payer-funded systems, like those of Europe). But in the end, any grouping system seemed to rely on a superficial judgment and, in any case, a regional geographical structure worked best. Accordingly, we have sections of the book covering countries in Africa and Western Asia (Part I), Eastern Asia and Southern Asia (Part II), South Eastern Asia and Oceania (Part III), The Americas (Part IV), and Europe (Part V). Although we all did a share of editing chapters across different regions, we each took primary responsibility for editing an allocation: Parts I and III (JB), Part II (YM), Part IV (JJ), and Part V (RM).

Identifying Our Readers and the Place of the Book in Context

This book is written for healthcare policymakers, bureaucrats, regulators, managers, clinicians, patients and patient groups, researchers, and those in the specialized healthcare media—in fact, all those interested in how health systems work from the top to the bottom of the system, and in-between, and how they can be improved. We hope readers all gain something from this book and enjoy what follows. We believe there is no other offering like it. Some books on health reform or quality and safety involve OECD member countries but do not represent developing or under developed countries. Other books deal with health reform but not quality and safety; and yet others focus on quality and safety but not health reform. We, instead, are able to present a constellation of chapters from as wide a group of countries as we could obtain given space restrictions, each expressing their answer to the key question of whether big-scale health reforms affect quality and safety, and if so, how and to what extent.

Having documented what we did to get to this point, there is only one final suggestion to our readers. We invite you to immerse yourself in a treasure-trove of fascinating and skilled writing from a cross-section of countries of the world, documenting their trials and tribulations in reforming, and seeking to improve, the quality and safety of care to their citizens. In human endeavors, it is hard to discern a topic that is more important to the world's present and future patients than to improve how health systems function.

PART I
Africa and Western Asia

Jeffrey Braithwaite

We open our account with Part I, an examination of Africa and Western Asia. The countries involved are a mix of lower- and higher-income countries, providing contrasts in health systems, reform efforts, and quality and safety initiatives. The countries are Ghana, Israel, Oman, and South Africa. In addition, unusually, compared with the rest of the book, we have a single chapter in this part covering seven countries—the Gulf States. They are brought together as their safety and quality issues are coordinated through the Health Ministers' Council in the Gulf Countries, involving efforts in Bahrain, Kuwait, Oman, Qatar, the Kingdom of Saudi Arabia, the United Arab Emirates, and the Republic of Yemen.

A key determinant of health governance and reform is per capita income. The wealth of the country is a major factor in the amount of resources available to provide for and pay the workforce, to build and maintain facilities and infrastructure, and tackle everything from basic community-level infections to child health, maternity service provision, and the like. Here we see the wide range of foci of the systems in this part, depending on those wealth differences. South Africa, a lower-income country, and Ghana, until recently relatively low, but now approaching middle-income levels, are both concerned with providing core services to the whole population, including dealing with issues of inadequate staffing and poor distribution of the workforce throughout the country, as well as tackling urgent problems such as maternal and child health, HIV/AIDS, and universal immunization.

Israel and Oman, with much more developed economies, are not lacking challenges; but in their cases many of the more fundamental issues facing South Africa and Ghana have been addressed. They, instead, can focus on figuring out how to tackle challenges such as improving the public availability of data, designing and introducing pay for performance models, and enhancing an already effective IT regime.

The chapter on the Gulf States nicely straddles this divide between rich and poor health systems, providing an interesting picture of how efforts are being coordinated across seven countries with widely disparate resource capabilities. Gross national income per capita in these states differs by a factor of almost 35—from $2,310 to $80,470 per person (purchasing power parity in international dollars). So across the Gulf countries, the problems differ enormously. Nevertheless, the Gulf States have recognized that there is much to be gained by sharing expertise, perspectives, and efforts in health reform and quality of care, and, as shown in the Gulf chapter in particular, there is much to learn in coordinating efforts and sharing ideas about creating safer systems and improved care for patients.

Chapter 2
Ghana

Sodzi Sodzi-Tettey[1]

Abstract

For more than a decade, Ghana has embarked on a number of health sector reform initiatives. These reforms have been aimed at improving access to quality healthcare and reducing financial risk, especially to the poor and vulnerable. The expectation is that these will contribute to bridging equity gaps and improving health outcomes. Through an evaluation of current reform initiatives, we portray their overarching impact on quality and safety. A brief historical account of the health system and its organization, current reform initiatives and their impact, the quality and safety landscape, and the future direction are tackled.

A Brief History of Healthcare Reform in Ghana

At independence from British colonial rule in March 1957, Ghana, under President Kwame Nkrumah, introduced free medical care. This was funded through general taxation. It marked a departure from the out-of-pocket payment schemes that characterized the pre-independence era. Subsequently, following stagnating economic fortunes, the Government, in 1972 and 1985 respectively, introduced low, and later significant, out-of-pocket payments at the point of service. The objective was to address stock outs of essential medicines and supplies. The Government's aim of a 15 percent recovery of recurrent expenditure in the 1985 out-of-pocket payment policy was achieved. This, however, introduced significant attendant inequities in access to care (Agyepong & Adjei 2008, Waddington & Enyimayew 1989). By 2000, and on the verge of national elections, public uproar against the out-of-pocket scheme, now christened "Cash and Carry," had peaked. This led to the center-right opposition New Patriotic Party (NPP) pledging to replace it with a National Health Insurance Scheme (NHIS), which it did subsequently.

---

1   The author would like to acknowledge the following: National Catholic Health Service, Professor Pierre Barker (Senior Vice President, IHI, Cambridge MA Clinical Professor, Gillings School of Global Public Health, UNC Chapel Hill, NC) and Dr Cynthia Bannerman (Deputy Director, Institutional Care Division, Ghana Health Service) for their senior technical guidance and Jacob Eyiah Ayetey (National Catholic Health Service) for research assistance.

Table 2.1   Demographic, economic, and health information for Ghana

Population (thousands)	25,366
Area (sq. km)*	227,540
Proportion of population living in urban areas (2011)	52
Gross Domestic Product (GDP US$, billions)^	40.7
Total expenditure on health as % of GDP	5.2
Gross national income per capita (PPP intl $)	1,910
Per capita total expenditure on health (intl $)	106
Proportion of health expenditure which is private	43
General Government expenditure on health as a percentage of total expenditure on health	57
Out-of-pocket expenditure as a percentage of private expenditure on health	67
Life expectancy at birth m/f (yrs)	61/64
Probability of dying under five (per 1,000 live births)	72
Maternal Mortality Ratio (per 100,000 live births) (2013)	380
Proportion of population using improved water and sanitation	87/14

Source: Unless otherwise stated data are for the year 2012 and taken from the World Health Organization 2014a. * Area from the World Bank 2014a. ^ GDP from the World Bank 2014b.

Notes: PPP is purchasing power parity, intl $ is international dollar which has the same purchasing power as US$ in the US.

Another set of major reforms occurred with the introduction of the Ghana Health Service and Teaching Hospital Act (1996), Act 525 (Government of Ghana 1996). This, in fact, led to the formation of the Ghana Health Service (GHS), which then became an "autonomous Executive Agency responsible for implementation of national policies under the control of the Minister for Health through its governing Council" (Ghana Health Service 2014). Through a number of partnership arrangements, the Ministry of Health coordinates the actions of the GHS and other agencies like the Teaching Hospitals, the Christian Health Association of Ghana (CHAG), the private self-financing sub sector, non-governmental, and civil society organizations (Ghana Health Service 2014).

These reforms have allowed for a clear separation of the policy formulation, resource mobilization, regulation, monitoring and supervisory functions of the Ministry of Health (MoH), and the actual implementation mandate of its service agencies. To drive the quality and safety agenda, some of these service agencies have dedicated clinical care units. A good example is the Institutional Care Division (ICD) of the GHS which has rolled out a suite of guidelines, standards, and protocols, and infection prevention control interventions aimed at improving facility-based care. At the regional level, the ICD is represented by a Deputy Director of Clinical Care.

Overview of the Health System Organization at the District, Sub-district and Community Levels

Ghana is divided into ten regions, each with a regional health directorate. The health system at lower levels complements the local Government structure where district, sub-district, and community levels have a district hospital, health centers, and Community Health Planning Services Compounds (CHPS), respectively (Figure 2.1).

A key strength of the Ghana health system is its ability to integrate public and faith-based facilities. At the district level, the distinction between the public and faith-based sectors is quite artificial. This partnership is no accident of history, but through careful design. Since 2003, this symbiotic relationship has been formalized in a Memorandum of Understanding between the MoH and CHAG (Ministry of Health & Christian Health Association of Ghana 2003). It makes provision for CHAG's management of Government-built hospitals and clinics, payment by Government to health professionals in CHAG facilities, access to essential supplies and drugs, and tax exemptions on medical equipment and supplies. Typically, CHAG places health facilities in rural and deprived communities, and shares routine service delivery data with the corresponding District Health Directorate. Government shies away from duplicating such district health facilities. More recently, to further strengthen the partnership at an operational level, a similar memorandum has been signed between GHS and CHAG that seeks to "regulate, institutionalize and exact desired operational performance and dynamics from these agencies" (Ghana Health Service & Christian Health Association of Ghana 2013).

Quality and safety weaknesses, however, exist in the sheer inadequacy of the health workforce, compounded by the inequitable distribution. A country case study on Ghana's human resource deficits, by the World Health Organization (WHO) and the Global Health Workforce Alliance (GHWA), showed that to achieve adequate staffing norm levels, the percentage increases across various cadres of staff would range from 69 percent (pharmacists) to 883 percent (X-ray technologists) (Global Health Workforce Alliance & World Health Organization 2006).

Significant transportation and communication challenges also remain in various parts of the country, thus compounding delays in reaching health facilities. This is in spite of Parliamentary approval for a €15.8 million loan for the purchase of 200 ambulances for the National Ambulance Service (NAS), in 2012, to improve referral and pre hospital care (Ghana News Agency 2012). Access to facilities also remains a weakness. Ghana has not achieved universal coverage in

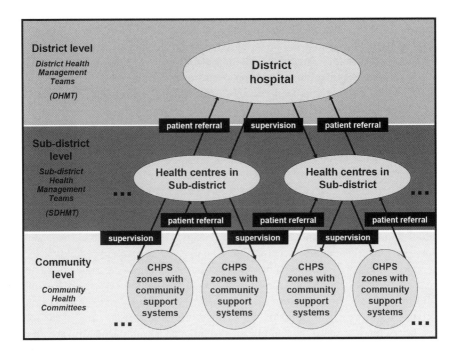

Figure 2.1   Organization of Ghana's district health system

Source: Nyonator 2005. In: Community-based Health Planning and Services (CHPS), The Operational Policy, A Ghana Health Service Policy Document, no. 20, May 2005.

the construction of CHPS. According to the Director General of the GHS, there is a current deficit of 2,500 CHPS compounds. Even if the Government were to successfully build 1,600 compounds as planned, only 64 percent of the current gap would be addressed. Other challenges pertaining to equipment and diagnostic weaknesses remain, although health managers confirm an ongoing National Medical Equipment Replacement Programme which has seen modern equipment being supplied to 40 district hospitals (Sodzi-Tettey 2014a).

Current Reform Initiatives

Ghana, like most developing countries, has inadequate numbers of health staff who are poorly distributed. The doctor to population ratio as of 2013 was 1:10,170—with wide regional disparities. While the capital Greater Accra region has a ratio of 1:3,178, the more deprived Northern and Upper West regions have 1:22,894 and 1:53,064 respectively (Ministry of Health Ghana 2014). Since 2011, Ghana's MoH has piloted the WHO's Workload Indicator of Staffing Needs (WISN). This has led to the development of a more evidence-based staffing norm that covers 74 percent of all categories of health professionals across the health system. With these workload-based staffing norms, the MoH hopes to better plan, implement, and monitor interventions to address inadequate staff numbers, inequitable distribution, and poor skills mix (Ministry of Health Ghana 2014).

Government has also expanded health training institutions with increased intake of health professionals. Recently, Ghana established a new University of Health and Allied Sciences (UHAS) through an Act of Parliament (Act 828, December 2011). UHAS is dedicated entirely to the training of health professionals and in 2012 commenced training of its first batch of students in nursing, midwifery, physician assistantship, public health, and allied health sciences (University of Health and Allied Sciences 2012).

Two major reforms of health sector pay policy in 2006 and 2010, coupled with the establishment of a college for postgraduate training of doctors, have contributed to stemming of the brain drain. While the Health Sector Salary Structure was implemented as a health sector-only initiative in 2006, the Single Spine Salary Structure (SSSS) was established in 2010 throughout the public sector to rationalize public sector pay, improve remuneration, and increase productivity. Today, the entire health sector has been migrated into the new SSSS pay structure. Of particular relevance to the health sector are two components of the policy: a) the market premium—which pays health workers a premium above the base pay on account of scarcity of skills, and b) inducement allowance to be paid to health professionals and others, working in deprived, or underserved areas. While the market premium has been implemented, the inducement component remains outstanding. With Government lamenting that the new pay policy has doubled the wage bill in less than a year, the future direction of the policy and its ability to meet its policy objectives remains unclear. The President has also called for a performance-based management system (Fair Wages and Salaries Commission 2010, Mahama 2012).

In 2003, Ghana's Parliament passed the National Health Insurance Act 650, aimed at removing cost as a barrier to quality healthcare. Since then, the scheme's provider payment mechanism has undergone a number of reforms to make it more efficient and effective. Starting with itemized fee-for-service, the country introduced the Ghana Diagnostic-Related Groupings (G-DRGs) payment method in 2008 and further reviewed it in 2012. In that same year (2012), the National Health Insurance Authority (NHIA) started piloting capitation for primary healthcare and outpatient services in one out of ten regions. Currently, plans are afoot to scale up the capitation policy to three new regions (Agyepong & Agyei 2008, Sodzi-Tettey 2014a, Sodzi-Tettey et al. 2012).

As of May 2014, the most significant proposed reform initiative in Ghana's health sector pertains to a Government policy to decentralize health to local Government. This move has the aim of improving equity, good governance, efficiency, access to services, and local participation. Diverse stakeholders are currently engaged in serious discussions aimed at tackling potential threats and limitations including "Monitoring and Evaluation capacity, clear regulatory framework, degree of autonomy, leadership and managerial capacity, availability and adequacy of human, financial, and other resources at decentralized levels" (Ministry of Health Ghana 2014, Ahwoi 2014). To address these anticipated challenges, Government has set up an Inter-Ministerial Coordinating Committee (IMCC) on Decentralization, chaired by the President. The IMCC has, in turn, set up a task force within the health sector to assist Government to address the anticipated required legal, structural, and functional arrangements and rearrangements (Ministry of Health Ghana 2014, Ahwoi 2014).

The Quality and Safety Landscape

Overall, current efforts to improve the quality and safety of healthcare are executed by the various agencies of Ghana's MoH and partner organizations. The Ministry has created an inter-agency leadership committee as a forum for improved communication and collaboration. The following agencies are represented: the GHS, CHAG, Teaching Hospitals, the NHIA, the National Blood Transfusion Service (NBTS), NAS, the Health Regulatory Institutions, and others.

Ghana has also adopted multiple approaches to improve the quality and safety of care. Broadly, these approaches include strengthening regulation of healthcare, introduction of quality assurance, and more recently, continuous quality improvement (QI) methods. Continuous QI has been implemented alongside the more traditional Quality Assurance approaches. In 2010, following initial individual regional-level peer-reviewed processes of hospitals, the Director General of the GHS directed all Regional Health Directorates to "institutionalize the Peer Review Mechanism and the District League Performance table and introduce schemes to encourage lower level managers to perform" (Clinical Care Division of the Volta Regional Health Directorate 2010).

To assist Ghana in accelerating the achievement of Millennium Development Goal 4 (MDG 4), to reduce child mortality, the National Catholic Health Service (NCHS), through its partnership with the Institute for Healthcare Improvement (IHI), formed 'Project Fives Alive!' (PFA!). PFA! is funded by the Bill and Melinda Gates Foundation. It has, since 2008, been implementing a large-scale Maternal Newborn and Child Health QI effort in collaboration with the GHS. As of May 2014, the Project has cumulatively been rolled out in all ten regions with almost 400 QI teams being formed in various health facilities. Significant improvements have been recorded in the continuum of care from early antenatal care through skilled delivery, post natal care and facility-based child mortality. The QI teams are developing and carrying out rapid cycle tests of innovative ideas within learning networks of their peers. Packages of effective interventions for improving child survival developed in earlier phases of the project are being rapidly scaled up. The project has also trained over 300 staff from the health system, including district managers in project sites, as Improvement Coaches to lead improvement processes (Project Fives Alive! 2013). Further, the GHS has rolled out a nationwide Leadership Development Programme to train various levels of management in problem-solving approaches.

The combined quality and safety approaches have thus been bi-directional—both top down and bottom up. In November 2013, the GHS, the NCHS, and IHI, represented by the PFA!, and USAid/Focus Region Project, collaborated to write a book on *Quality and Patient Safety*. This book will be used by QI teams constituted by facility managers to diagnose their own system and process failures which can be addressed systematically using innovative solutions generated by frontline staff. Methods to improve quality and safety have thus witnessed a fair mix of the well-known Juran triad—"Quality Planning, Continuous Quality Improvement and Quality Control" (Juran 1989).

With 14 psychiatrists, eight medical assistants, three clinical psychologists (in public service), no occupational therapists, 600 psychiatric nurses, (with a 4,000 gap), the quality and safety challenges in mental healthcare for the population of 24 million are formidable. Even so, the passage of Ghana's acclaimed Mental Health Act 846 (2012), offers a glimmer of hope as it indicates a focusing of high-level attention on this sector. The Act creates a new Mental Health Authority with the express object of promoting a holistic, culturally appropriate, integrated and specialized mental healthcare nationwide (Sodzi-Tettey 2012).

In May 2010, the last case of guinea worm disease was confirmed in Ghana. Free of guinea worm disease for almost four years, Ghana is on the verge of international certification for stopping the transmission. An international certification team is expected in the country in July, 2014, to assess public and health sector awareness of the disease, the cash reward instituted for reporting incidents of hanging worms, and the provision of safe potable water in endemic areas. To achieve this, however, the country must bridge the 20–30 percent public awareness gap that currently remains pertaining to the proportion of the population that knows about the GHC 200 (US$73) cash reward instituted for the reportage of a hanging worm. In 1989, Ghana established a guinea worm eradication program, which developed national surveillance systems and facilitated the provision of potable water in endemic areas (Ministry of Health Ghana 2014, Sodzi-Tettey 2014b).

HIV prevalence among pregnant women aged 15–24 years is currently at 1.2 percent compared to 3.6 percent in 2000 (Ministry of Health Ghana 2014, Ghana Health Nest 2014). Ghana's relative success in the management of HIV traces its roots to the establishment of the national Ghana AIDS Commission (GAC) in 2002 (by an act of Parliament 613) as a supra Ministerial and multi-sectored body chaired by the President. GAC is thus the highest policymaking body on HIV/AIDS. At the 2014 Annual National Health Summit, the MoH identified worsening counseling and testing, as well as treatment for adults, as shortfalls to be tackled (Ghana Aids Commission 2014, Ministry of Health Ghana 2014).

Socio-political, Economic and Technological Forces Influencing Reform Initiatives

Ghana has been a peaceful and stable democracy since 1992, holding six successful elections that have witnessed changes in Government. With each election cycle has come political party manifestoes with express intentions for transforming the health fortunes of the citizens. Typically, the decision to implement a risk-pooling health-financing model to replace payment at the point of service delivery was announced in the run up to the 2000 national elections, as a campaign policy initiative of the opposition, NPP. The NPP subsequently won power, leading to the introduction of the NHIS in 2003 (Agyepong & Agyei 2008).

Similarly, the establishment of the new UHAS in 2012 was a political campaign promise of the ruling National Democratic Congress (NDC) Government in its 2008 manifesto. Further, Ghana's landmark Mental Health Act, hailed for its community-oriented approach, was passed in 2012 in fulfillment of a manifesto pledge by the NDC Party. The current move to decentralize the country's health sector is also firmly rooted in constitutional stipulations, specifically Article 240 (2) (d) of Ghana's 1992 Constitution and Government policy decision to restore the health sector, according to local Government expert Professor Kwamena Ahwoi, "to the Decentralization by Devolution Schedule …" (Ahwoi 2014). The country's competitive partisan political process has therefore served, perhaps inadvertently, as a catalyst for the kinds of policy initiatives that touch, and seek to address, the core health concerns of the populace.

With the commencement of offshore oil production in the Jubilee fields, in December 2010, coupled with significant existing natural and mineral resources, Ghana's economy was reputedly the fastest growing in the world in 2011 at 15 percent (Central Intelligence Agency 2014). Ghana's economy has since been rebased, with the country being declared a lower middle income (LMIC) country. In this context, a rigorous public debate has begun on funding the country's healthcare. In 2010, the Ghana Medical Association recommended the investment of some oil revenues to sustain the health insurance scheme (Winful 2010).

Technology has also played its part with various, somewhat uncoordinated, attempts to implement mobile health solutions in areas of the country. Vodafone, a mobile network in Ghana, established a doctor-to-doctor network that enabled doctors to communicate at no cost in order to improve patient care through enhanced consultations and better referral-related communication (World Health Organization 2011a).

A former Ministerial Advisor on Health Systems Strengthening, Dr Frank Nyonator, draws attention to an innovative program, "Mobile Technology for Community Health," (MoTeCH, implemented in Ghana through a GHS partnership with the Grameen Foundation and Columbia University). MoTech The Program improved maternal and child health services through mobile technology. Specifically, it stimulated demand by providing relevant information to pregnant mothers while addressing supply side issues through notification of midwives and nurses of pending and past due dates of clients.

Finally, for purposes of providing accurate, timely, and complete data for decision making and strategic guidance at various levels of the health system, the GHS has rolled out the web-based District Health Information Management Systems (DHIMS2) (Nyonator 2013). The GHS, in collaboration with partners like PFA! and MalariaCare/USAid, have rolled out a nationwide data quality improvement (DQI) initiative to improve the completeness, timeliness, and accuracy of this national data system. The DQI protocol requires data officers to cross-check data as reported in the DHIMS2 with source data verified from folders retrieved from health facilities.

Impact of Reform Initiatives

We will now scan high-level in-country data to illustrate the nature and extent of some of the reform and improvement processes at national, regional, and local levels.

Relative to the country's 1990 baseline performance in MDG-4, overall deaths of children less than five years old reduced by about 30 percent to current levels of 80 deaths per 1,000 live births (Ghana Health Service & Ghana Statistical Service 2008). Typical of other countries, the greatest progress has been with infants and young children, whereas progress for newborns has stagnated. Maternal mortality rates have also experienced a 50 percent decline to current levels of 350 deaths per 1,000 live births. Coverage for any attendance at antenatal care stands at 95 percent, while skilled delivery is recorded at 57 percent, and about 68 percent of women received a post natal check up from health professionals within 48 hours of delivery (Ghana Health Service & Ghana Statistical Service 2008).

Similar improvements were observed in the sites of PFA!, which has currently scaled up its QI approaches nationwide to assist accelerating the achievement of MDG-4. With evidence of improvements in early antenatal care, skilled delivery, and post natal care, the continued stagnation of neonatal mortality begs the question of the quality of facility-based care. This reflection is now the focus of a national newborn strategy being currently drawn up under the guidance of the GHS and other partners like UNICEF, WHO, Path, Jhpiego, and PFA!.

Within the NCHS, hosts of PFA!, 32 hospitals, have over a four-year period (2009–2013), reduced facility-based under five deaths by 27 percent using QI approaches in collaborative learning networks. Similarly, facility-based under five deaths in the Upper East and Upper West regions have reduced by 32 percent, and 36.5 percent respectively between September 2009 and September 2013. While overall under five deaths have not reduced in the Northern region, deaths within the 12–59 month age group have decreased by 39 percent within the same time period (Project Fives Alive! 2013).

Nationwide, PFA! has, over the past five years, built a potential critical mass of capacity in QI that may promote sustained improvements in outcomes. Since July 2008, over 3,712 frontline health workers have been provided training in QI methods as part of improvement learning collaboratives. The 400 QI teams formed have benefited from over 2,693 on-site supportive site visits by a combined team of project staff who are trained Improvement Advisors and health staff trained as Improvement Coaches. The 320 plus Improvement Coaches were trained using a rigorous interrupted ten-week training curriculum and includes district directors, deputy directors of clinical care, deputy directors of public health, physicians, public health nurses, and other leaders of QI teams leading various QI initiatives within their respective systems and sub-systems.

For better management of the claims processes, the NHIA has established Claims Vetting centers and a Clinical Auditing department. Cases bordering on questionable professional practices are routinely referred to professional groups, like the Ghana College of Physicians and Surgeons, to factor into training and continuing medical education programs.

The above achievements have been facilitated largely by the clear health system priorities. This clarity enables stakeholders to align quickly. The generation of real-time data for decision making and strategic direction as per DHIMS2 has been most beneficial (Nyonator 2013). Further, the infusion of continuous QI approaches and its adoption, especially within the NCHS as a turnkey strategy, has helped to provide a systematic approach to pursuing improvement by liberating the creative potential of frontline workers with active management support. Today, the NCHS has proceeded to use continuous QI methods and tools to significantly reduce health insurance claims losses in their facilities, in addition to introducing learning collaboratives within some of its nursing and midwifery training institutions to improve student pass rates.

Remaining Challenges for Reform Initiatives

Key challenges include sub-optimal coordination of the activities of multiple development partners. It is not uncommon to find different development partners, working in similar care pathways, competing in the same geographic space. This has prevented optimization of resources and achieving national coverage for certain essential services. It is encouraging that, recently, leadership within the GHS has begun to assert itself more strongly in this regard. Secondly, greater intersectoral collaboration will provide significant leverage for improving health outcomes.

The infrastructural gap continues to be massive and the current retooling of the health system ought to be encouraged and accelerated with attendant equipment maintenance training. The goals of the new Single Spine Pay policy are laudable. It is, however, deeply worrying that with almost 90 percent of health sector budgets reportedly going into salaries and emoluments, inequitable distribution of health workers continues to remain a serious challenge.

Future Direction

Variations in regional performances on various indicators have been recorded. The Upper East region for example, its classification as a deprived region notwithstanding, has, at this point, achieved 65 percent reduction in child mortality with higher than average skilled delivery rates of 67.5 percent, and a nurse to population ratio of 1:715, which is better than the WHO recommended ratio of 1:800. It is important, therefore, for the health system to be more deliberate about creating a platform where best practices from high-achieving regions can be shared. Such an initiative is more imperative given the nationwide stagnation observed in certain care pathways (Ministry of Health Ghana 2014).

Dwindling donor support, especially with the attainment of LMIC status, poses new fiscal challenges. This calls for the Ministry to better assert its oversight and coordinating role in order that multiple partner resources will be better aligned to achieve true national coverage. Hopefully, after July 2014, Ghana will be officially spared the tag of being a transition state for guinea worm disease and elevated to a guinea worm free state.

With the establishment of the Mental Health Authority, it is hoped that the dreams for transformation within the sector, through the attraction of resources, the creation of integrated care with a motivated workforce, and supportive population, will be realized. With the establishment of a Non-Communicable Disease (NCD) unit within the GHS, the development of National Cancer Registers, and ongoing pilot tests of cervical cancer screening programs, the health system is expected to increasingly strengthen its capacity to tackle the present NCD burden.

What perhaps is lacking at this point is a coordinated National Quality Strategy spearheaded by the MoH. Such a strategy would better link up policy initiatives to management action in allocation of resources, for execution of continuous QI projects by motivated frontline staff at all levels.

Chapter 3

The Gulf States

Tawfik AM Khoja and Abdelrahman A Kamel

Abstract

This chapter highlights the efforts undertaken by the Health Ministers' Council in the Gulf countries in the field of patient safety, given that the Gulf Cooperation Council (GCC) was one of ten organizations to prioritize patient safety since 2005. Current activities in the GCC countries, as well as collaborative efforts with regional and international organizations, are highlighted with the aim of understanding efforts designed to help disseminate the concept, propagate the culture, and support the promotion of patient safety in all aspects of the healthcare systems. Future perspectives are discussed and recommendations are made in an effort to overcome underlying challenges in this vital field.

Background

GCC States constitute a regional community with commonalities including religion, language, population, geography, values, as well as history, traditions, economic sources, and social and cultural circumstances. The Gulf States are (at the time of writing): Bahrain, Kuwait, Oman, Qatar, Saudi Arabia, the United Arab Emirates, and the Republic of Yemen. Unifying their efforts, these states have faced multiple challenges, and considerable developmental demands.

The Health Minister's Council (HMC) for GCC States was established in 1397H[1] (1976G) to encourage collaboration between member states in the field of health, and to join in the global effort for better achievements in health, quality of care, and patient safety. The Gulf States based their health mission on the following principles:

- Common development and coordination between the members states in the preventive, curative and rehabilitation sectors.
- Identification of key directions in health and science with the aim of unifying priorities for adoption of a common executive program amongst the Gulf States, including: healthcare quality and patient safety, health planning, improving health system performance, quality assurance, primary healthcare, family health, environmental health, and health education.

---

1   The Hijri year is the Islamic calendar system. Gregorian years are in brackets.

- Assessment of the existing systems and strategies in the health field to provide examples of successful initiatives within the Gulf States for modeling and spread to other member states.
- Conducting field surveys and research to identify areas of common interest to the Gulf States.
- Procurement of safe and efficient pharmaceutical products, hospital consumable products, and high-quality equipment with appropriate prices accessed through a central group purchase program. Establishment of a central registration of pharmaceutical products and companies is encompassed in the aim.

Table 3.1   Demographic, economic, and health information for the Gulf States

Population (thousands) (total excluding Oman)	67,965
Area (sq. km)* (total excluding Oman)	2,791,450
Proportion of population living in urban areas (2011) (range excluding Oman)	32–99
Gross Domestic Product (GDP US$, billions)^ (total excluding Oman)	1,534
Total expenditure on health as % of GDP (range excluding Oman)	2.2–5.5
Gross national income per capita (PPP intl $) (range excluding Oman)	2,310–80,470
Per capita total expenditure on health (intl $) (range excluding Oman)	118–1,805
Proportion of health expenditure which is private (range excluding Oman)	16.4–72.7
General Government expenditure on health as a percentage of total expenditure on health (range excluding Oman)	27.4–83.6
Out-of-pocket expenditure as a percentage of private expenditure on health (range excluding Oman)	52.2–98.7
Life expectancy at birth m/f (yrs) (range excluding Oman)	62–79/65–80
Probability of dying under five (per 1,000 live births) (range excluding Oman)	7–60
Maternal Mortality Ratio (per 100,000 live births) (2013) (range excluding Oman)	6–270
Proportion of population using improved water and sanitation (range excluding Oman)	55–100/ 53–100

Source: Unless otherwise stated data are for the year 2012 and taken from the World Health Organization 2014a. * Area from the World Bank 2014a. ^ GDP from the World Bank 2014b.

Notes: PPP is purchasing power parity, intl $ is international dollar which has the same purchasing power as US$ in the US.

Introduction

Historical Developments

"First do no harm" is a well known saying, but similar sentiments are reflected in many works in most cultures. The Almighty Allah in the Holy Quran says "… and if any one saved a life, it would be as if he saved the life of the whole people." Prophet Mohamed, Peace be upon him, said: "Whoever practice Medicine without any previous experience, he is guarantee" and "Allah like that when one performs a work, he make it perfect."

Avoiding harm is challenging, as recognized by the World Health Organization (WHO):

> Health care interventions are intended to benefit patients, but they can also cause harm. The complex combination of processes, technologies and human interactions that constitutes the modern health care delivery system can bring significant benefits. However, it also involves an inevitable risk of adverse events that can — and too often do — happen. (World Health Organization 2002, p. 1)

Therefore it is not surprising that patient safety is considered a cornerstone of patient rights in the healthcare system, and quality management a key mechanism for ensuring quality of care. Achieving this can be particularly challenging, however, in developing nations.

The impetus for reform in the Gulf States included: the need to stimulate improvement of the quality of healthcare delivered, so as to strengthen community confidence in healthcare institutions, reduce unnecessary costs and wastages, increase efficiency, provide credentials for education, internships, and other training programs, and potentially protect against law suits. Reforms are also designed to facilitate acceptance by, and funds from, third-party payers.

Dating from May 2001, several important strategic resolutions were made by the HMC for GCC. Key policy decisions include the introduction of quality improvement measures and accreditation programs within the organizational structure of the health system. The aim is to imbue these initiatives, and the knowledge derived from them, into the educational and training programs for workers. As well as to monitor progress through the introduction of relevant criteria and standard indicators of the efficiency, effectiveness, and quality of health services in all facilities (resolution 3 at the 51st conference held in Geneva, 2001, and resolution 11 at the 52nd conference in Riyadh, 2002). It was also agreed that such measures would require oversight by a specialized department located in the higher level of the organizational structure of the ministry.

At the 57th conference "patient safety" was adopted an important priority of the quality of health (resolution 5, Geneva, 2004). A Gulf Working Team was also proposed to review activities relating to infection control.

The position of patient safety as a top priority for decision makers was strengthened with the establishment of a "Gulf Task Force," tasked with establishing the executive plan and the guidelines for following up different aspects of patient safety, with a specific emphasis on reducing rates of medical errors, malpractice, and nosocomial infections (resolution 3, 58th conference, Muscat, 2005). To this end, effective cooperation with the World Alliance for Patient Safety, and integrated coordination with the WHO Eastern Mediterranean Regional Office (EMRO), would also be strengthened.

More Recent Developments

In 2005, it was determined that the, previously separate, Quality Assurance and Patient Safety programs would be joined to form a single entity entitled "Healthcare Quality and Patient Safety" (resolution 3, 59th conference, Geneva, 2005). Over the next few years, the regional strategy for patient safety was further unified and more work was undertaken towards the reporting of medical errors and risks.

In line with this progress, it was agreed that HMC for GCC, along with related establishments, should constructively participate in launching a "Safe Surgery Saves Lives" initiative, as an important strategic move (resolution 10, 65th conference, Geneva, 2008).

By 2009, there was endorsement by the Saudi Criteria for Accreditation of Health Facilities as a Gulf standard and increased encouragement for national authorities to be formed, responsible for accreditation with trial implementation in each state of the Arab Accreditation Instrument in a hospital (200 beds at least) and five primary healthcare centers. The HMC for GCC also urged member states to adopt and give effect to constructive participation in the international campaign to control disasters "Disaster—safe hospitals" (67th conference, Geneva).

There were other, associated measures. It was also identified, for example, that drug manufacturers and vaccine exporters to GCC should follow WHO criteria and recommendations for pharmacovigilance.

In summary, the key strategic directions for health systems in the Gulf Region were:

- development of health services according to the priorities of each country;
- setting unified quality and patient safety strategies at the level of the Gulf Region;
- sustaining and integrating of healthcare at all levels;
- giving effect to the Joint Gulf work in improvement of health sector performance;
- coping with recent international progress in the field of health services, improvements, policies, and initiatives development;
- setting and developing rules and regulations for good, quality medical practice;

- setting and developing the accreditation system for improving medical practice in Gulf health establishments;
- moving forward to realize decentralization, as well as financial and administrative independence, for health establishments in GCC countries.

The Current Situation

The Gulf States acknowledge that they face unique challenges. Currently, some of the most important reasons for developing quality improvement strategies include:

- unacceptable variation in performance, practices, and outcomes;
- weak levels of effectiveness and efficiency in provision of health services due to wastefulness, deficiencies, or misuse of health services;
- erosion of trust resulting from weak performance, malpractice and errors;
- recipients' dissatisfaction with services;
- inequality in distribution of health services;
- commonly-occurring medication errors and interventions, for which the evidence is poor;
- decay and diminution of trust and satisfaction among the public, as well as among health service providers;
- inability of local communities to bear the cost of health services;
- high expectations of consumers.

The policy direction taken by the HMC has been aimed at addressing these challenges. The progress of each country is listed in the Table 3.2 overleaf.

Current Reform Initiatives

Recent strategic directions in patient safety have been led by the Supreme Council (Their Majesties, Highnesses and heads of State of the GCC), in consultation with the Ministers of Health in the Council States, and informed by the experience of the Kingdom of Saudi Arabia with regards to the introduction of the Central Council for Accreditation of Health Facilities. In 2012, they endorsed implementation of the resolution taken by the "Supreme Council for Cooperation Council States" in its 32nd session, held in Riyadh (2011) for development of health services to match international standards, and in particular:

- Endorsement of the Saudi standards for Accreditation of Health Facilities as Gulf reference standards.
- Assigning the Gulf Committee for Healthcare Quality and Patient Safety to study the possibility of recognition of the Saudi Central Council for Accreditation of Health Facilities as a Gulf Reference Center.

Table 3.2   Situational Analysis of Patient Safety in the Gulf countries

	UAE	Bah.	KSA	Om.	Qa.	Ku.	Ye.
National Committee	N	Y	Y	N	N	N	N
Related Committee	QI & E-Gov.	QI, IC	IC, QI	QI, N.Acc., Med. Errors	QI, N.Acc.	QI, N.Acc.	QI
National Program	N	Under way	Under Way	Under way	Under way	Under Way	N
Basic Indicators	Task force	Y	Y	Y	JCI	Y	N
Questionnaire	Current situation	Report medical errors	Current situation	N	Evaluation	Denmark tool, reporting events	N
Activities:							
IC	Y	Y	Y	Y	Y	Y	Y
Environment	N	Y	Y	Y	Y	Y	N
Cl. Practice	Y	Y	Y	Y	Y	Y	Y
Medication	Y	Y	Y	Y	Y	Y	Y
Equipment	Y	Y	Y	Y	Y	Y	N
Patient Safety procedure	N	Y	Health specific, job descrip.	Y	Flagging system	N	N
Reporting system	N	Edu. & improv.	N	N	Y	N	N
Incorporation into P. rights	N	N	N	Y	Y	N	N

Notes: Y = Yes, N = No, N.Acc. = National accreditation body, QI = Quality Improvement, IC = Infection Control, JCI = Joint Commission International, E-Gov. = Electronic Government, UAE = United Arab Emirates, Bah. = Bahrain, KSA = Kingdom of Saudi Arabia, Om. = Oman, Qa. = Qatar, Ku. = Kuwait and Ye. = Yemen.

Other key policy decisions included: endorsement of the "Gulf strategic Plan for Healthcare Quality and Patient Safety—revised, 2011/2016," to be implemented in the Council States; endorsement of the "Gulf Executive Plan for Infection Control—The next five years 2011/2016," to be implemented in the Council States; urging the member states to establish centers of excellence in patient safety (similar to the Gulf Center for infection control, and with reference to the Gulf Center for Evidence-Based Medicine); encouraging the inclusion of patient safety and healthcare quality concepts, notably the WHO Patient Safety Curriculum, within the educational curricula at all levels, and calling upon the countries to establish the "International Patient Safety Forum" under the supervision of WHO.

Resolution 2 at the 73rd conference (Geneva, 2012) encompassed two main strategic goals. The first was agreement on holding a Gulf Workshop on "Mechanism of implementation of the WHO Curriculum on Patient Safety," and creating a road map for implementation with participation of Gulf health and academic leaders from ministries of health and high education in the Council States, the Executive Board of the HMC, the Regional office of the WHO Eastern Mediterranean Region, and international experts taking part in the scientific curriculum.

Second, it involved strengthening the activities of patient safety in all primary healthcare facilities according to the recommendations and outcomes of the International Consultative Meeting, "Patient Safety in Primary Care Institute" (2012) held in the WHO Headquarters in Geneva.

Although it was agreed that the "Saudi Central Council for Accreditation of Health Facilities" would be used as a guide for reference for the Gulf Center, according to the "Guideline Criteria for Evaluation and Accreditation of Gulf Reference Collaborating Centers," emphasis was placed on the fact that each country of the Council has the right to choose the National, Gulf or International Accreditation System appropriate to their healthcare system and existing facilities (resolution 4, 74th conference, Manama, 2013).

At the same conference, a research proposal was agreed upon to gain knowledge about the culture of patient safety in the Gulf States. A national team was established, with a unified conception and funding plans (resolution 5).

The Quality and Safety Landscape

1—Declaration of Kuwait for Patient Safety

Endorsed by resolution 3 of the 58th conference of the HMC (2005), the purpose of this declaration is to ensure that the Gulf's healthcare systems take major strides and are able to respond to changing needs of both the community, and the individual, and to anticipate safety health needs. The aim is to be proactive, rather than simply reactive to events. The most important goals of the declaration are:

- To develop integrated national patient safety programs, with clear targets to ensure the safety of patient care at all levels and activities, to all healthcare services.
- To facilitate a culture of safety, through better reporting and information systems, assisting the systematic monitoring, analysis, and improvement of patient outcomes.
- To build awareness and understanding of healthcare safety, improved early identification, and management of risks in patient care.
- To involve consumers in improving healthcare safety and improve communication between patients, physicians, and nurses.
- To support and professionally develop all healthcare staff, to deliver safe patient care.
- To enhance and support the research activities for patient safety, and develop centers of excellence at national levels.

2—Jeddah Declaration on Patient Safety

Endorsed by resolution 2 of the 68th conference, as a platform to be implemented in the Council States, the Gulf Committee for Patient Safety and Quality was assigned the task of transforming the Jeddah Declaration into an integrated work method for implementation, follow up, and measurement within the framework of re-updating, and improvement of the Gulf plan for patient safety. The Council States were asked to adopt the call of Jeddah Declaration on Patient Safety to reduce the prevalence of adverse events by 50 percent within 10 years (2010–2019).

The Jeddah Declaration focused on the following:

- It called for the establishment of international reference bodies for patient safety to undertake many responsibilities: classification and definitions of patient safety terminologies, dissemination of patient safety culture, setting database for study, and follow up of current situation and collaboration with related international, regional, and local authorities.
- It requested member countries to initiate national programs on patient safety and promote the concept of patient safety to the highest level of leadership, and to increase awareness.

3—Issuance of the "Glossary of Patient Safety" Textbook

The world alliance for patient safety launched the *Glossary of Patient Safety* textbook as one of the top ten international patient safety activates in 2005. The director general of the Executive Board of the Health Ministers' Council for GCC States (author of this chapter, Professor Tawfik Khoja) is the editor in chief, and key persons from the WHO and Imperial College London shared resources in reviewing the text and updating the third and fourth editions (Khoja, Kamel & Rawaf eds 2011). This text remains unique in its concept, view, and content, and has been distributed free of charge all over the globe to enhance advocacy and commitment towards patient safety.

4—Leadership Training and Capacity Building in Patient Safety

At the first GCC workshop on Quality Assurance in Primary Health Care (PHC) held in Muscat (2003), 41 indicators were agreed on; 13 structure indicators, 16 process indicators, and 12 outcome indicators. The experience of countries implementing quality measures and indicators was reviewed at the second meeting in Kuwait at the end of the year, and the first group of 12, primary health indicators for GCC countries were developed. A final evaluation of the indicators took place in Abu-Dhabi in 2009.

Key to patient safety was the declaration of Riyadh for Counterfeit Medication, at the GCC Drug Quality Symposium held in Riyadh (2007). It concluded that national pharmacovigilance infrastructure would require:

- developing a network of single points of contact per sector;
- developing a network of official Medicines Control Laboratories, and specific counterfeit expertise;
- defining regional and national priorities, based on risk analysis.

Another significant move in the support of enhanced patient safety was the United Arab Emirates' Declaration for the "Inauguration of the Patient Safety Friendly Healthcare Facilities Initiative" (Dubai, 2007). The aims of this declaration were to encourage sound medical practice on the part of all concerned bodies, hospitals, and health authorities in the Eastern Mediterranean Region. The project included an overview, mission, and specific objectives, in addition to a work plan at the national and international levels, as well as methods and a program for setting criteria and indicators of performance.

Nursing was recognized as a central element to improved patient safety in 2007 and medical errors were examined in Bahrain in 2009. The latter included reference to the WHO initiatives in Patient Safety:

- Safe Surgery Save Lives (SSSL);
- Learning from Error;
- Patients for Patient Safety (PfPS);
- research into patient safety.

Implementation: Barriers and Solutions

The WHO has listed several of the challenges faced by developing countries and countries in economic transition. The probability of adverse events is much higher, for example, than in industrialized nations, for many reasons. Key ones include:

- the poor state of infrastructure and equipment;
- unreliable supply and quality of drugs;
- shortcomings in waste management;
- inappropriate infection control policies implementation;
- poor performance of personnel because of low motivation or insufficient technical skills;
- insufficient or lack of continuous professional development programs;
- under-financing of essential operating costs for health services.

Recently the GCC oversaw the regional launch of the WHO curriculum on Patient Safety, held in Oman (2012). It has been recognized that making an evidence-based change in practice involves a series of action steps, and a complex, nonlinear process. Increasing staff knowledge about a specific evidence-based patient safety, and passive dissemination strategies, are not likely to work, particularly in complex healthcare settings.

Many Gulf strategies that seem to have a positive effect on promoting the use of evidence-based practice include, audit and feedback, use of clinical reminders and practice prompts, opinion leaders, change champions, interactive education, mass media, educational outreach and academic detailing, and promotion of the key characteristics of care delivery (for example, leadership, learning, and questioning). The senior leadership, and those leading these improvements in the Gulf States, are keenly aware of change as a process, and want to continue to encourage and teach peers about improvements in practice, usually through evidence-based guidelines.

Prospects for Success and Next Steps

The Strategic Gulf Plan for Health Care Quality & Patient Safety 2011–2016, derives its elements from the various endorsed executive plans and tables set during the meetings of the Gulf Committee for Healthcare Quality and Patient Safety. This document is considered a comprehensive guiding plan for the next five years, and has the authority of executive by-laws for the general plan. Each Gulf country will set its national operational action plans in the light of the elements included in this plan, and within a bound timeframe (usually annual or biannual) in such a way that it expresses the higher (optimal) level of the required criteria and infrastructure for each country. Due to the variation in geography and in available resources, it is necessary to recognize the differentiable capacities of the different states at any given point. Nonetheless a unified direction has been agreed upon.

Vision

The promotion of healthcare quality and patient safety in the health facilities of Cooperation Council States.

Mission

Continuous improvement of healthcare quality and patient safety, through setting strategic plans to support quality and patient safety activities, developing quality and patient safety standards and criteria within health facilities, and implementing training and education plans. As well as the continuous development towards unification of Cooperation Council States, to help cope with and support the development of their health systems, in fulfillment of the needs and expectations of the service beneficiaries and providers.

Healthcare Quality

General objective
The institution and application of quality systems in the health facilities of Cooperation Council States.

Strategic objectives

- setting national programs for quality systems;
- setting and implementation of Gulf indicators for healthcare quality;
- building national capacities in the field of quality;
- setting a system for quality auditing.

Patient Safety

General objective
The institution and implementation of patient safety systems in the health facilities of Cooperation Council States.

Strategic objectives

- an analytical study on the current situation of patient safety in healthcare facilities;
- setting executive national programs for patient safety;
- setting and implementing patient safety Gulf standards;
- strategic objectives;
- building national capacities in the field of patient safety;
- establishment and support of medical errors reporting system;
- adoption and implementation of patient safety solutions;
- adoption and giving effect to international and regional initiatives in the field of patient safety.

Current Achievements

It is recognized that a major key to success will be moving toward a culture of safety. To move from a culture of blame towards a culture of safety, change is necessary. The development of a culture of safety has three stages:

Stage 1: Emphasis is on complying with regulatory standards and meeting technical requirements.
Stage 2: Good safety performance is seen as an organizational goal and valued as being important.
Stage 3: The culture of safety permeates the organization and there is an emphasis on continuous improvement.

Table 3.3   Status of each nation against objectives

Executive Activities	UAE	Bah.	KSA	Om.	Qa.	Ku.	Ye.
Strategic Objective I							
Preparing an instrument for current situation analysis of Patient Safety in health facilities.	Yes	No	Yes	Yes	Yes	No	
Implementation of the analytical study.	No	No	Yes	Yes	Yes	No	No
Presentation and discussion of the national results to develop a unified Gulf report.	No	No	Yes		No	No	
Strategic Objective II							
Establishment of an endorsement dept / committee for patient safety within the organizational structure of the Quality Dept at the central level.		Yes	Yes	Yes	Yes	Yes	Yes
Setting an endorsed and documented strategic, executive plan for patient safety.	Yes	Yes	Yes	Yes	Con.	Yes	Yes
Setting patient safety policies.	Yes		Yes	Yes	Under study	Yes	Under study
Development of indicators to measure patient safety in healthcare facilities.	Yes	Yes	Yes	Yes	Yes	Sitting	No start
Strategic Objective III							
A) Gulf Standards for Patient Safety in Hospitals							
Finalization of the Gulf standards for patient safety in hospitals.	No	No	Yes	Yes	Yes	Yes	No
Experimental application of the draft standards.	No	No	Yes	Yes	Yes	No	Yes
Endorsement and circulation of the Gulf standards for patient safety at hospitals.	No	No	No	Yes	Yes	No	Yes
Application of the Gulf standards for patient safety.	No	No	Yes	Yes	Yes	No	
B) Gulf standards for Patient Safety in Primary Health Care							
Preparing Gulf standards for patient safety in Primary Health Care.	Under study	No	No	Yes	Yes	Yes	Yes
Experimental application of the draft standards.	No	No	No	Yes	Yes	No	
Endorsement and circulation of the Gulf standards for patient safety in PHC	No	No	No	Yes	Yes	No	
Application of the Gulf standards for patient safety at PHC	No	No	Yes	Yes	Yes	No	
Strategic Objective IV							
Developing qualification and training programs in patient safety.	Yes	Yes	Yes	Yes	Yes	Yes	
Utilization of available qualifying programs in the Council States.	No	No	No	Con.	Yes	Yes	

Table 3.3   Status of each nation against objectives *concluded*

Executive Activities	UAE	Bah.	KSA	Om.	Qa.	Ku.	Ye.
Introduction of patient safety concepts within the educational curricula in the health education institutions.	Under study	Yes	Yes	Yes	Yes	Yes	Yes
Strategic Objective V							
Setting a specific policy for registration and reposting systems of medical errors.	Yes	Yes	Yes	Yes	Con.	Yes	No
Enacting legislations and laws necessary for the support of reporting system.	No	No	Yes	Yes	No	Yes	No
Setting mechanisms and tools of notification in health facilities.	Yes	Yes	Yes	Yes	Yes	Yes	No
Developing mechanisms of root analysis for causes of errors, and setting necessary corrective procedures.	Yes	Yes	Yes	Yes	Con.	Yes	No
Strategic Objective VI							
Developing a national executive plan for application of patient safety solutions.	No	Yes	No	Yes	No	Yes	Yes
Setting policies for each of the patient safety solutions.	No	Yes	No	Yes	No	Yes	No
Training staff on application of patient safety solution policies.	No	No	No	No	Yes	Yes	No
Development and application of mechanisms of follow up and monitoring.	No	Yes	No	No	Yes	Yes	No

Notes: Same country abbreviations as for Table 3.2.

What Next?

Critical to the future of quality and safety in the Gulf States will be effective partnerships. Health practitioners, leaders, and managers should collaborate with each other to develop and evaluate interventions designed to support a healthy work environment. This will require interdisciplinary teams to develop positive working relationships that contribute to safe and effective care by reducing errors, and creating a more supportive work environment. Each individual in the health system has a responsibility to contribute to the continuous improvement of his or her work environment and, thus, improve patient safety. Significant improvements will require the development of a patient safety research culture in all healthcare institutions and facilities, as well as the primary healthcare sector, through ministries of health, the academic community, and civil society. With these measures, the Gulf States will be able to perform continuous evaluation and updating of the Gulf plan for patient safety, according to the international and regional changes and developments.

Conclusion

The Gulf States have thoughtfully formulated principles, framed declarations, and made recommendations in the recent past in order to structure reforms designed to improve quality of care and patient safety. Progress is being made, but there is recognition that there is a long journey ahead.

Chapter 4

Israel

Eyal Zimlichman

Abstract

Recent years have seen a surge of reform initiatives aimed at improving quality and patient safety in Israel. Within the last four years the Ministry of Health (MoH) has set down a policy infrastructure that includes a quality measures program, accreditation of hospitals, a nationally coordinated infection control program, a national patient experience survey, the establishment of a national program for electronic health information exchange, and other policy initiatives. With these steps, Israel seems to have closed the gap with other leading developed countries. In this chapter we will outline the challenges and opportunities for initiating successful quality and patient safety reform in Israel and attempt to discern which of the initiatives are already showing evidence of their success. Finally, we will recommend what future steps are needed to further advance quality and patient safety on a national level.

Background

The healthcare system in Israel is one of contrasts: social foundations yet highly competitive market, low-cost spending (half the average of Organization for Economic Cooperation and Development (OECD) countries) yet continuously improving population health outcomes, and high-quality community healthcare services, with hospital care trying to catch up. The reforms that have helped shape this unique system stem back to the foundations of the State of Israel, although the last 20 years have seen a new set of reforms centered around: equity, patient rights and patient-centric care, national measurement at the community level, and now also at the hospital level, and national quality and patient safety initiatives aiming to cover the gap with leading developed countries.

Throughout these past 20 years, and particularly the past four years, a set of legislations and policies set by the Government and MoH have reshaped the healthcare landscape, with the improvement of quality and safety in mind. This was started by setting the responsibilities of the providers and the rights of the patients as a national law in the mid-1990s and expanded to include the setting of national quality measures, monitoring safety, accreditation of hospitals, and tying financial incentives to quality and safety milestones.

Table 4.1   Demographic, economic, and health information for Israel

Population (thousands)	7,644
Area (sq. km)*	21,640
Proportion of population living in urban areas (2011)	92
Gross Domestic Product (GDP US$, billions)^	257.6
Total expenditure on health as % of GDP	7.5
Gross national income per capita (PPP intl $)	28,070
Per capita total expenditure on health (intl $)	2,239
Proportion of health expenditure which is private	38.3
General Government expenditure on health as a percentage of total expenditure on health	61.7
Out-of-pocket expenditure as a percentage of private expenditure on health	65.3
Life expectancy at birth m/f (yrs)	80/84
Probability of dying under five (per 1,000 live births)	4
Maternal Mortality Ratio (per 100,000 live births) (2013)	2
Proportion of population using improved water and sanitation	100/100

Source: Unless otherwise stated data are for the year 2012 and taken from the World Health Organization 2014a. * Area from the World Bank 2014a. ^ GDP from the World Bank 2014b.

Notes: PPP is purchasing power parity, intl $ is international dollar which has the same purchasing power as US$ in the US.

Israel instituted two landmark laws that have fundamentally impacted the patient–provider relationship: the National Health Insurance Law, in 1995, and the Patient's Rights Law, in 1996. Among other things, the former ensured universal health insurance coverage for all citizens while providing a free choice of health plans. The result was to increase the role of patients as consumers in a competitive market. Equally important was the Patient's Rights Law, the goals of which were to ensure caregiver professionalism and quality, and to protect the dignity and privacy of patients (Israel 1996).

Introduction

In this chapter we will describe the healthcare initiatives that have played out in Israel and establish the relationship between those initiatives and the quality and safety of healthcare, emphasizing what has worked, what hasn't, and what needs to happen in the future to attain the highest quality and patient safety to its citizens.

The broader healthcare system stems from social foundations set in place when the State of Israel was established in 1948. As a result, the current structure is primarily tax-funded, based largely on state activities. Universal coverage is provided to all citizens and permanent residents through a national health insurance system that allows the insured to choose a health plan. The four non-profit, competing health plans (Clalit, Maccabi, Meuhedet, and Leumit) must provide their members with access to a benefits package that is specified in the national law, also providing community healthcare services to all citizens (Rosen & Samuel 2009). Although there are a few private hospitals, most acute care beds and long-term inpatient facilities are operated by the Government, and the Government sets the level of per capita financing that all four health plans receive. Clalit (the largest health plan that insures roughly 50 percent of the population) is the only health plan to run its own general hospitals, operating about one-third of the general hospitals in the country.

The Current Situation

Israel's healthcare system faces many quality and safety challenges, most are shared by all other developed countries, yet some are more pronounced for Israel. While quality of care in the community has been demonstrated through the National Quality Indicators program, demonstrating a continuous improvement for many indicators (Jaffe et al. 2012), the level of quality and safety for Israel's hospitals has been mostly unknown. With the overcrowding in hospitals and continuous budget cuts, as well as the ongoing lack of monitoring and supervision by the state, this lack of knowledge, regarding level of quality and safety, has been a concern for policymakers. Some of the other challenges include transitions between the hospitals and the community, caring for the aging and the chronic disease populations, and transforming the system to being more patient-centered.

Charged with the responsibility to reform Israel's healthcare system and address the above mentioned challenges is the Government, specifically the MoH. Yet, much of the initiatives impacting quality and safety have originated from the health plans that have individually set the agenda ahead of national policy. Such is the case with setting a national program of quality indicators for the community (and later for hospitals), large-scale patient experience surveys, and policy for the accreditation of general hospitals. Within the Israeli healthcare system another key player is the Israeli Medical Association (IMA) which represents the physicians in Israel and acts both as a workers union, and in setting and overseeing professional standards for physician's specialization programs. This duality poses a potential for conflict between representing the physician's interests and ensuring high quality and safety. This will be discussed in more detail later in this chapter.

Reform Initiatives

Recent years have seen a surge of policy initiatives all aimed at increasing quality and patient safety. The Patient's Rights Law (1996) had set the expectations for high-quality, safe, and patient-centered care. The law explicitly defined the rights and obligations of patient–provider relationships, and epitomized the shift from a paternalistic model of care to a patient-centered one emphasizing patient autonomy. Specifically, the Patient's Rights Law addressed important issues such as informed consent for treatment, provider–patient shared decision making, the right for a second opinion, and more. In this, Israel was a true pioneer in an era preceding the Institute of Medicine reports in the United States (US).

Measuring quality on a national level started a few years later. In 2004, the Israel National Institute for Health Policy and Health Services Research launched the National Program for Quality Indicators in Community Healthcare in Israel (QICH), a program that began in 1999 as a Ben-Gurion University research project (Jaffe et al. 2012). With the intention of being able to compare across countries, indicators were based on existing international measures, mostly from the Healthcare Effectiveness Data and Information Set (HEDIS), of the National Committee for Quality Assurance (NCQA), in the US. With all four health plans cooperating and supporting the program, it was considered a success from its early days. Measuring quality of care in hospitals started much later with the MoH stepping in and filling the gap only in 2013. The National Program for Quality Indicators in Hospitals currently (as of early 2014) includes 22 process indicators, of which ten are for general hospitals, six for psychiatric hospitals, and six for geriatric long-term care hospitals. The program currently enjoys the cooperation of all hospitals who submit data to the MoH, yet, challenges stemming from differences in clinical and administrative systems as well as diagnosis and procedure coding still need to be worked out before the data are considered valid enough to allow comparisons and public reporting.

The current focus of the MoH on ensuring higher quality and safety in hospitals was not limited to measuring quality, but has also recently expanded to a national hospital accreditation reform. In Israel, no national accreditation system existed prior to 2012, although the MoH conducted audits for the purpose of relicensing hospitals, and the Scientific Council of the IMA conducts audits for residency and fellowship programs. Clalit Health Services was the first to initiate a hospital accreditation program, contracting with the Joint Commission International (JCI). This has prompted the MoH to consider and then embrace the JCI as the national accreditation body for all general hospitals, with aims of expanding to non-general hospitals in the near future. The MoH has set the JCI accreditation certification as a pre-condition for relicensing of general hospitals, starting in 2015. With more than half of Israeli general hospitals already accredited by the JCI, this has brought about a major change in terms of implementing quality and safety evidence-based practices.

Key reforms are also taking place, aspiring to enhance the patient experience. The MoH has recently set priorities in improving availability, equity, lingual, and cultural accessibility of services. Yet, well ahead of new national policy, again, local initiatives have set the patient-centered care agenda. First through pilots and demonstrations, and later through a comprehensive program, all four plans now actively assess the patient experience as part of a comprehensive service-oriented roadmap, and have integrated patient experience into their organizational goals. Following the National Health Insurance Law, national surveys on experience of care were sponsored by the MoH and the health plans. They were conducted by the Myers-JDC-Brookdale Institute in Jerusalem, biannually (Brammli-Greenberg et al. 2011), via telephone surveys of a representative sample of adult residents. Although survey results are published, the impact on consumer behavior is unclear. Yet, the surveys most likely have had some effect on both the macro level (policy), as well as the micro level (service). One initiative attributed to the surveys were the MoH issued regulations regarding notifications on copayments and supplemental insurance, which translated to increased publication and dissemination of relevant regulations by the health funds (Gross 2006).

Measuring and comparing patient experience with hospital care in Israel is more sporadic, and results of surveys are rarely available publically (Siegel-Itzkovich 2012, Midgam LTD 2011). A 2011 survey comparing all Government-owned hospitals on patient experience of care was criticized in the media as not addressing the right questions and not being adequately transparent (Linder-Gantz 2012). With that in mind, the MoH has recently committed to institute ongoing, publicly reported, national surveys for patient experience aimed initially at acute-care hospitals, starting in 2013/2014, and later other inpatient settings and community care.

Other reform initiatives seeking to improve quality and safety have focused on preventing hospital acquired infections (HAIs) through first establishing a program for collecting and reporting national data from all hospitals on the prevalence and incidence of multidrug resistant organism acquisitions and central-line associated blood stream infections through the National Center for Infection Control (Schwaber & Carmeli 2014). Furthermore, to improve adherence to guidelines issued by the MoH, a financial incentive initiative, tied to implementation of a hospital infection control program, was launched in 2014.

Lastly, policy aimed towards improving data sharing across providers and across the continuum of care has meant the initiation of an electronic health information exchange program. While this was officially enacted in 2014, and is set to include all patients across the country by 2015, this initiative is based on a program launched by Clalit Health Services ten years earlier called the "Ofek" program ("horizon" in Hebrew). To improve the information flow within the network of Clalit community care and hospitals, in 2005, Clalit launched the "Ofek" system of hospital community on-line medical records (Frankel et al. 2013). The same system is now in the process of expanding to include all four health plans and all hospitals in the country—an ambitious project that will place Israel as one of the only countries with a country-wide health information exchange system.

The Quality and Safety Landscape

The quality and patient safety landscape is being shaped within the MoH by the office of Director General, Professor Ronni Gamzu. In the past, the lack of a formal structure and leadership in regard to safety and quality from the Ministry led to a situation in which many stakeholders were drawn into the vacuum. Among them, of course, the health funds have always played a major role, with the IMA and some of the professional societies active mostly through supervision and accreditation of training programs and clinical policy setting (guidelines). Patient safety was promoted mostly through the liability and risk management lens. For example, a Government agency (Inbal) provides legal support and insurance to Government hospitals to reduce medical malpractice claims through risk management activity within hospitals. A more comprehensive patient safety strategy was lacking prior to the recent reforms that have embraced the JCI and have set specific patient safety goals.

Recent actions by the MoH have drawn some criticism from hospitals and health funds due to, what was sometimes conceived as, increased control by the regulator and more bureaucracy. For providers, in a reality of shrinking budgets and mounting debts, the demands included in quality and safety reforms drew increasing concerns regarding the ability to execute them without additional resources. The IMA and the physician's union, in reaction to accreditation requirements, specifically dealing with continuous evaluation and re-credentialing of physicians, have also expressed their concern that it compromises physician's interests, instructing physicians not to cooperate with the new JCI regulation requirements on physician evaluation. One needs to stress that in Israel no real re-licensing regulations exist for physicians, whether in the form of a continuous medical education (CME) like system, or other. These issues were being negotiated at the time of writing of this book. Despite these obstacles, implementation of the accreditation program was progressing according to the timeline set by the MoH.

The Impact of the Reform Efforts on Quality and Safety of Care

As quality and safety reforms push forward in Israel, early evidence of its impacts are starting to emerge. Compared to other countries, Israel has traditionally enjoyed comparatively high population health indicators. Life expectancy at birth is relatively high compared to other OECD countries at 81.8 years in 2011, compared to the average for the 34 OECD countries at 80.1, or to the US at 78.7 (Organisation for Economic Cooperation and Development 2013a). Infant mortality, another indicator frequently used to compare across countries, is lower in Israel (3.5 deaths per 1,000 live births) than the average for OECD countries (4.1), and compared to the US (6.1). In some of the other indicators used by the OECD, like mortality following acute myocardial infarction (AMI) and stroke, Israel performs better than the average for OECD countries, but below the US (for AMI Israel 7.1 per 100 admissions, OECD 7.9 and US 5.5; for stroke Israel 6.3, OECD 8.5, and US 4.3). A clear improvement, which could be attributable to some of the policy initiatives and strengthening of the community services in Israel, is a significant reduction in asthma and *chronic obstructive pulmonary disease (*COPD) hospital admissions between 2006 and 2011 (from 90 per 100,000 population to 61.4 respectively for asthma, and from 285 to 229 respectively for COPD). Taken together, the high performance considering relatively low healthcare spending, these results have raised the attention of health policy experts (Chernichovsky 2009) and have gained praise from the OECD, especially concerning the community health services (Organisation for Economic Cooperation and Development 2012).

The National Program for Quality Indicators in the Community, launched in 2004, allows comparison of performance indicators across countries. As Rosen et al. (2011) have found, in a comparative analysis of adherence to standards of care between Israel and the US, Israel achieves comparable quality on several primary care indicators and more rapid quality improvement. While for adherence to screening standards Israel was lagging behind the US, in adherence to standards for care of diabetes patients, the compliance in Israel was higher. In terms of intermediate outcomes achieved, in Israel the rate of uncontrolled diabetes was lower (13.3 percent vs. 31.0 percent in the US patients with A1c Hb (Glycated hemoglobin) above 9 percent) and the rate of controlled hypertension was higher (66.8 percent vs. 31.7 percent respectively with systolic blood pressure under 130 mmHg) (Rosen et al. 2011).

Furthermore, when comparing quality indicators in the community longitudinally, a significant improvement can be seen in many of the indicators. Jaffe et al. (2012) have done a comparison across three years (2006–2009) and demonstrated an overall improvement, especially in proper documentation, and to a lesser extent in other indicators such as primary prevention measures and documentation of cardiovascular risk (Jaffe et al. 2012). It is believed that the connection between the launch of the National Program for Quality Indicators in the Community and the improvement in the performance is causative. The health funds have taken seriously the quality measurement and have invested in improvement programs and re-structuring, as well as tracking their performance.

For most of the other reforms initiated in the last 3—4 years it is still too early to evaluate which have been successful and which have not. With the JCI accreditation already achieved by over half of the general hospitals in the country, one can assume quality improvements, or at least the infrastructure for quality and patient safety, is being set in place. Specifically for HAIs, national coordination of efforts to prevent multidrug resistant organism acquisitions was successful in substantially reducing nosocomial carbapenem-resistant enterobacteriaceae (CRE) acquisition in acute and long-term facilities (Schwaber & Carmeli 2014). Lastly, the rapid implementation across the country of the "Ofek" health information exchange program has already improved quality by reducing duplicate and unnecessary blood tests and imaging in medicine departments where adoption has been adequate (Nirel et al. 2011).

Implementation: Barriers and Solutions

Standing in the way of the much needed improvements in quality and patient safety are a few obstacles and barriers, of which most would be generic to other, developed countries, while some would be more specific to Israel. Limited resources—both human and physical—would probably be conceived as the foremost obstacle in many countries. Especially by US, but also by European hospital's standards, Israeli hospitals are considerably under staffed. While staffing ratios in intensive care units (ICUs) in Israel are usually one nurse for two or three patients, in the US ICUs would usually have a nurse per hospitalized patient. This gap would be even larger for general ward staffing ratios—both for nurses and for physicians. Since evidence shows that staffing ratios are linked to improved outcomes for patients, specifically proper infection control efforts, in-hospital complication prevention, and mortality (Shekelle 2013, Penoyer 2010), Israel is at a disadvantage compared to other OECD countries in this regard.

Several opportunities currently exist in Israel for quality and patient safety improvement. First, it is the current MoH administration, which has placed quality and patient safety as the upmost priority, initiating policy and regulations and enhancing control over quality and safety. While still in office, it is likely that more reforms will be initiated and infrastructure will be put in place to sustain quality and patient safety as we move forward. The hospital accreditation program, and commissioning of the JCI to accredit hospitals in Israel, can also be viewed as an opportunity for continued quality and patient safety improvements in hospitals. Finally, Israel's healthcare system enjoys the advantage of a strong information technology infrastructure and having a national system for data exchange (Lejbkowicz et al. 2004, Peterburg 2010). As the healthcare system moves ahead to addressing current and future challenges, this would certainly play a major role in enhancing quality and patient safety (Zimlichman & Bates 2012).

Prospects and Next Steps

Where else should the Israeli healthcare system turn in order to improve quality and patient safety for its citizens? A logical next step to the national measurement programs for quality, safety, and patient experience, would be public reporting of measures across the country (both hospitals and the community), followed by a pay-for-performance (PFP) incentive program, similar to the value-based purchasing policy set up in the US just recently (VanLare & Conway 2012). Of course, public reporting, which is currently planned for launch in the immediate future, should help, but only after there is sufficient confidence in the metrics and the ability to appropriately compare between providers. The PFP program should include quality metrics (including re-admissions as a motivator to enhance continuity of care and reduce hospital utilization), avoidance of hospital acquired conditions, patient experience, and also implementation of health information technology (HIT) components. Any PFP program should be based on the principal that the top performing percentage (however determined) will get an incentive, while the bottom would pay a penalty on reimbursement, which should work as a zero-sum gain for the MoH and the Government in terms of expenses. National surveys assessing patient experience, developed now for acute care hospitals, should expand to include all levels of care, with an emphasis on care transitions as well as assessing levels of patient engagement (Zimlichman, Rozenblum & Millenson 2013).

Additionally, harnessing HIT to promote patient safety is pivotal because it extends to all providers. This is especially important for domains with robust evidence such as implementation of medication safety systems—computerized physicians order entry and bar-coding systems in particular. With the high adoption rate of electronic health systems (Lejbkowicz et al. 2004, Peterburg 2010) Israel could make significant strides on this in a relatively short time. Implementing an incentive and penalty program similar to the Meaningful Use program in the US, where providers gain financial incentives and avoid a penalty for implementing certain HIT components or functionalities (Blumenthal & Tavenner 2010), could further develop the HIT infrastructure towards improvement in quality and safety. In Israel's case, this would be more critical for hospitals at this point.

Conclusion

Israel has made substantial reform efforts in the last few years, yet much still needs to be done to push quality and patient safety forward on a national scale. Although some countries have had a substantial head start in creating national quality and patient safety infrastructure and policy, Israel has the potential to catch up fast. Policymakers need to learn what has worked and what has not in other countries, and better understand what is still needed. Harnessing HIT to promote patient safety holds much promise and could present Israel with an opportunity to turn the tide.

Table 4.2   Healthcare reforms undertaken in Israel to improve quality and patient safety

Year	Reform	Details	Quality Domains
1995	National health insurance law	Ensured universal health insurance coverage for all citizens while providing free choice of health plans.	Equity, patient-centeredness
1996	Patient's rights law	Defines the rights and obligations of patient-provider relationships, epitomizing the shift from a paternalistic model of care to a patient-centered one emphasizing patient autonomy.	Safety, effectiveness, equity, timeliness, patient-centeredness
2004	Quality indicators in community healthcare*	A national quality measures program for community services with the participation of all four health funds. Launched by the Israel National Institute for Health Policy and Health Services Research.	Effectiveness, equity, timeliness, efficiency
2007	National program (and center) for infection control	Collecting and reporting national data from all hospitals on the prevalence and incidence of multidrug resistant organism acquisitions and central-line associated blood stream infections.	Safety, effectiveness, efficiency
2012	Accreditation of general hospitals (followed by psychiatric and geriatric hospitals)	Commissioning the Joint Commission International as the national accrediting body for general hospitals and setting an accredited status as a pre-condition for relicensing of hospitals starting 2015.	Safety, effectiveness, equity, timeliness, patient-centeredness, efficiency
2012	National hospital quality measures program	Including (as of early 2014) 22 process indicators for general, geriatric and psychiatry hospitals collected centrally through hospital reporting and aimed for public transparency.	Safety, effectiveness, timeliness, efficiency
2013	National patient experience survey	MoH to institute ongoing, publicly reported, national surveys for patient experience aimed initially at acute-care hospitals, starting in 2013/2014, and later other inpatient settings and community care.	Equity, timeliness, patient-centeredness
2014	Electronic health information exchange program	A nation-wide hospital-community health information exchange program that will allow data sharing across providers and across the continuum of care.	Safety, effectiveness, patient-centeredness, efficiency
2014	Quality improvement incentives program	Focusing on both infection control and emergency department structure and waiting times will provide funding to hospitals that are meeting MoH standards.	Safety, effectiveness, timeliness, patient-centeredness, efficiency

Note: * National program not yet an MoH regulation or law.

Chapter 5

Oman

Ahmed Al-Mandhari

"As it is well known that a healthy mind is in a healthy body, health should be a right of every citizen. Since July 1970, we have decided to attach a high priority to the development of health of the Omani people."

HM Qaboos Bin Said
Sultan Oman (Ministry of Health Oman 2010a)

Abstract

Healthcare systems are dynamic as they deal with human life. Quality and patient safety are essential dimensions; however, globally, healthcare systems are facing challenges that put them at risk of regressing in terms of improving quality and patient safety. Therefore, many countries around the globe have taken active steps towards reviewing their healthcare systems and enabling them to identify strengths, weaknesses, opportunities, and threats which can impact on quality and patient safety. This chapter will shed light on the reforms the Omani system has undertaken since its establishment in 1970, focusing on the impact of these reforms on quality and patient safety.

Background

Current Reform Initiatives

The Omani healthcare system, like other systems, has witnessed an increase in community demand for services, thus putting it under continuous pressure. The Ministry of Health (MoH), being the main healthcare provider, has taken major steps in reforming its system including the *Vision 2050* that has short-, medium-, and long-term targets for improving the standards of services. Other providers, such as Sultan Qaboos University Hospital (SQUH) with the College of Medicine and Health Sciences (COMHS), and the Military Medical Services, have taken similar steps including enrolling in an international accreditation process and introducing of new medical curricula.

Table 5.1   Demographic, economic, and health information for Oman

Population (thousands)	3,314
Area (sq. km)*	309,500
Proportion of population living in urban areas (2011)	73
Gross Domestic Product (GDP US$, billions)^	78.1
Total expenditure on health as % of GDP	2.6
Gross national income per capita (PPP intl $)	25,320
Per capita total expenditure on health (intl $)	810
Proportion of health expenditure which is private	19.6
General Government expenditure on health as a percentage of total expenditure on health	80.4
Out-of-pocket expenditure as a percentage of private expenditure on health	61.3
Life expectancy at birth m/f (yrs)	74/78
Probability of dying under five (per 1,000 live births)	12
Maternal Mortality Ratio (per 100,000 live births) (2013)	11
Proportion of population using improved water and sanitation	93/97

Source: Unless otherwise stated data are for the year 2012 and taken from the World Health Organization 2014a. * Area from the World Bank 2014a. ^ GDP from the World Bank 2014b.

Notes: PPP is purchasing power parity, intl $ is international dollar which has the same purchasing power as US$ in the US.

Current Efforts to Improve the Quality and Safety of Healthcare

As part of the current reforms in the country, the MoH has taken steps toward improving quality and patient safety. Provision of high-quality services was explicitly stated as one of the goals in the sixth and seventh five-year plans (2006–2010 and 2011–2015) (Ministry of Health Oman n.d., Ministry of Health Oman 2010a). Objectives included establishing and developing quality management systems in healthcare services, ensuring the safety of patients and healthcare workers, and training and qualifying a national Omani cadre to lead the quality assurance and improvement programs in their regions. These have led to several actions including establishing quality and patient safety bodies supervising quality and patient safety activities at the hospital, health services directorate, and the ministry headquarter levels. Furthermore, the MoH created several task-force committees that are responsible for reviewing the current situation of certain services such as emergency, obstetric and gynecology, and intensive care services, as well as planning the way forward. Similarly, SQUH and COMHS have worked toward improving quality and patient safety through gaining accreditation from international bodies such as Accreditation Canada International (ACI), and the accreditation of the COMHS by the Association for Medical Education in the Eastern Mediterranean Region (AMEEMR).

Economic, Political, Socio-cultural, and Technological Forces Influencing These Reform and Improvement Efforts

Like many other reforms, healthcare system reforms in Oman have faced competing forces. Top of the list of progressive forces is the strong, political commitment, and high priority accorded to the health and education sectors by His Majesty Sultan Qaboos bin Said, as reflected in many of his speeches (Ministry of Health Oman 2010a). Other essential positive forces are the cultural and economic stability compared to many other countries in the region. For example, investments have been considerable: MoH total expenditure proportional to percentage of governmental expenditures increased from 3.0 percent in 1980 to 4.5 percent in 2012. Similarly, MoH expenditures per capita (RO) increased from 28.0 RO in 1980 to 133.1 RO in 2012. Another important force is the sustainable increase in the production of the national workforce cadre. For example, the number of post-diploma nursing graduates increased from 50 in 1998 to 246 in 2012 (Ministry of Health Oman 2012). Similarly, the number of general nursing graduates increased from 52 in 1984 to 554 in 2005, and 485 in 2011 (Ministry of Health Oman 2012). Furthermore, links with international bodies such as the World Health Organization (WHO), have added value to the system. For example, with WHO technical support, Oman managed to launch the Expanded Immunization Program (EPI) which led to a reduction in the prevalence of childhood communicable diseases (Ministry of Health Oman 2002).

The system has also faced reactionary forces that have negatively impacted on these reforms. One of these is the unstable political status in the Middle East, which discourages many skilled healthcare professionals from joining the healthcare systems in the Gulf Countries. Another factor is competing regional and international markets for skilled healthcare professionals, which constrains the budget of the system. For example, there were 6.8 percent, 5.6 percent, and 6.4 percent salary rises in one of the Gulf Countries in the years 2010, 2011, and 2012 respectively (GulfTalent 2012). This is complicated by the high dependence on expatriate medical personnel, with the challenges of differences in culture, medical practices, and patient care. In addition, such personnel are subject to high turnover as they view their work in the Gulf countries, as a learning experience for international exposure, and later move back to their home countries, or developed markets, for higher paid jobs (Alpen Capital 2011). Furthermore, increased prevalence of lifestyle-related diseases, such as diabetes and hypertension, puts pressure on health reforms in terms of redirecting resources from other programs to the management of these diseases. For example, a study showed that the age-adjusted prevalence of diabetes among Omanis aged 30–64 reached 16.1 in 2000, compared with 12.2 in 1991 (Al-Lawati et al. 2002). Notably, the International

Diabetes Federation reveals that Oman is among the top 12, globally, for diabetes prevalence among citizens aged 20–79, with a prevalence rate of 13.4 percent (Alhyas, McKay & Majeed 2012). Such high prevalence is compounded by the fact that the average cost of these lifestyle-related ailments is higher and extends over a longer term than other conditions, leading to higher healthcare-related spending (Alpen Capital 2011). Furthermore, coupled with the increasing cost and Government spending in healthcare service, was the introduction of new modalities of interventions. The effects of these have been reflected in the WHO report that highlighted an increase of Government spending from 56.4 percent in 2000 to 60.5 percent in 2008 (Alpen Capital 2011).

Introduction

Brief Historical Background to Reform

The history of healthcare reforms in the country begins in 1970, the year in which His Majesty Sultan Qaboos took over the leadership of the country. That year witnessed the establishment of the MoH, which was followed, in 1976, by the introduction of the first five-year national plan (1976–1980), which had five year targets, reviewed annually. The first three plans were generally service extension plans, aiming to establish accessible, affordable, acceptable healthcare services to all members of the community. For example, the period 1981–1990 witnessed the introduction of EPI, the establishment of the College of Medicine & Health Sciences, the introduction of National Women & Children Care Plan (NWCCP), the introduction of the national residency programs for physicians, and decentralization of the health administration.

The subsequent plans (1990–2013) continued building infrastructure with special attention to delivering high standards of healthcare to the community. For example, based on many situational analyses carried out with the support of international experts, MoH introduced several public health programs such as, the Malaria Eradication Program (MEP) in 1991, which was followed by a 97.2 percent reduction in the incidence of malaria cases for the period 1991–2005 (Ganguly et al. 2009), and screening programs for certain diseases like congenital hypothyroidism (Elbualy et al. 1998, Ministry of Health Oman 2010b). It also introduced the autonomous hospital initiative, which allowed regional hospitals to plan and run their budgets. In 2013, the MoH introduced its *Vision 2050*, with its major reform of the healthcare system in the country, allocating resources to hit targets in the curative, preventive, and rehabilitative domains of the system. This was linked with the targets developed by the other providers in the country such as SQUH and the Military Medical Services. This period also witnessed the review of both the medical and paramedical curriculums, aimed at improving the quality of graduates from these programs, as well as raising some of the programs up to bachelor and master levels. Also, it witnessed the establishment of the Research

Council, tasked with drawing strategic plans with regard to the country's need for research, including in the field of healthcare, thus supporting service development.

The national reforms that have been undertaken have added value to the outcome of healthcare services at both community and individual levels. One of the indicators of such positive impacts is the accessibility of services, reflected in the number of primary healthcare facilities which increased from 19 in 1970 to 192 in 2012 (Ministry of Health Oman 2012). Another indicator is the reduction of registered communicable diseases such as polio, measles, and malaria. For example, the number of notifiable measles, at all ages, fell from 3,675 in 1985 to three cases in 2012 (Ministry of Health Oman 2012). In addition, the annual parasite incidence of malaria per 1,000 population decreased from 2.188 in 1994 to 0.006 in 2012 (Ministry of Health Oman 2012). Information Technology (IT) was also efficiently introduced which led to the addition of electronic patient records in all institutions. Based on such success stories, the system has been ranked by WHO as number eight in the world in terms of providing the best overall healthcare (World Health Organization 2000). Such rankings reflect the strong impact of the reforms on the quality and patient safety.

The Current Situation

The healthcare system is composed of the primary, secondary, and tertiary levels which provide free healthcare for all citizens and expatriate Government employees through purpose-built institutions located throughout the country. The rest are user-pays or funded by employer paid insurance schemes. The MoH is the main provider of healthcare services, supported by other Government institutions providing services at the three levels including, SQUH, the Military Medical Services, the Royal Oman Police Medical Services, the Royal Court Medical Services, and the Petroleum Development of Oman Medical Services. The private sector is developing and participating in providing services at the three levels through hospital and clinics dotted throughout the country.

The system has faced strengths and weakness that affect service delivery. One of the strengths is that Omani staff represents a good percentage of the total number of employees and this proportion is increasing. For example, in 2012 Omani nurses in the MoH institutions represented 66 percent out of the total nursing staff compared to 12 percent, in 1990 (Ministry of Health Oman 2012). Similarly, the numbers of Omani pharmacists out of the total number of pharmacist employed in the MoH represented 80 percent in 2012 compared to 21 percent in 1990 (Ministry of Health Oman 2012). Furthermore, having well-established public health programs has helped maintain high coverage rates of immunization for childhood communicable diseases such as tuberculosis and polio. For example, Bacillus Calmette–Guérin (BCG) and polio vaccination coverage increased from 54 percent and 19 percent in 1980, to 100 percent and 98 percent respectively in 2012 (Ministry of Health Oman 2012). Furthermore, access to services has improved, as reflected by the average number of antenatal care visits which increased from 4.25 percent in 1980, to 6 percent in 2012 (Ministry of Health Oman 2012). However, the system is experiencing weaknesses that are deterring its successes. For example, there is a shortage of staff in certain specialties such as obstetrics and gynecology, intensive care, and anesthesia. Such shortages, along with a lack of beds for these specialties in the tertiary hospitals, has negatively impacted on quality and patient safety.

In addition to these stated strengthens and weaknesses, the system is facing other challenges. These include, but are not limited to, developing and maintaining a culture that supports the concept of quality and patient safety among staff at all times, developing knowledge and skills of the staff, ensuring continuous provision of essential medications, attracting and retaining competent staff, and creating and maintaining a trustful partnership with patients and community members.

The list of participants in the healthcare system is long. However, there are key participants who play a major role in initiating and monitoring the reform efforts. One key participant is the community, as its members live with the day-to-day outcomes of such reforms. Furthermore, it is well known that healthcare systems should be community and patient focused, thus their participation in system development has became noticeable in the last few years. Another participant that has been recently introduced is the "Shura Council" (The Lower House), in which its members are free and politically supported to raise and discuss any issues related to the healthcare system, either with the individual decision makers, or during the council meetings. In addition, the "State Council" (The Upper House), plays a similar role in terms of reviewing the strategic plans of the systems, reviewing the budget allocated for such plans, and making recommendations accordingly to the Ministerial Council.

Similarly, Oman Medical Specialty Board (OMSB) and Oman Medical Association (OMA) have an input in initiating and monitoring the progress of the reforms. For example, OMSB looks after developing and implementing career and professional development plans for physicians working in the system. Although OMA is relatively new to the system, it witnessed major improvements in the last few years in terms of numbers of professional societies under its umbrella, as well as the number of registered physicians. The association also played a major role in the process of developing *Vision 2050*. In addition, the association supported the MoH in developing the medical bylaw. Lastly, the State Audit Office plays a major role in terms of assessing the adherence of the institutions to the rules and regulations, thus ensuring efficient and effective use of allocated resources.

Detail of Current Reform Initiatives

Vision 2050 is one of the major reforms of the MoH. Its main focus includes strengthening primary healthcare, coupled with an increased awareness in Omani society through health promotion, intersector collaboration, and improving tertiary care facilities. Also, its focus is to get the best value for the money invested in the health sector. Furthermore, the vision aims to improve accessibility to the services by setting up 10,000 health centers, to meet increasing demand from its growing population and expanded urbanization (Oman Observer 2013). As one of the outcomes of this reform, the MoH announced the development of the Sultan Qaboos Medical City, which is expected to cost $1.5 billion.

Other healthcare providers, such as SQUH, have taken similar steps by inviting international experts to participate in the review process of the hospital strategic plan. Its main focus is to incorporate new strategies, in line with the *Vision 2050*, that will help in meeting the expanding demand of the teaching, research and clinical services of the hospital. This is coupled with expansion of the stock of infrastructure of the hospital systems such as buildings and human resources as well as its administrative structure.

The current reforms are also encouraging the private sector to invest in the system through new "medical cities," as well as developing a number of small hospitals. For example, the International Medical City in Salalah is considered the largest private sector investment. It covers an area of 866,000 square meters, which includes a healthcare complex, a healthcare resort, an educational facility, and a 530-bed multi-sociality hospital. Although these facilities will serve the Omani population, the private sector seeks to attract patients from around the world as medical tourism grows.

The Quality and Safety Landscape

As the main provider of healthcare services, the Under Secretary of Health Affairs, in the MoH, is responsible, with the support of the other two undersecretaries, for quality and patient safety improvement. At the meso level, he is supported by the health authorities in the governorates. Such authorities supervise and monitor implementation of quality and patient safety plans. They further report their recommendations to the decision makers at the ministerial level with regard to the status of quality and patient safety based on regular data collection such as infection control or medication use. Other Government institutions (for example, SQUH) have their own system of implementing, supervising, and monitoring quality and patient safety improvements. For example, SQUH have a Medical Advisory Committee, composed of all heads of clinical departments and chaired by a professor from the COMHS. Its tasks include, developing policies and procedures for ensuring high-quality patient care, and advising on resource requirements to provide high-quality healthcare. At micro levels, the health authorities and hospitals have quality management and patient safety departments that supervise and monitor quality and patient safety activities. These are linked directly with the highest leadership of the institution, to ensure smooth reporting and implementation of improvement recommendations.

There are other committees and authorities that have indirect links with monitoring quality and patient safety. For example, the regional primary medical and technical committees and the higher medical committee are responsible for investigating alleged medical errors. Findings of investigations, and system curative and preventive recommendations, are reported to the MoH and other Government healthcare institutions for implementation.

Other stakeholders are involved in different ways. At the macro levels, the MoH is invited on a regular basis to the discussions of "Shura Council." Dialogue is based on questions raised by members of the council on various healthcare issues such as accessibility, affordability, safety, continuity, and technical aspects. Similarly, the State Council invites decision makers from the MoH during its regular discussions of the healthcare system. Both are involved in reviewing the system's strategic planning. Following these discussions, these bodies provide political support for the system to get the needed resources. Furthermore, the system takes the input from these bodies into consideration for many issues, such as directing resources to some of the health needs in the community.

Detail of the Impact of These Reform Efforts on Quality and Safety of Care

Many initiatives have been taken up by the system in targeting quality and patient safety. For example, the most recent reform initiative taken by the MoH, the strategic *Vision 2050*, is a comprehensive plan that targets improving the quantity and quality of healthcare services provided. Another key reform initiative is the review of the medical and paramedical bylaw, which is aimed at having a self-governing rules and regulations dedicated to healthcare professionals, and reviewing and upgrading of nursing and other paramedical curricula carried out by the MoH.

Other providers have initiated similar reforms. For example, the COMH introduced its new medical curriculum in 2008 which seeks to improve the quality of its graduates. In addition, the college gained international accreditation from the AMEEMR, which is expected to add value to improving quality of under and post-graduates. Similarly, SQUH witnessed improvement in quality and patient safety following ISO certification in 2005, and the hospital is also heading toward ACI. In addition, having electronic patient records, since 2006, has added value to improving quality and patient safety. Similarly, the OMSB seeks international accreditation of its residency programs, which ultimately improves the quality of graduates and thus provides better quality and safe services.

Reviewing the reform efforts that have been taken, there are several efforts that have successfully driven Oman towards improving quality and patient safety. One of these is the five-year plans adopted since 1976, which have helped improve various dimensions of quality and patient safety. Accessibility for the public to the services is reflected in the number of facilities available. For example, there were 65 hospitals in 2012, compared to two hospitals in 1970. Similarly, the number of nurses per 10,000 people has increased from 5.6 in 1975 to 43.1 in 2012 (Ministry of Health Oman 2012). Acceptability of services by the public has improved due to a successful public awareness program which led to increased utilization of these services. For example, immunization against measles increased from 10 percent in 1980 to 100 percent in 2012. Similarly, the effectiveness of various programs is reflected in decreased prevalence of Protein Energy Malnutrition (PEM) among children below the age of five years from 128 in 1995 to 4.6 in 2012 (rate per 1,000 children under 5 years) (Ministry of Health Oman 2012). Furthermore, immunization programs have led to a polio-free country for the last 15 years (Ministry of Health Oman 2012). The Infant Mortality Rate has also decreased from 118 deaths per 1,000 live births in 1970 to 9.5 in 2012 (Ministry of Health Oman 2012). Continuity of care has improved which was evidenced by the increase in the average number of antenatal care visits made by pregnant mothers during the period 1980–2012. These success stories, ultimately, have led to overall improvement in quality and patient safety. High political support, visionary leadership, community understanding and support, international collaboration and support, and availability of resources, were the driving forces for such successes.

Implementation Barriers and Solutions

Similar to other initiatives, quality and patient safety faces several barriers that can impede success. These can be system or individual oriented. The list for both is long, however, the most common system barriers are: lack of up-to-date policies and guidelines for managing certain diseases, shortage of skilled staff, shortage of equipment, difficulty of creating and maintaining a supportive culture to quality and safety, lack of clear description of staff rights and responsibilities, shortage of beds in critical areas like Intensive Care Units, lack of patient and family engagement in care, lack of a central incident reporting system with insufficient data analysis, feedback, and intra- and inter-institutional sharing of lessons learned, lack of regular quality monitoring systems, and difficulty in maintaining staff in the quality and patient safety departments.

On the other hand, individual barriers include, lack of leadership skills among some staff at low and middle management positions, and lack of personal commitment towards one's profession and professional development.

Like other improvement initiatives, there are opportunities which facilitate the implementation of quality and patient safety improvement initiatives. Enablers include supportive leadership at the various levels of the system, existence of core values that are widespread among professionals, widespread IT use, availability of the state of art facilities with highly qualified and skilled staff in the tertiary-level hospitals, easy access to the facilities mainly at the primary healthcare level, and successful experiences at the regional and nationals levels (for example, with the malaria eradication program), which have boosted the motivation of staff to seek improved performance.

Implementation opportunities that have facilitated implementation of quality and patient safety improvement initiatives include: a supportive and understanding community reflected in the implementation of many public health programs such as the EPI and MEP, prospects of utilizing the IT system to improve incident reporting and learning, the efficient and effective utilization of the mortality and morbidity data that would help in identifying strengths and weakness of the system, and the efficient and effective utilization of available data, to assess levels of quality and patient safety such as those collected by the infectious disease reporting system.

Prospects for Success and Next Steps

Although the system has undergone several reform initiatives, still more needs to be done to achieve safe and high-quality services. On one hand, funding to the system needs to be increased, directing better resources to some of the regional hospitals which are located in densely populated governorates. Although primary healthcare in Oman is a success, given the challenges the system is facing in terms of increasing prevalence of non-communicable diseases, further development is needed with regard to providing adequate resources, particularly competent staff, and diagnostic facilities.

Coordinated efforts among all providers need to be developed, in order to avoid unnecessary duplication of services as well, as to strengthen some services with expertise from all providers (such as solid organ transplantation). Also, more needs to be done to improve the active participation of the community in the development and implementation of strategic plans. In addition, other parties need to be actively involved in the development of a supportive culture, such as the media, and judicial system, thus helping to improve trust between the health system and the community.

For future successful implementation of reforms there are some essential levers. One of these is the political support for promoting the health of the community. In Oman this facilitated getting extra resources. Furthermore, a clear vision by leaders will make all those involved in service delivery head towards the same target. Another important aspect is developing professional bodies that help in protecting, promoting and maintaining the health and safety of community members through making sure that doctors and paramedical staff follow appropriate standards of medical practice.

The reforms are promising, with short-, mid-, and long-term targets. Great human and material resources have been identified and stakeholders are working together to secure these resources. International experts from developed systems have been invited to review these reforms and positive critiques have been provided. The different domains of the reforms are planned to be completed on time. Overall, the improvements to be achieved by these reforms are expected to be seen by 2020.

Conclusion

Healthcare reform is an essential step to be taken in order to improve quality and patient safety. However, as it is challenging to ensure success, it must be done in a well planned manner. Oman's healthcare system has undergone multiple reforms over the last 44 years. Improving quality and patient safety is at the heart of these reforms and targets identified have been achieved, as reflected in various quality and patient safety indicators, which have captured improved accessibility, acceptability, efficiency, effectiveness, safety, and efficacy. High-level leadership and political support have played a major role in making these reforms successful. However, there remain lessons to be learned from less successful initiatives the system has experienced, which can help Oman continually improve its strategies for future reforms.

Chapter 6
South Africa

Stuart Whittaker, Carol Marshall, and Grace Labadarios

Abstract

During the period 1994 to 2013, South Africa experienced dramatic changes within its health services. Having inherited a fragmented and highly inequitable health system, an early aim of the African National Congress (ANC) Government was to establish a national health system that incorporated both the public and private sectors and offered universal coverage. There have been many barriers to achieving this aim, including insufficient professional staff, inadequate leadership, management, and governance of the health service, and a high burden of disease. Government has responded to these challenges at many levels, with a particular focus on improving the quality of healthcare services. The National Health Amendment Act was passed by Parliament in 2013, resulting in the establishment of the Office of Health Standards Compliance (OHSC). The Office will regulate the quality of health services using a set of National Core Standards (NCS).

Background

Summary of Current Reform Initiatives in this Country

South Africa is a nation of diversity reflected in 11 national languages representing at least as many cultures in a population of 51.8 million (Statistics South Africa 2011a). Around 70 percent of the population relies on the public sector for provision of health services (Statistics South Africa 2011b). Table 6.2 summarizes some key figures on health financing in South Africa in 2012.

South Africa was the birthplace of the primary care approach, which was implemented by Sidney and Emily Kark in Pholela in the 1940s (Tollman 1994). However, subsequent political events did not promote the further development of what is now accepted as the preferred system of healthcare delivery.

During the apartheid regime (1948–1994), the health system was fragmented into three chambers (White, Indian, and Black and Colored) with separate budgets and widely disparate levels of service and outcomes. These historical policies contributed to the wide variations in life expectancy, health outcomes, access to health services, and the quality of services observable in the population of today.

Table 6.1   Demographic, economic, and health information for South Africa

Population (thousands)	52,386
Area (sq. km)*	1,213,090
Proportion of population living in urban areas (2011)	62
Gross Domestic Product (GDP US$, billions)^	384.3
Total expenditure on health as % of GDP	8.8
Gross national income per capita (PPP intl $)	11,010
Per capita total expenditure on health (intl $)	982
Proportion of health expenditure which is private	52.1
General Government expenditure on health as a percentage of total expenditure on health	47.9
Out-of-pocket expenditure as a percentage of private expenditure on health	13.8
Life expectancy at birth m/f (yrs)	56/62
Probability of dying under five (per 1,000 live births)	45
Maternal Mortality Ratio (per 100,000 live births) (2013)	140
Proportion of population using improved water and sanitation	95/74

Source: Unless otherwise stated data are for the year 2012 and taken from the World Health Organization 2014a. * Area from the World Bank 2014a. ^ GDP from the World Bank 2014b.

Notes: PPP is purchasing power parity, intl $ is international dollar which has the same purchasing power as US$ in the US.

Table 6.2   Health financing in South Africa in 2012

Indicators	**2012**
GDP	US$384.31 billion
Total health expenditure	9% GDP
General Government expenditure on health as a percentage of general Government expenditure	13% General Government expenditure
Donor funding for health	2% Total health expenditure
Private expenditure on healthcare	52% Total health expenditure
Private health insurance	81% Private expenditure on healthcare 42% Total health expenditure
Out-of-pocket expenditure	14% Private expenditure on healthcare 7% Total health expenditure
NGOs serving households	2% Total health expenditure

Source: World Health Organization 2014b

Legislation and policy since 1994 (see Table 6.3 below) have demonstrated Government commitment to establishing a health service which meets the basic needs of all South Africans by pooling the use of public and private resources. However, a major barrier to achieving this goal is the poor quality of service delivered in many health facilities in South Africa, especially but not only in the public sector. Consequently, legislation and policy have provided a focus on quality of care and debate around the exact model to follow in securing safe quality health services has continued for several years. The table below provides a summary of health-related legislation and policy since 1994.

Table 6.3   Health-related legislation and policies in South Africa since 1994

Year	Government Policy Document	Summary
1994	Reconstruction and Development Programme	Stated the intention to establish a national health system.
1996	Constitution of the Republic of South Africa	Section 27—Right of access to healthcare services for all.
1997	Transformation of the Health System White Paper	Policy objectives with implementation strategies to achieve universal health coverage.
2003	National Health Act	Legal framework for a structured uniform health system in accordance with the Constitution.
2009	Ten Point Plan	Ten priorities to be addressed during 2009—2014 including leadership, quality, human resources, and infrastructure.
2010	National Service Delivery Agreement	Charter to improve the population's health status.
2010	Re-engineering of Primary Health Care in South Africa—Discussion document	Identified three priorities: primary healthcare outreach teams, strengthening of school health services and district-based Clinical Specialist Teams focusing on maternal and child health.
2011	National Health Insurance Green Paper	Outlined four key interventions to implement National Health Insurance, including, transformation of the health service provision and delivery, overhaul of the healthcare system, radical change of administration and management, and re-engineering of primary healthcare.
2011	National Health Amendment Bill	Parliamentary process regarding new regulator; extensive public hearings
2011	Human Resources for Health South Africa	Strategic plan to meet human resource requirements for required improvements in the health service to improve access to healthcare for all and improve health outcomes.
2011	National Development Plan	Plan to eliminate poverty and reduce inequality by 2030; includes the provision of quality health services.
2013	National Health Amendment Act	Enabled establishment of the OHSC; signed into law July 2013, promulgated September 2013.

With the transition to democracy in 1994 health was, in part, overshadowed by competing priorities. The deterioration of health outcomes and lack of progress towards the United Nations Millennium Development Goals (MDGs) has been well documented (Lawn & Kinney 2009). This was principally due to the failure of successive Governments to provide an adequate response to HIV/AIDS and the policy of AIDS denialism during the period 1999–2009 (Chigwedere et al. 2008). However, during this time more than 1,300 additional Primary Care Clinics were provided, improving access to care in previously underserved areas (Chopra et al. 2009).

The year 2009 saw a change of Government in which Aaron Motsoaledi, appointed as Minister of Health, implemented measures to ensure the provision of adequate treatment for those infected with HIV, alongside many additional healthcare reforms. The impact of these reforms is discussed below. The National Health Insurance (NHI) approach to healthcare financing gained increasing prominence during this time and in 2011 the Green Paper on NHI was released, aiming to ensure universal healthcare coverage for all South Africans.

The Current Situation

South Africa's quadruple burden of disease is well documented, consisting of HIV/AIDS and tuberculosis (TB), maternal and infant mortality, Non-Communicable Diseases (NCDs), and violence and trauma. The Government has responded and continues to respond to these challenges. Since 2009, health outcomes in South Africa have shown improvement in several areas. In particular, the implementation of anti-retroviral treatment (ART) and prevention of mother to child transmission (PMTCT) programs have contributed to the increase in life expectancy from 57.1 in 2009 to 61.3 in 2012 (Dorrington, Bradshaw & Laubscher 2012). Case detection for TB has improved from 61 percent in 2005 to 69 percent in 2011 (World Health Organization 2014b). Smear negative cure rates have improved (Churchyard et al. 2014). Maternal and infant mortality still leave much to be desired, although improvements are being shown especially for infant mortality (Dorrington, Bradshaw & Laubscher 2012).

As in other developing nations, South African health policy has focused on the MDGs, particularly those relating to HIV and TB. Consequently NCDs received relatively less attention from national policy makers. However, following the United Nations General Assembly in 2011, South Africa developed a strategic plan for the prevention and control of NCDs, which was released in 2013 (Human Sciences Research Council 2013).

A major contributing factor to the deterioration in quality of health services and the difficulties implementing programs to improve quality of care has been weaknesses in leadership at healthcare facilities. This has been acknowledged and steps are being taken to address these deficiencies (Department of Health

Republic of South Africa 2011a). The Academy for Leadership and Management in Healthcare was launched in November 2012 (Bateman 2012a). The Academy is responsible for defining the competencies required for leadership and management in the healthcare sector, accreditation of institutions to providing training in these competencies, ensuring that appointed managers and leaders have the required competencies, and monitoring the impact of these interventions (Maja 2012). In several provinces, many Chief Executive Officers have been replaced by more appropriately trained individuals (Health Systems Trust 2014).

An additional contributing factor has been the recognized lack of accountability in the public system. This is addressed in part by the NCS (Department of Health South Africa 2011b), which set out what is required from managers of health establishments. These requirements provide indicators which can be used to monitor health establishments and their managers. Over time, the effects of these provisions should deliver improvements in quality of care.

South Africa has a shortage of trained clinical staff (Department of Health Republic of South Africa 2011a). In 2012, the Health Professions Council of South Africa reported a total of 30,728[1] medical practitioners licensed to practice in South Africa. Of these, 66 percent were registered as general practitioners and 34 percent as specialists. Sixty-two percent of general practitioners and 42 percent of specialists were employed in the public sector (Econex 2013). Doctors employed in the public sector can also provide services to the private sector, under the controversial Remuneration for Work Outside the Public Sector (RWOPS) system (Bateman 2012b). This practice exerts further strain to an already overburdened public sector health service and compromises supervision of junior staff; it is under review by the National Department of Health.

In 2013, 260,698 nurses of all grades were registered with the South African Nursing Council (South African Nursing Council 2014). Recruitment and retention of staff is challenging for many reasons (Padarath et al. 2003). Rural recruiting difficulties are further compounded by historical disadvantage in provision of facilities and health workers. In consequence, staff in rural areas frequently lack relevant skills and experience, resulting in patient harm (Ministerial Task Team 2012).

Multi-level interventions have been introduced to improve the quality of services. At a clinical level, national policy targeted both health systems strengthening and specific disease groups. Health systems strengthening is being addressed by implementation of the NCS, which target both clinical service delivery and systems, and processes that underpin service delivery. Programs

---

1 The number of doctors in the private sector has been estimated from accounts submitted to medical insurance schemes by Econex (2013). The estimation process for the total number of doctors takes account of doctors who work both in the public and private sectors.

targeting specific diseases included TB, HIV/AIDS, malaria, PMTCT, and maternal and child health amongst others.

National guidelines for hospital management of clinical conditions have been updated and distributed (National Department of Health South Africa 2012, National Department of Health South Africa 2006). National priority conditions have been identified including TB, HIV/AIDS, maternal, and child health amongst others and the NCS require establishments to perform clinical audits to demonstrate adherence to these guidelines. Annual Performance Plans (APPs) are being developed for each district, which include outcome-related targets aligned with national priority programs, such as reduction in maternal mortality (Department of Health Republic of South Africa 2013).

Clinical aspects of care are supported by clinical governance interventions. Hospital, district, and provincial morbidity and mortality meetings are required to allow for in-depth analysis of cases and provide a platform to share learning acquired during the investigation of these cases.

To support implementation of the NCS, the OHSC has developed a quality improvement manual detailing methods of implementing, monitoring, and evaluating quality improvement activities. At present, training in these techniques and support to facilities in their implementation, is provided mainly by Non-Government Organizations (NGOs). The OHSC works closely with these NGOs to coordinate their activities, learn from their experience, and share best practice.

Clinical supervision is provided to clinical staff. This is intended to take the form of regular, formal visits to smaller facilities with documentation of findings and responses, although operational challenges limit the anticipated effectiveness. The NCS require evidence that these visits are undertaken, properly performed, and the data collected responded to appropriately. A further layer of clinical governance is provided by the District Clinical Specialist Teams (DCSTs) which were instituted as part of the re-engineering of primary care. The purpose of these teams is to improve the quality of healthcare and health outcomes for mothers, newborns, and children. A full team should comprise of four doctors and three nurses, although recruitment is not yet complete. The doctors include a family physician, a pediatrician, an anesthetist, and an obstetrics and gynecology specialist. The nurses include an advanced midwife, advanced pediatric nurse, and advanced primary care nurse. The team provides guidance, support, and oversight to clinical staff in each district. They are responsible for monitoring and evaluation of services delivered and improvement of these services where necessary (Ministerial Task Team 2012). Although the primary focus of these teams is maternal and child health services, it is anticipated that the benefits of their activities and interventions will spill over into the remaining services.

Summary of Current Efforts to Improve the Quality and Safety of Healthcare

Accreditation

In 1995, Council for Health Service Accreditation of Southern Africa (COHSASA) was registered as a not-for-profit organization to implement quality improvement and accreditation in South African hospitals. COHSASA was accredited by the International Society for Quality in Health Care (ISQua) in 2002; reaccredited in 2006 and 2010, and is a partner organization of the National Department of Health assisting with the development and implementation of the NCS. COHSASA has implemented a quality improvement approach in a limited number of facilities in South Africa over the past 19 years with some success. Since 1995, 109 private facilities, 86 public facilities, and 33 not-for-profit facilities in South Africa have achieved accreditation using COHSASA standards, many facilities achieving accreditation more than once. Implementation of COHSASA hospital standards in hospitals in *KwaZulu-Natal* province was associated with decreased perinatal mortality rates (Pattinson 2013). COHSASA's approach differs from that of its international peers in that it has a policy of encouraging gradual improvements in hospitals. Methods used have included facilitation components in its program to assist healthcare staff to understand and implement standards. In addition, a system of graded, step-wise recognition of improvements was introduced to provide momentum and encouragement towards accreditation. This allows for recognition of the progress made in facilities that have achieved substantial compliance with the standards, in particular demonstrating achievements in strategic leadership, service provision, and the ability to evaluate performance. Such an achievement represents a vast amount of effort by facility staff and the graded recognition program allows for official recognition of this by means of a certificate.

Facilities frequently do not comply with the majority of the accreditation standards, particularly when entering the program for the first time. In such cases the NCS are ideal in assisting these facilities to meet basic quality and safety requirements.

Patient safety with associated medico-legal implications is a problem in South Africa. The Australian Adverse Incident Monitoring System (AIMS) has been implemented in the Free State province during the period 2008–2013 with beneficial effects. An example of the impact of the program is the improvement in maternal mortality directly attributable to it. Data captured and analyzed in the AIMS database indicated that a lack of transport for maternity cases was a major contributory factor to maternal mortality. In response, the Free State provincial Department of Health (DoH) purchased additional emergency vehicles dedicated to maternity transport with a significant decrease in maternal mortality in the ten-month period following the intervention (Schoon 2013). A system with similar monitoring and evaluation capabilities implemented at a national level holds promise for similar improvements in patient care.

Following closure of the AIMS program in 2013, COHSASA redesigned the patient safety information system for the South African setting in-house. This program provides a computerized system for the voluntary reporting of adverse events and near misses by hospital, primary care, and medical emergency staff to a call center where trained medical professionals capture and analyze the incidents. Incident details are captured in less than seven minutes. Serious incidents are instantly relayed to a named contact person to ensure an immediate response. Online reports are provided to assist staff in managing adverse events and near-misses.

Public Sector Change and Accountability/Consequences

The public sector is not an easy sector to hold to account, either at the level of individual staff members, or managers, leading to the highly centralized authority that now exists, where many decisions are taken (or not taken) very far away from where problems are detected. There is also a fairly widespread situation where resource allocation decisions are not taken in the same forum as service delivery planning. Where resource limitations are critical to poor quality, a debate on "what the country can and should afford" becomes central. However, improvements in resource allocation will not necessarily provide additional capacity within the health system. At present much inefficiency is evident in the health system, for example, misallocation of available resources relative to workload, unacceptably high levels of fraud and theft, top heavy management and administration structures, and an excessively hospi-centric and specialist focus in the delivery of healthcare.

Overview of the National Core Standards (NCS)

The aim of the NCS is to reflect the South African policy context based to a large extent on existing legislation, policies, guidelines, and protocols, many of which are specific to the DOH and define the standards of healthcare and managerial responsibilities that managers are expected to meet in health establishments. The standards provide proactive guidance to health establishments in the provision of holistic quality of care with the aim of ameliorating risk within the healthcare system and a strong focus on acceptability of care, as well as safety, reliability, and accessibility/availability. Measures have been defined for each standard to determine the level of compliance as well as the potential severity of the impact of non-compliance and the likelihood of a risk occurring; these have been used to assess compliance in about 15 percent of all establishments in the country as part of a "mock" exercise in preparation for regulation. Following an evaluation of a healthcare establishment, a report is produced on site, accompanied by a quality improvement plan template that lists all measures with non-compliance and provides space for the facility to add its action plan.

Further refinements are planned with the aim of making available reports which provide direction and support for quality improvement initiatives, and to develop a real-time monitoring and early response system that will allow shortfalls in quality and safety to be recognized early and, where possible, prevented.

Establishment of the Office of Health Standards Compliance (OHSC)

In September 2013 the OHSC was established to regulate the quality of services in the public health sector, protecting and promoting the health and safety of service users. The OHSC is a single national body, independent of the NDoH, with three primary functions. The first is "certification" as a regulatory function (certification awarded following achievement of a predetermined level of compliance with NCS). Secondly, the OHSC is responsible for ongoing inspections to ensure maintained compliance with prescribed norms and standards. Thirdly, it must receive and respond to complaints from the public including through providing operational support to and Ombudsmen placed within the office but reporting independently to the Minister of Health. The responsibility for improvement interventions and systems required to ensure the implementation of, and compliance with, the NCS, will remain with the DOH at national and provincial levels.

Preparing for Regulation

Using regulatory powers to impact positively on the system is a powerful tool in part because it sends a strong signal regarding the importance that Government attaches to a particular issue and its readiness to use its coercive powers to ensure that there are indeed consequences for those who persistently fail to read this signal and act accordingly in the interests of the beneficiary. However regulation is not always coercive—the signal for change can be effective without getting to the point of punitive measures through enacting a more developmental approach of disseminating information and guidance, and giving time for corrective measures to be put in place. This requires the regulator to use their powers and independence where this becomes necessary and to be seen as acting on behalf of the user of the regulated services, not as protecting or covering up poor performance by the provider. Any recommendation to close an establishment, for instance, should always be weighed against the decreased access to services that will inevitably result.

To ensure that the regulatory process is effective and efficient, procedural regulations are being drafted setting out how the system will work as a whole. The NCS are being extensively reviewed to determine their appropriateness for regulation. In addition, the measurement and reporting tools described above are now also being subjected to rigorous review and refinement to ensure consistency, relevance, and accuracy. The aim is to understand and control the areas of greatest risk to patient safety and the acceptability of care.

There are also opportunities for improvement under the National Health Insurance Scheme. The link to NHI funding will effectively introduce a "pay for performance" aspect to the work of the OHSC in certifying health establishments as compliant. It is critical that its work is scientifically sound and seen as credible and accurate. This link to financing will, however, bring a whole range of new challenges—the legal challenges to the decisions of the Office will inevitably increase and the risk of "undue influence" on the inspectors to ensure a good outcome may also be seen.

Conclusion

Since 2009, many gains have been made in health including an increased life expectancy, improved TB outcomes, increased access to anti-retroviral drugs, and some improvement in infant mortality.

However, weak leadership remains a barrier to the provision of quality services, which may be overcome by the work of the National Academy of Leadership and Management in Health. While recognizing that errors may, and unfortunately do, happen in such a complex system as healthcare, it is important that all possible efforts are made to reduce these, while simultaneously providing an environment conducive to staff cooperation with investigations into adverse events. In this light, it is critical that those responsible for ensuring that the service delivery platform is effective and efficient are equally held to account when this proves not to be the case.

The OHSC is being established to regulate the quality of health services, using the NCS to improve the quality of care and reduce risk in healthcare establishments. Both financial and administrative support is being provided to ensure that the organization can function effectively.

In summary, a solid platform is being built which has the potential to facilitate the delivery of quality healthcare services for the South African public and enable the provision of universal health coverage.

PART II
Eastern Asia and Southern Asia

Yukihiro Matsuyama

Part II takes up our themes in Eastern and Southern Asia, with representation from China, Hong Kong, India, and Japan. The contrasting health systems, and the reform combinations which they represent, provide very useful insights into global health reform trends. China and India have unrivaled large populations, with over 1.3 billion and 1.2 billion citizens respectively. The task of managing these systems is unmatched in human history. Both have placed priority on health reforms to improve access to healthcare services, while Hong Kong and Japan are competing for first place in world average life expectancy, contributed to by different types of health systems, with universal access.

The progress of health reform is influenced by each health system's governance structure. The population of Hong Kong is slightly over seven million, and its health system seems to be functioning well, comparatively. This size of population allows for a sharply focused set of reforms and improvement initiatives.

On the other hand, China and India are working towards more effective governance mechanisms to address disparities in healthcare. Japan lacks effective governance over its public health insurance system, and its healthcare delivery system is proportionally more private than public by comparison with others in the region. For example, there are over 3,000 insurers, most of which are too small to manage, effectively, the risk of increasing healthcare costs. Japan is having to meet, more rapidly than other countries, the serious problem of an aging population, and its demand for healthcare services. China and Hong Kong will increasingly face this problem over the next ten years.

All this suggests that each country should work on patient safety and quality issues, not only in acute care, but also in chronic, and long-term care. And perhaps having a series of regional meetings, for the purpose of working together on common issues from the standpoint of systems with differing structures and improvement initiatives underway, is necessitated by the publication of this book. Learning together at the national level can be very productive.

Chapter 7

China

Sun Niuyun

Abstract

Safeguarding people's rights to and interests in health is integral to China's socioeconomic development. Establishing a healthcare system in line with public demands and China's level of socioeconomic development, focused on constantly improving the quality and performance of the system, are the current goals of Chinese healthcare. It is a common challenge for all countries to strike a balance between the improvement of quality and the control of costs. In pursuing this goal, China is promoting comprehensive healthcare reform. It is accelerating improvements to its universal medical insurance system, strengthening and improving the essential drug system, and the new operating mechanisms of grassroots health facilities. It is also actively promoting public hospital reform and equality in essential public health services. The Government has developed the medium- and long-term strategic plan for the development of the health service industry, with the goal of covering the entire lifetime of people with wide-ranging services within a rational structure, constantly increasing health resources, reducing service costs, and improving service quality.

Background

The recent round of healthcare and pharmaceutical system reform in China was planned in 2006 and launched in 2009. The reform focused on the improvement of the healthcare delivery system (including public health services and medical services) and the improvement of the medical security system supported by a comprehensive, top down reform of the healthcare system (CPC Central Committee & State Council 2009). The objectives and measures were designed in accordance with the contemporary Chinese socioeconomic development and the demand for healthcare. China is the most populous country in the world with an estimated total population of 1.38 billion (World Population Review 2014), about one fifth of the global population, and is the second largest economy in the world; however, its health resources remain inadequate. China's per capita health expenditure in 2010 was US$219, lagging far behind the world average of US$941; China had 14.6 physicians and 15.1 nurses per 10,000 people, ranking it internationally as 117 and 145 respectively. China also has an unbalanced distribution of health resources

Table 7.1   Demographic, economic, and health information for China

Population (thousands)	1,390,000
Area (sq. km)*	9,327,490
Proportion of population living in urban areas (2011)	51
Gross Domestic Product (GDP US$, billions)^	8,227.1
Total expenditure on health as % of GDP	5.4
Gross national income per capita (PPP intl $)	9,040
Per capita total expenditure on health (intl $)	480
Proportion of health expenditure which is private	44.0
General Government expenditure on health as a percentage of total expenditure on health	56.0
Out-of-pocket expenditure as a percentage of private expenditure on health	78
Life expectancy at birth m/f (yrs)	74/77
Probability of dying under five (per 1,000 live births)	14
Maternal Mortality Ratio (per 100,000 live births) (2013)	380
Proportion of population using improved water and sanitation	92/65

Source: Unless otherwise stated data are for the year 2012 and taken from the World Health Organization 2014. * Area from the World Bank 2014a. ^ GDP from the World Bank 2014b.

Note: PPP is purchasing power parity, intl $ is international dollar which has the same purchasing power as US$ in the US.

between urban and rural areas. Quality health resources were concentrated in urban areas. In 2011, the number of registered physicians (including assistant physicians), nurses, and beds per 10,000 populations in urban areas was 49, 30, and 32.9 respectively, while in rural areas this was 20, 13.3, and 9.8 respectively (World Health Organization 2013a, Ministry of Health of the People's Republic of China 2012, National Bureau of Statistics of China 2012). With reference to the current aggregate and distribution of health resources in the healthcare system reform, the Government has focused, in the short term, on providing basic healthcare in the form of public goods to each citizen, ensuring basic healthcare, and guarantees that each citizen would have equal access to basic care.

Since the introduction of market economy, China's GDP has increased from US$60.036 billion in 1978 to US$8.553 trillion in 2012 (calculated by current exchange rate), with the average annual growth rate of 15.7 percent (nominal GDP growth). China's health financing has also increased with the rapid growth of GDP over the past 30 years or so. The proportion of total health expenditure against GDP has constantly risen from 3.02 percent in 1978 to 5.15 percent in 2011. The increase of funding has contributed to the improvement of healthcare provision and quality. However, the example of other countries has demonstrated clearly that more investment in healthcare is not necessarily better, and we should seek to control irrational and unproductive expenditure growth. Improving quality, while containing costs for better efficiency of input and output at the macro level, is the core rationale of China's reform. Although the short-term goal of the reform is to ensure that all the population has access to healthcare, the long-term goal is to establish a system focused on universal health coverage and the use of the health service industry as an important engine for sustainable socioeconomic development.

Introduction

The Government is committed to improving the healthcare system from the perspective of delivery and security.

From the 1950s to the late 1970s, the Government adopted centralized management of the healthcare system and established a three-tier network covering both urban and rural areas. China's health professional training system focused on secondary education, which cultivated a large number of primary care professionals. "Barefoot doctors," who were rural residents and medical professionals without formal medical training, also provided strong support to the system in rural areas (Ministry of Health of the People's Republic of China 2012). During this period, national health resources rose and the rural healthcare system witnessed rapid development. With the development of a market economy in China since the 1980s, the amount and efficiency of health resources continued rising due to continuous emancipation of medical productivity, access of social capital in the delivery system, the introduction of competitive mechanisms, and growing autonomy of health facilities. Since the outbreak of severe acute respiratory syndrome (SARS) in 2003, China started to reflect on its input in public health. Tens of billions of central and local Government Renminbi (RMB) has now been invested to strengthen the disease prevention and control facilities and improve the two-tier healthcare network in urban areas and three-tier network in rural areas. More recently, the Government is pursuing comprehensive reform of grassroots health facilities, and improving urban and rural grassroots healthcare networks.

China's medical insurance system can be dated to the 1950s when the Government set up the free medical care system (FMC) in Government institutions, the labor protection medical care system (LPMC) in urban areas, and cooperative medical care system (CMC) in rural areas. By the end of the 1970s, the LPMC covered over 200 million citizens, the FMC over 50 million citizens, and the CMC 90 percent of administrative villages in China. China was applauded by the World Health Organization (WHO) as "an economically-poor country that provided healthcare comparable to that of a developed country" (Song 2009). After ushering in the market economy system in China, state-owned enterprises underwent reforms. People's communes, where rural residents cooperated with each other, were terminated, and the LPMC and rural CMC shrank rapidly. The original medical security system collapsed in the early 1990s and the financing burden was transferred to health facilities and individuals. In order to alleviate the burden among its citizens and establish a security system in line with its socioeconomic development, China gradually established the urban employee basic medical insurance system (UEBMI) in 1998, new rural cooperative medical system (NCMS) for peasants in 2003, and urban resident basic medical insurance system (URBMI), for urban residents with informal employment and unemployment in 2007. After the initiation of the new reform, accelerating the establishment of the medical security system remained one of the priorities for the Government. By the end of 2011, 1.305 billion people were covered by these three basic medical insurance systems (Figure 7.1). In 2012, China put forward the idea of establishing a major disease insurance system, on top of the three basic medical insurance systems, aiming to further strengthen the bottom of the system.

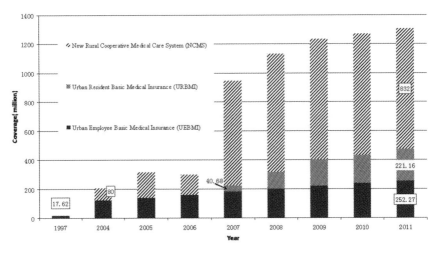

Figure 7.1   Coverage of the three basic medical insurance systems, 1997–2011

Source: National Bureau of Statistics of China 2012, State Statistics Bureau & Ministry of Human Resources and Social Security 2003, State Statistics Bureau & Ministry of Human Resources and Social Security 2010, Ministry of Human Resources and Social Security of China 2012, Ministry of Human Resources and Social Security of the People's Republic of China 2013.

Current Status

The medical security system and healthcare delivery system have been established in line with China's socioeconomic status, demographic structure, and epidemiological profile. China is increasing its input in healthcare and gradually optimizing the financing structure in the reforms. The contribution of Government, society, and individuals to health expenditure was 30.7 percent, 34.6 percent, and 34.8 percent respectively in 2011 (Figure 7.2).

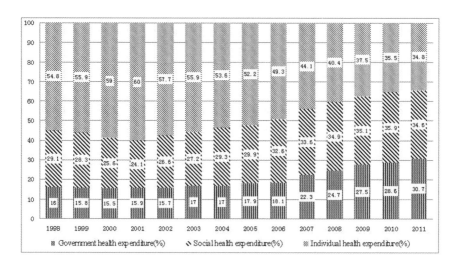

Figure 7.2   Changes in the constituent ratio of China's total health expenditure, 1998–2011

Source: National Bureau of Statistics of China 2012.

Meanwhile, improvements have been realized in health outcomes and the performance of the system, reflected by the major indicators of national health. The health of Chinese citizens is high compared to other developing countries. Per capita life expectancy increased from 35.0 in 1949 to 74.8 in 2010. The maternal mortality rate and under-five mortality rate were 24.5 per 100,000 and 13.2 percent respectively in 2012 (Table 7.2 and Figure 7.3).

Table 7.2   Improvement of health outcomes in China since 1999

	1991	2001	2010	2011	2012
Under-five mortality rate (%)	61	35.9	16.4	15.6	13.2
Maternal mortality (1/10,000)	80	50.2	30	26.1	24.5
Antenatal examination rate (%)	66.5	90.3	94.1	N/A	N/A
Maternal hospital delivery rate (%)	50.6	94.1	97.8	N/A	N/A

Source: National Bureau of Statistics of China 2012.

Currently, China's medical security system is composed of UEBMI, URBMI, and NCMS, supplemented by major disease insurance for urban and rural residents, free medical care for the civil servants, enterprise supplementary medical insurances and commercial medical insurances, and urban and rural medical aid.

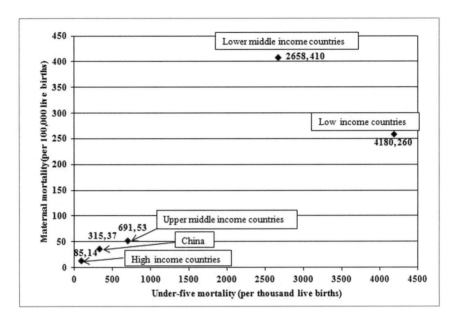

Figure 7.3   Maternal mortality and under-five mortality in China, and in other countries in the world, 2010

Source: World Health Organization 2013a, National Bureau of Statistics of China 2012.

Establishment and improvement of the medical security system has alleviated the burden on Chinese residents and optimized the financing structure of the system.

China's healthcare system consists of the public health service delivery system and the medical service delivery system. Public health services, focusing on disease prevention, are provided by professional public health facilities. Medical service, focusing on disease treatment and rehabilitation, are provided by urban and rural health facilities at various levels. By 2012, China had 950,297 health facilities, including 23,170 hospitals, 912,620 primary health facilities, and 12,083 professional public health facilities; 9.119 million health professionals, including 4.937 million hospitalists (54.1 percent), 3.437 million primary care providers (37.7 percent), and 670,000 professional public health providers (7.3 percent) (National Health and Family Planning Commission, People's Republic of China 2013). Even with the continuous improvement of the system and growing health resources, China still faces an unbalanced, inverted-triangle distribution of health resources: professionals with higher academic degrees, new technologies, and capital are concentrated in developed areas and large cities, while at grassroots areas, rural areas, and underdeveloped areas health resources are short. This forestalls improvement of the entire system and denies urban and rural residents equal access to healthcare.

Current Reform Plans

The current reform focuses on accelerating the spread of the basic healthcare system, consolidating the new operating mechanisms of grassroots health facilities, promoting public hospital reform, and coordinating and pushing forward reform to healthcare-related industries (CPC Central Committee & State Council 2013a).

As for the medical insurance system, the focus has shifted from expanding coverage to improving quality. China will continuously consolidate and expand the coverage of basic medical insurances (BMIs), highlighting the coverage of migrant workers, employees hired by non-public economic organizations, "flexible employees," retirees of bankrupt enterprises, and employees of less profitable enterprises. It is also committed to increasing Government subsidy for URBMI and NCMS to above 360 RMB, per person, each year, and increasing the reimbursement rate of inpatient expenses to around 75 percent by 2015. It is trying to improve the management and service of the three BMIs, including promoting real-time settlement of BMIs and medical aid, and improving the management, supervision, and risk prevention mechanism of BMIs funding, in order to prevent overdraft. China is promoting the establishment of a hierarchical care system that leads the patients to primary facilities for care of minor diseases by enhancing the reform of the medical insurance payment system, developing payment policies encouraging visits in primary facilities, and encouraging traditional Chinese medicine.

As for the delivery system, China plans to continuously deepen the comprehensive reform of primary facilities, improve the networking of urban and rural primary facilities, and ensure that over 95 percent of primary facilities meet publicized standards by 2015. China is encouraging patients to make service contracts with community doctors, aiming at improving the hierarchical care system. Meanwhile, it is accelerating the establishment of the general practitioner system by training over 150,000 general practitioners for primary facilities, in order to meet the target of more than two general practitioners per 10,000 urban residents by 2015 (CPC Central Committee & State Council 2013a). China is also gradually establishing new operating mechanisms for public hospitals that guarantee public welfare, motivate enthusiasm, and ensure sustainability.

Reform efforts in all health-related areas are coordinated. The efforts include, improving the equalization of basic public health services, adjusting and optimizing health resource structure, encouraging the development of private health facilities, innovating mechanisms for the training and use of health professionals, pushing forward the reform of pharmaceutical production and distribution, accelerating health informatics, strengthening regional information platforms, promoting mutual sharing of health information, and improving health supervision mechanisms.

Current Status in Reform of Healthcare Quality and Patient Safety

Healthcare quality and safety is associated with cost-effectiveness, accessibility, responsiveness, efficacy, equality, and patient-centered care. China has conducted multiple rounds of the reform to improve quality and safety in these domains.

The universal medical security system that is being forged is an important pillar in the continuous improvement of quality. Medical insurance provides necessary resources to support healthcare quality improvement and patient safety, and facilitates people's enjoyment of fair and equal access to basic care. Meanwhile, China is gradually setting up incentive and supervisory mechanisms for healthcare delivery, based on reform of the payment systems, in order to draw the attention of public and private health facilities to the cost-effectiveness of care, standards execution, and quality. By improving the payment system of medical insurance and establishing a hierarchical care system, China is pushing forward new mechanisms for care delivery and supervision.

Healthcare has the property of a public good. The Government and health administration departments (such as the National Health and Family Planning Commission and local health departments) have gradually established a series of quality assurance and improvement systems to ensure the safety, effectiveness, equality, and availability of healthcare provided by health facilities. Firstly, to obtain market access, public and private health facilities, health professionals, and medical technologies must meet certain standards, thus laying a solid foundation for quality assurance. Secondly, a quality control system has the objective of developing practice rules and evaluation systems that healthcare providers should follow when providing healthcare. China is regulating healthcare providers based on a series of measures including laws, regulations and rules, diagnosis, treatment and nursing standards, specifications and methods, hospital accreditation, and healthcare evaluation. It is seen as important for the Chinese Government to manage the healthcare industry and for health administration departments to manage hospitals. Thirdly, China has set up an inspection and supervision system to ensure effective execution of laws, regulations, standards, common practices, and other practicing rules in the healthcare industry. Fourthly, China is gradually establishing a healthcare monitoring and early warning system based on information systems. These systems of healthcare quality and safety are not perfect, but they are priorities for the next steps towards improvement.

As in other countries, the most significant challenge for China to constantly improve healthcare quality is to strike the balance between quality improvement and cost control commensurate with current socioeconomic development levels. Constant improvement of quality depends on strong material support. Development of advanced technologies and application of new materials, drugs, diagnostics, and therapeutics contributes largely to the improvement of quality and the ensuring of patient safety, but they are also main drivers of continuous increase of expenditure. It is unrealistic to emphasize healthcare quality without consideration of the cost of care. No country is able to support an unrealistic healthcare quality improvement system. China is trying to engender its reforms by applying and promoting appropriate technologies and drugs, strengthening grassroots healthcare, improving health professionals' awareness of quality improvement, and promoting the transformation of health seeking behavior and health concepts of its people.

Furthermore, with the economic development, improvement of the social welfare and security system, and ageing of population in China, imbalance between demand and supply of healthcare has emerged, exerting a severe impact on the improvement of quality. On one hand, there are growing demands for healthcare: from 1.286 billion visits in 2000 to 6.27 billion visits in 2011, and the number of patients receiving inpatient care has increased from 35.84 million in 2000 to 150 million in 2011. On the other hand, the workload of health professionals has increased by nearly 50 percent and the bed utilization efficiency and rotation rate kept on rising from 2000 to 2011 (Ministry of Health of the People's Republic of China 2004, Ministry of Health of the People's Republic of China 2012). Demand witnessed rapid growth with the gradual improvement of the medical insurance system and the aging of the population. As a result, health professionals suddenly had heavier workloads, which could mean greater medical risks and pressure on healthcare quality.

Reform Obstacles and Solutions

Improvements and guarantees of quality are closely associated with the service delivery capacity of the system, the security of the medical insurance systems, and the incentives and restrictive mechanisms on healthcare demand and supply.

Publicly-owned health facilities remain the main supplier in China's health service system and Government grants only account for a small proportion of hospital revenue, and fail to provide adequate compensation to hospitals. Consequently, hospital operations mainly depend on service revenue. As a result, public hospitals in urban areas, aiming to expand their hospitals' scale and increase profit, have inadequate incentives to improve healthcare quality. Grassroots health facilities lack the foundation to improve healthcare quality. They have shortages of health professionals and only have low-level technologies and management.

Disparities in healthcare insurance systems and regional differences create gaps in medical security, inequality of healthcare and low-level social benefit. Meanwhile, the lack of effective incentive and restraint mechanisms between the Government, medical insurance organizations, and hospitals, also impedes quality improvement.

Furthermore, the quality assurance system still needs further improvement. Firstly, China might strengthen its legal system underpinning healthcare quality. It lacks legislation on patient safety. Further improvement of the management systems and operational guidelines to report quality and safety incidents are also needed. Secondly, China could also move to establish a quality safety evaluation system. It could set up the quality-oriented performance evaluation system from the perspective of Government supervision and insurance payment. Thirdly, China also might set up a monitoring and early warning system, based on information technologies (Sun 2012), and provide better evidence supporting decision making in patient safety assurance and management. In addition, risk control measures could be strengthened. Finally, embedding a culture of patient safety with the participation of the entire society should be promoted, effective doctor–patient communication mechanisms need to be established and medical risk sharing mechanisms improved.

Overall, China is gradually deepening its health reform to improve healthcare quality and performance of the entire healthcare system. The State Council of China has issued a medium- and long-term plan for the development of the health service industry with the goal of covering the entire lifetime of people with wide service scope and rational structure (CPC Central Committee & State Council 2013b). The plan requires the joint efforts of the Government agencies for health, medical insurance, finance, development, and reform, in easing market access, optimizing planning and guarantee of land use, optimizing investment and financing guidance, improving fiscal, taxation, and pricing mechanisms, and guiding and ensuring sustainable growth of health service consumption. Alongside this, there is also the need to improve laws, regulations, standards, and supervision on health services in order to empower the healthcare delivery system, strengthen health management, improve health insurance, gradually expand the health supporting industry, and optimize a favorable environment for the development of the health service industry.

Conclusion

The reform and development of healthcare in China represents a shift from a disease-oriented to universal health-oriented healthcare system. This depends on cooperation across the system, at all levels. Reforms are moving forward through the efforts of health professionals, hospital managers, medical insurance staff, policymakers, and researchers. In the final analysis, there are three factors to be considered. Firstly, the Government should enhance its input, at a rational rate, to the healthcare system in order to provide necessary resources to improve the quality and efficiency of healthcare. Secondly, continuous reform of the healthcare system should be promoted, in order to enhance the capacity of the healthcare system, especially by strengthening the comprehensive reform of the grassroots healthcare system. Meanwhile, the risk sharing capacity of the healthcare system should be strengthened for the mitigation of economic risks for patients. Thirdly, it should motivate the public to improve their own health management and health literacy, for better doctor–patient relations and control, and eliminate negative factors; internal or external, influencing better health for everyone. These measures can help inject new vitality to the socioeconomic transition and development of China.

Chapter 8

Hong Kong

Eng Kiong Yeoh and Hong Fung

Abstract

Hong Kong has adopted a unique approach in reforming healthcare so as to improve quality and safety. The key reform initiative involved corporatization of the public hospitals by setting up the Hospital Authority (HA) in 1990. The statutory organization is charged with the responsibility of introducing governance and management reforms in the public hospital system and to improve quality and safety of the public healthcare services. The reform led to initial success, with increased public confidence and demand for public healthcare services. In recent years, the Hong Kong Government has started to use the HA as a platform to introduce further reform initiatives to engage the private sector, including various public–private partnership (PPP) initiatives and hospital accreditation. The HA plays a central role in these reform initiatives.

Background

The healthcare system in Hong Kong has evolved from the colonial system developed under British rule prior to 1997. Primary care is mainly provided by private medical practitioners, many of whom are in individual practices. Secondary and tertiary care is mainly provided in the public hospitals. In the pre-HA era, the public hospital system was made up of 19 Government hospitals and 25 "subvented" hospitals, operated by 17 different non-government or charitable organizations (Hutcheon 1999). The latter received different forms of subvention from the Government and had different governance and management systems. Quality of care in the "subvented" hospitals was generally regarded as lower than that in the Government hospitals, which, on the other hand, were overcrowded with patients.

In 1990, the HA was set up as a statutory body to manage all the public hospitals. The purpose was to put all public hospitals operated by the Government and the 17 non-government organizations under one governance arrangement and introduce management reforms so as to improve the quality of care. This has become the most important reform to the healthcare delivery system so far. Subsequent to the setting up of the HA, the Government has also introduced several rounds of public consultation on reforming healthcare financing with the aim to improve the long-

**Table 8.1		Demographic, economic, and health information for Hong Kong**

Population (thousands)	7,187
Area (sq. km)	1,104
Proportion of population living in urban areas	na
Gross Domestic Product (GDP HK$, billions)^	263.2
Total expenditure on health as % of GDP (2010–2011)	5.1
Gross national income per capita (PPP intl $) ^	52,260
Per capita total expenditure on health (HK$) (2010–2011)	13,302
Proportion of health expenditure which is private (2010–2011)	51.3
General Government expenditure on health as a percentage of total expenditure on health (2010–2011)	48.7
Out-of-pocket expenditure as a percentage of private expenditure on health	-
Life expectancy at birth m/f (yrs)	81/87
Infant Mortality rate (per 1,000 live births)	1.6
Maternal Mortality Ratio (per 100,000 live births) (2012) *	2.2
Proportion of population using improved water and sanitation	-

Source: Unless otherwise stated data are for the year 2013 and taken from the Government of the Hong Kong Special Administrative Region (HKSAR) 2014. * From previous year's edition.^ GDP and GNI from the World Bank 2014b and 2014c.

Notes: PPP is purchasing power parity, intl $ is international dollar which has the same purchasing power as US$ in the US.

term financial sustainability. There has been very little progress on reform on this front except for some minor reforms to public hospital fees.

As part of its governance and management reform agenda, the HA has introduced systems and initiatives to improve quality and promote patient safety in the public hospitals. These include clinical governance structures, clinical information systems, clinical audit systems, performance management systems, incident management systems, and patient engagement activities. Based on the HA experiences, the Government has also introduced programs and activities to promote quality and safety in the private sector, using the HA as a platform. The reform initiatives have had some initial successes but scaling up will be an upcoming challenge.

Public confidence and support for public healthcare remains high in Hong Kong, leading to a perennial problem of extremely high demand for public healthcare services. While public healthcare is basically funded from general revenues, long-term financial sustainability has been a concern of the Government. However, public expectation of the quality of public healthcare services continues to grow and there are high political expectations on the Government to further invest and increase funding to public healthcare.

Introduction

Hong Kong's health system is characterized by a dominant public hospital sector, while primary care is predominantly provided by the private medical practitioners (Figure 8.2). The public hospitals, 42 in number, with over 27,400 hospital beds in 2014 (Census and Statistics Department HKSAR 2013a, Hospital Authority 2014), are managed by the HA, a statutory organization set up by the Hong Kong Government in 1990 as a major reform initiative for improving the quality of public hospital services. The HA provides 88 percent of the hospital beds in Hong Kong while the other 12 percent is provided by 11 private hospitals, with just over 4,000 hospital beds (Census and Statistics Department HKSAR 2013a). Within the public hospital system, the HA also runs specialist outpatient clinics and general outpatient clinics; however, visits to public hospitals only contribute around 30 percent of all outpatient visits (Figure 8.2). The remaining services are largely provided in the private sector, which also includes the Chinese medicine practitioners.

The setting up of the HA has been the most significant reform to the healthcare delivery system in Hong Kong. Not only has it transformed the delivery of public hospital services, but it has also become the platform for the Hong Kong

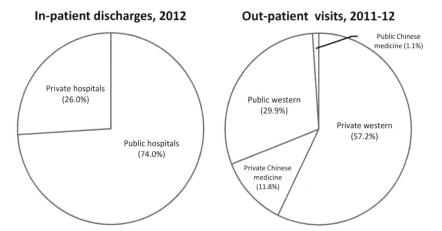

Figure 8.1   Public and private healthcare services (%) in Hong Kong

Source: Census and Statistics Department HKSAR 2013a, Census and Statistics Department HKSAR 2013b.

Note: Inpatient discharges included deaths in the hospitals. Outpatient visits referred to doctor visits during the 30 days before the date of survey.

Government to introduce other health system reform initiatives including, inter alia, integration of primary and secondary care, new service models for chronic disease management, patient empowerment programs, incorporation of Chinese medicine, development of electronic health records, PPP, an incident management system for patient safety, and an accreditation system for both public and private hospitals. This chapter reviews the evolutionary and central role of the HA in assuring quality and safety of healthcare, and transforming the healthcare delivery system in Hong Kong.

Healthcare Reforms in Hong Kong

The Hong Kong health system is underpinned by the policy "no one is denied adequate healthcare through lack of means." Public hospitals are heavily subsidized, with 91 percent of the budget coming from Government funding, supported by general revenues. Fees in public hospitals are HK$100 (US$12.90) per day, for the acute hospitals and HK$68 (US$8.70) per day, for the rehabilitation hospitals, which have not been adjusted for over a decade (Hong Kong Special Aministrative Region 2003). The per diem charges cover all medical expenses, including major surgeries and intensive care. The fee for specialist outpatient visits is HK$100 for the first consultation, reducing to HK$60 for subsequent visits, plus a charge for drugs at HK$10 per item (Hong Kong Special Aministrative Region 2003). The fee for general outpatient visits, providing primary care to the poor, elderly, and chronically ill patients, is HK$45 per visit, with no additional drug charge. Fee charging in public hospitals is determined by Government, ensuring affordability of services to the public. In 2010/11, Government expenditure in healthcare accounted for 49 percent of the total health expenditure (Food and Health Bureau HKSAR 2013).

On the other hand, private healthcare is largely funded on a fee-for-service basis, which accounted for 35 percent of total health expenditure in 2010/11 (Food and Health Bureau HKSAR 2013). Hospital care is supported by voluntary private medical insurance as well as medical benefits provided by employers, which account for 7.4 percent and 7.2 percent of the total health expenditure respectively (Food and Health Bureau HKSAR 2013). On the whole, Hong Kong spent around 5.1 percent of the GDP on healthcare in 2010/11 (Food and Health Bureau HKSAR 2013), with the public and private expenditure each contributing about half of total expenditure.

Public hospitals in Hong Kong were plagued by challenges including overcrowding, poor quality of care, low staff morale, and high staff turnover in the 1980s. In order to bring about major reforms, the Government set up the HA in 1990 as a statutory organization to manage all the public hospitals. The HA was conferred the autonomy to set up its own systems to recruit and retain healthcare professionals, improve staff morale, and reduce turnover, improve quality of care through efficient use of resources. At the same time, the HA was accountable to the

Government and the legislature for the use of public funds. The reforms brought about by the HA were characterized by the following:

- Change in governance structure—with separation of the Government's role as steward of the system, management of public hospitals is governed by an independent board, which incorporates community participation in the monitoring and decision making in the provision of public hospital services.
- Devolution of management responsibility and accountability to the hospital level—with setting up of governance structures to make sure hospitals would be more responsive to patient needs and professional aspirations at the local level.
- Building of a patient-centered culture—with cross-functional clinical management teams focusing on development of clinical services to improve the quality of care provided to patients.
- Development of systems to allow flexible use of resources, recruitment and deployment of manpower, as well as fair and transparent allocation of resources.
- Strengthening capacity of the hospital system by rationalizing the planning of hospital facilities, supported by information systems to guide decision making.
- Extensive staff engagement in strategy formulation, service development, business planning and management of day-to-day hospital operations, supported by leadership and management training and development.

The HA's reform measures in the 1990s met with great success. There was increased public satisfaction and demand for public hospital services. Private hospitals started to complain about losing patients to the public sector. The Government was concerned about the long-term sustainability of public healthcare, with much increased demand on top of the rapidly aging population. It was recognized that a complementary reform in healthcare financing was needed in order to address the fragmentation of the healthcare system and redress the interface between public and private healthcare. Several rounds of reports from expert consultants and public consultations have been introduced over the past two decades. Reform processes are ongoing, with the Government's current efforts aimed at developing and promoting a partially subsidized voluntary insurance scheme to supplement current healthcare financing, recognizing that all proposals requiring mandatory contributions had been rejected by the public in the past.

Since 2000, the Government has made use of the HA as a platform for bringing in further reforms to the healthcare delivery system. The first of such reform initiatives, in 2003, was for the HA to take over from the Government all public general outpatient clinics for primary care. The public general outpatient clinics serve mainly the poor, the aged, and chronically ill patients who cannot afford to see private doctors. There are 73 clinics covering the whole territory (Hospital

Authority 2014). The reform allowed the integration of care between primary and secondary care in the public system for these vulnerable groups of patients.

Most importantly, through this HA reform platform, the Government has started a series of PPP initiatives to address problems of accessibility in public healthcare, either due to gaps in the provision of healthcare facilities in specific locations or long waiting times arising from increased demand (such as cataract surgeries and radiological examinations). The Government sees PPP as a contractual arrangement involving the private sector in the delivery of public services. Based on a partnership approach, the responsibility for the delivery of services is shared between the public and private sectors, both of which bring their complementary skills to the enterprise (Hong Kong Special Administrative Region Government 2008). The PPP initiatives were supported by the sharing of electronic patient records built up by the HA's very successful clinical information systems.

The Quality and Safety Landscape

In regard to assuring quality and safety of care, the HA has developed systems, putting in place structures and processes, to address the six dimensions of quality according to the Institute of Medicine in the US (Institute of Medicine Committee on Quality of Health Care in America 2001). These include:

- Equity—The Government's policy of "no one should be denied of adequate healthcare through lack of means" is reflected in the fee charging policy on public healthcare services. Patients on social security are exempted from all hospital fees in the public hospitals and clinics. In addition, a second safety net, the Samaritan Fund, provides subsidy to means tested patients who cannot afford certain "self-financed" items, mainly medical consumables such as disposable catheters for cardiac intervention not covered by public subsidies in public hospitals. The HA regularly reviews the criteria for establishing "self-financed" items and funding for operating the Samaritan Fund, which is partially supported by Government funding as well as charities. The mechanism ensures adequate protection of the public from financial risks arising from catastrophic illnesses and medical treatment.
- Efficiency—Efficiency of the system is assured through structured processes of strategy review, annual plan, and performance management. The annual planning process has incorporated mechanisms for the benchmarking of costs and manpower, casemix adjusted activity funding, program budgeting, and pay for performance on quality and clinical outcomes. The public hospitals are organized into seven clusters based on geographical locations and accessibility by public transportation. Cluster Chief Executives are appointed to account for the hospital operations and performance. The HA Head Office has evolved into the role of an "internal purchaser" or "commissioner," setting corporate policies and systems to

ensure accountably, value-for-money, efficiency, and cost-effectiveness of the services provided in public hospitals.

- Efficacy—Specialty Coordinating Committees were set up with broad participation from specialist clinicians from the public hospital system to provide advice to the HA on service development, quality assurance and training, and development of medical specialists. These committees promote and ensure an evidence-based approach to the development of services and quality assurance. A mechanism for safety in the introduction of technology was also initiated on the assessment and control of new medical technology in the public hospitals, allowing the systematic introduction of new medical technology based on scientific evidence of safety, efficacy, and cost-effectiveness. A strategic approach also ensures the timely acquisition and distribution of new and advanced medical technology to keep Hong Kong healthcare abreast of international development.
- Safety—The HA first enhanced its clinical governance structure and processes in the late 1990s to strengthen the accountability of clinical management teams. A comprehensive risk and incident management system has been put in place to systematically identify and address patient safety risks, strengthen reporting of incidents, including sentinel events, support openness and transparency in the handling of incidents for staff, patients and the public, build competencies in conducting root cause analysis, develop a just culture, and establish corrective measures to protect patient safety. A corporate-wide approach for auditing the surgical outcomes of patients who have undergone major surgical operations provides opportunities for the surgical teams from all hospitals to annually review any system problem that might affect the clinical outcomes of patients and also learn from best practices.
- Timeliness—The HA addressed the challenge of increased demand through: establishing structured systems of triage and prioritization based on the urgency of the healthcare needs of the patients, making access and waiting time information transparent to the public and patients, setting open performance standards and targets, developing guidelines and protocols to streamline referrals, coordinating care between primary and secondary care providers, facilitating cross-regional use of extra capacities, and initiating PPP programs to reduce long waiting lists. The multiplicity of strategies and initiatives, adopted on a corporate and coordinated basis, help to ensure speedy responses of the system to the urgent needs of patients on the one hand, and reasonable waiting times within public expectation on the other.
- Patient-centeredness—Apart from conducting regular patient satisfaction surveys, the HA has established mechanisms to engage patient group representatives in extensive areas of decision making. Patient groups are consulted and involved in the setting of policies on drug formulary and self-financing items, development of strategic frameworks for patient care services, annual planning and allocation of resources, as well as governance

of hospitals. At the local level, hospitals have all developed structures and processes to strengthen patient relations and engagement. Patient feedback and complaints are addressed according to the corporate guidelines and standards. A patient charter was introduced to promote understanding on the rights and responsibilities of patients in the relationship between the healthcare workers and the patients.

As the HA evolves to become the Government's platform for healthcare reforms, it also spearheads the development of systems to provide reference and to promote quality and safety of care in the private hospitals as well as that provided by private medical practitioners. Such development has taken place along three main directions:

- Performance management—Performance management of the private medical practitioners is supported by various PPP initiatives, which include programs for electronic patient record sharing, cataract surgery, primary care provision in under-provided districts, management of chronic diseases (hypertension and Diabetes mellitus), hemodialysis, radiological investigation, and patient empowerment. These initiatives represent the Government's proactive attempt at strategic purchasing, with the aim of promoting integration between the public and the private sectors, addressing under-met demand in the public sector, enhancing patient access and choice of providers, and ensuring sustainability of the healthcare system. Standards are established on clinical guidelines and protocols, patient records, as well as clinical outcome monitoring and evaluation.
- System benchmarking—Through the Department of Health, as the licensing authority, private hospitals are now required to establish systems to promote patient safety and the management of medical incidents including sentinel events similar to the systems established in the public hospitals. There is a requirement for timely reporting, open disclosure, and investigatory procedures by root cause analysis.
- Hospital accreditation—Under the direction of the Government, a common hospital accreditation program has been established since 2009 for both the public and the private hospitals, based on the Australian Council of Healthcare Standards' accreditation program. The program not only provides a common framework for continuous quality improvement in the public and private hospitals in Hong Kong, but also serves as a platform for the sharing and learning of good practices among hospitals, thus enhancing the mutual understanding among the healthcare workers coming from both sectors.

Under the corporatization of the public hospital system, parallel reforms were also initiated in the public health system. The Government, through the Department of Health as its executive arm, is in the driving position on many initiatives to strengthen system performance as well as to enhance the quality of healthcare. These include strengthening regulations and monitoring on the manufacture and sales of pharmaceuticals, setting up of the Chinese Medicine Council to regulate the registration of Chinese medicine practitioners, licensing of Chinese medicines traders and registration of proprietary Chinese medicines, setting up of the Academy of Medicine to standardize the training of medical specialists leading to specialist registration, and setting up of the Center for Health Protection for the prevention and control of diseases, especially in the prevention of infectious diseases and responses to major outbreaks.

Impact of Reform Efforts on Quality and Safety of Care

Hong Kong continues to enjoy improving trends in key health indices. In 2012, the life expectancy was 80.7 years for males and 86.4 years for females; the infant mortality rate was 1.5 per 1,000 live births; the age standardized death rate of 3.2 per 1,000 standard population, dropped from 6 per 1,000 standard population in 1981 (Centre for Health Protection 2014). The age-standardized death rates of the top five leading causes of death all show decreasing trends, except that for pneumonia (Table 8.2). In August 2013, Bloomberg ranked Hong Kong as the most efficient healthcare system in the world, according to a weighted summation of life expectancy and healthcare costs (Bloomberg 2013) (Table 8.3).

Table 8.2   Age-standardized death rates per 100,000 standard population of top five leading causes of death in Hong Kong

Causes of death	2001	2012
Malignant neoplasms	133.5	106.2
Pneumonia	32.4	42.0
Diseases of heart	52.3	43.0
Cerebrovascular diseases	34.4	22.5
Chronic lower respiratory diseases	22.9	13.1

Source: Centre for Health Protection 2014.

Table 8.3   Top three ranking of healthcare systems

	Hong Kong	Singapore	Japan
Efficiency score	92.6	81.9	74.1
Life expectancy	83.4	81.9	82.6
Healthcare cost			
% of GDP per capita	3.8%	4.4%	8.5%
US$ per capita	$1409	$2286	$3958

Source: Bloomberg 2013.

In regards to patient safety, reform initiatives focusing on engaging frontline healthcare workers in developing a safety culture, enhancing safety systems, promoting safe practices, and preventing adverse incidents, have led to much improvement in terms of a reduction in sentinel events and the occurrence of errors. Education on patient safety has been incorporated into the curriculum of undergraduate, postgraduate, and specialist training for all medical, nursing and allied health students, and trainees. There is a growth of awareness among healthcare workers of how patients can be protected through a systems approach to care and the adoption of safe practices in day-to-day work. Patient safety has also become a key consideration in the further development of clinical information systems and design of healthcare facilities.

Among the six dimensions of quality, overcrowding and long waiting time in public hospitals continue to bring tension to the system. During the winter "surge" months, compounded by the effects of seasonal influenza epidemics, bed occupancy rates in the medical wards of the public hospitals often fluctuates between 100–120 percent (Lo 2014). Patients have to wait for hours in the accident and emergency departments if they are triaged as non-urgent cases or waiting for admission. Waiting lists for consultations in the specialist outpatient clinics of public hospitals continue to grow and require intensive efforts of operational management to keep them under control. These efforts include the control of referrals, diversion of patients to primary care, and shifting of patients to clinics with less demand or shorter waiting lists. Waiting lists for some elective surgeries, in particular joint replacement surgery, are long and require the allocation of additional resources to the hospital clusters every year through the annual planning process.

In the private sector, quality and safety systems in hospitals are much improved through benchmarking of the systems with those in the public hospitals, participation in the hospital accreditation program, and regular inspection by the Department of Health. Standards among the private medical practitioners in primary care remain highly variable. The number of private medical practitioners participating in the PPP programs only makes up a small proportion of all those working in the private sector and primary care. There is a lack of mechanisms to monitor and assure quality and safety in these settings.

Barriers and Solutions

The healthcare system in Hong Kong continues to face the challenges of (1) the dichotomous public and the private systems that creates demand for public hospital services when quality improves, (2) integration between primary and secondary care, especially when primary care is mostly provided by the private medical practitioners, and (3) integrated provision of health and social care in addressing the healthcare needs of the aging population and chronic disease burden. There is no effective regulatory mechanism for managing demand and keeping a balance between public and private healthcare at present, except for waiting lists and waiting times in the public services, thus compromising the aspects of quality in terms of timeliness or accessibility, leading to public dissatisfaction. Making price adjustments has not been a feasible option for political reasons. There is an imminent need to develop strategies using different policy instruments to meet these three challenges. The proposal to develop voluntary medical insurance, subsidized and regulated by the Government with standard and transparent benefit packages and pricing, is one option being considered.

Another major barrier to ensuring quality and safety of care in the current system is the overall shortage of healthcare workers, not only doctors and nurses, but also the support workers (including care assistants). Since 1997, medical graduates from the Commonwealth countries can no longer practice in Hong Kong without passing the licentiate examination and going through internship training. These measures have drastically reduced the supply of doctors from overseas countries. The shortfall in supply was further aggravated by the downward adjustment in medical and nursing student numbers at the downturn of the economy following the Asian financial crisis and the severe acute respiratory syndrome (SARS) epidemic. In recent years, the Government has increased the number of medical and nursing students to be produced by the tertiary institutions. The supply of the nursing workforce has stabilized and improved. The long lead time in the training of doctors would take several more years before the estimated shortfalls are met. This affects the quality of care, especially in addressing the waiting times and the expectations of the public. There is an imminent need for Hong Kong to recruit more doctors from overseas to meet gaps in services.

Reforms to primary care predominantly provided by private medical practitioners can only take place incrementally, and must cope with obstacles and resistance. General practitioners or non-specialists working in the private sector maintain a position against mandatory continuous medical education. There are reservations in relation to the Government's initiative of introducing the electronic health records, shared by both the public and the private medical practitioners and hospitals. The ordinances that govern the private sector are outdated and are currently being reviewed by the Government. Enforcement of regulations by the Department of Health needs to be strengthened, in particular the imposition of sanctions and penalties for non-compliance. Alternative strategies to provide incentives for change are needed.

The Way Forward

The Government is ultimately responsible for ensuring quality and safety in the healthcare system. Musgrove (1996) suggested four key Government tools for influencing the private sector and the overall healthcare system, which include direct provision of services, financing, regulation and mandate, and provision of information. In Hong Kong, the Government has exercised a unique approach of corporatizing all public hospitals under the HA to bring about governance and management reforms for improving the direct provision of services. Further strengthening of the existing system would require:

- Developing supplementary medical insurance to strengthen healthcare financing and provide mechanisms for achieving a balanced healthcare system involving both the public and the private sectors.
- Updating regulatory mechanisms, expediting the roll-out of the hospital accreditation system, and strengthening the enforcement of regulations to ensure quality and protect patient safety.
- Extending strategic purchasing of services from the private sector through the HA platform which is targeted to: (i) addressing the primary and secondary care "disconnect," (ii) enhancing opportunities for engaging the resources in the private sector, and (iii) ensuring better performance management of both public and private components of the healthcare delivery system.

Conclusion

Most health systems in the world are mixed public and private systems. The World Health Organization suggests Governments should have the stewardship responsibility to ensure the health of the population, protect the citizens from financial risks, and ensure public satisfaction with the healthcare services (World Health Organization 2000). The Government stewardship role should include the assurance of quality and safety in healthcare services. The Hong Kong Government has initiated the first reforms in corporatizing the public hospitals with the setting up of the HA, through which to introduce governance and management reforms, and subsequently used the HA as a platform for introducing reforms to influence and promote the performance of the private sector. However, it is evident that reforms on the provider side alone are not enough. One important quality dimension, timeliness and access to care, continues to be a problem in the delivery of public healthcare, while mechanisms for assuring quality and safety in the private sector remain inadequate. It is necessary to enhance multiple complementary reform strategies that include financing, regulation, and other mechanisms for enhancing Government influence in order to meet health system objectives and goals.

Chapter 9

India

Girdhar J Gyani

Abstract

Healthcare is one of the key pillars of any democratic society; the other two being education and the environment. Government is duty bound to ensure the well-being of the population through frameworks of governance built around these pillars. Health reforms are characterized by four elements: accessibility, availability, affordability, and safety. Quality in healthcare and patient safety are two faces of the same coin. Quality is generally driven by market forces (that is, by way of open competition). However, when supply is limited, as compared to demand, quality takes the back seat. Healthcare in India is at this stage. Healthcare is expected to be regulated, as it affects the well-being of the common person, but with the Government short of resources, and dependent on the private sector, the enforcement of regulation has become difficult. Today, when the private sector has about an 80 percent share in healthcare expenditure, Government is highly reliant on the private sector to provide healthcare, even for its own welfare schemes. In such circumstances the key way to promote quality is to drive change through payers, and at the same time, empower the community to demand quality. This chapter highlights key aspects of India's journey and current status in this area of healthcare reform.

Background

The National Rural Health Mission (NRHM) was launched as a major healthcare reform in 2005 (Ministry of Health and Family Welfare India 2011), as a part of the common minimum program of the Government of India with the goal "to promote equity, efficiency, quality and accountability of public health services through community driven approaches, decentralization and improving local governance." The mission sought to provide accessible, affordable, and quality healthcare to rural populations, an especially vulnerable and underserved population group in the country. The mission aimed to achieve an infant mortality rate (IMR) of 30 per 1,000 live births, maternal mortality rate (MMR) of 100 per 100,000 live births, and a total fertility rate of 2.1 by 2012.

In line with NRHM, the Government has also launched the National Urban Health Mission (NUHM) as a new sub-mission under the over-arching National

Table 9.1   Demographic, economic, and health information for India

Population (thousands)	1,240,000
Area (sq. km)*	2,973,190
Proportion of population living in urban areas (2011)	31
Gross Domestic Product (GDP US$, billions)^	1.858.7
Total expenditure on health as % of GDP	4.1
Gross national income per capita (PPP intl $)	3,910
Per capita total expenditure on health (intl $)	157
Proportion of health expenditure which is private	66.9
General Government expenditure on health as a percentage of total expenditure on health	33.1
Out-of-pocket expenditure as a percentage of private expenditure on health	86
Life expectancy at birth m/f (yrs)	64/68
Probability of dying under five (per 1,000 live births)	56
Maternal Mortality Ratio (per 100,000 live births) (2013)	190
Proportion of population using improved water and sanitation	93/36

Source: Unless otherwise stated data are for the year 2012 and taken from the World Health Organization 2014. * Area from the World Bank 2014a. ^ GDP from the World Bank 2014b.

Notes: PPP is purchasing power parity, intl $ is international dollar which has the same purchasing power as US$ in the US.

Health Mission (NHM). Under the Scheme the following proposals have been approved:

- One Urban Primary Health Center (U-PHC) for every 50,000–60,000 people.
- One Urban Community Health Center (U-CHC) for five to six U-PHCs.
- One Auxiliary Nursing Midwife (ANM) per 10,000 people.
- One Accredited Social Health Activist (ASHA) for 200 to 500 households.

In order to improve the quality of health services, the Government has adopted the Clinical Establishment Act (Ministry of Health and Family Welfare India 2010), with the objective of creating uniform regulatory framework for the entire country. Likewise, a national accreditation system under the name NABH was launched in February 2006, and, to date, more than 200 hospitals have been awarded certificate of accreditation.

Aspects which have been incorporated in NRHM and NUHM reflect that the role of social determinants in health outcomes must be recognized and addressed. Specifically, the role of infant, child, and adult nutrition, literacy, particularly amongst girls, and access to clean drinking water have a direct correlation to maternal, new-born, and infant health.

Until 2008, only a small fraction of total expenses were pre-paid and most were out-of-pocket payments. According to the national health account study in 2009, the percentage of private out-of-pocket expenditure has decreased from 92.2 percent in 2000 to 78 percent in 2009. As the state Governments' insurance schemes are planned for launch, it is expected that 50 percent of the population will gain coverage under some or other insurance scheme by 2015.

Introduction

At the time of Indian independence, in 1947, only 8 percent of modern medical care was provided by the private sector. Limiting the need for private practitioners was one of the recommendations of the seminal 1946 report on the Health Survey & Development Committee (BHORE Committee). The preamble of the BHORE committee report began with the opening line: "No individual should fail to secure adequate medical care because of inability to pay for it." The social obligation for the Government to ensure the highest possible health status for its population, and as part of this to ensure that all people have access to quality healthcare, has been recognized by a number of key policy documents. The policy direction "health for all" became the stated declaration of the Government of India, with the adoption of the National Health Policy statement of 1983. Further to this, the health policy of 2002 provides for the need to (a) increase the total public health expenditure from 2 to 3 percent of GDP, and (b) strengthen the role of public sector in social protection against the rising cost of healthcare and the need to provide comprehensive packages of services.

The Constitution of India incorporates provisions guaranteeing everyone's right to the highest attainable standard of physical and mental health. Article 21 of the Indian constitution guarantees protection of life and personal liberty for every citizen. The Supreme Court of India has held that the right to live with human dignity, enshrined in Article 21, derives from the directive principles of state policy and therefore includes protection of health. Further, it has also held that the right to health is integral to the right to life and the Government has a constitutional and moral obligation to provide healthcare facilities to every individual. Keeping this in view, India launched its flagship program for providing healthcare to the rural population, known as National Rural Health Mission (NRHM) on April 12, 2005. Rural areas have a three-tier system: a sub-center per 5,000 people with one male and one female worker, a primary care center (PHC) per 30,000 people with a medical doctor and paramedical staff, and a community health center (CHC) per 100,000 people with 30 beds and basic specialists. Urban areas have a two-tier system: a basic freestanding health post for every few thousand people, and an urban health center per 100,000 people attached to a general hospital.

This chapter provides, in reasonable detail, the reforms in healthcare initiated by the Government independently and with public–private partnership (PPP). The chapter brings out, in quantifiable terms, the outcomes from these reforms, and also provides details about the effectiveness of regulations and accreditation in driving quality and safety in this vital sector.

The Current Situation

Contrary to the recommendations made by the BHORE committee, the private sector now dominates the provision of personal care (except in selected health programs). More than 70 percent of all outpatient and 50 percent of all inpatient care is being delivered by the private sector, despite the public health system having a vast network of facilities capable of providing accessible, affordable, and quality healthcare (Table 9.2)

Table 9.2   Public health system facilities

Sub Centers	148,124
PHCs	23,887
CHCs	4,809
Sub-divisional Hospitals	985
District Hospitals	613

The NRHM program has engaged 884,000 community health volunteers, known as Accredited Social Health Activists (ASHA) (National Rural Health Mission 2013), as links between the community and health systems. Further, about 31,000 patient welfare committees have been set up involving community members in all district hospitals.

Key health issues in India are the poor IMR and MMR. According to Dr Devi Shetty, an office bearer of the Association of Healthcare Providers India (AHPI) (a peak body encompassing over 10,000 hospitals across the country), India has only 27,000 gynecologists compared to 42,855 in the United States of America (US). Most of them live in cities. The IMR is 40 per 1,000 in India, compared to 6.4 per 1,000 in the US, and the MMR in India is 200 per 100,000, compared to 12.7 in the US. In order to effectively overcome these challenges, India needs at least 150,000 gynecologists. India has one pediatrician per 18,367 children, compared with 1 per 1,769 in the US, and there are only 20,000 practicing pediatricians in India, compared to 60,000 in the US. In regards to anesthetists, India has one anesthetist per 30,000 people, compared to six per 30,000 people in the US, and the country has only 40,000 practicing anesthetists, compared to 48,000 in the US. India also has one radiologist per 100,000 of the population, compared to ten for the same number of people in the US.

India has about 9.5 million deaths a year. Cardiovascular diseases account for nearly 27 percent of these; and infectious and parasitic diseases accounts for nearly 20 percent. Other major causes of death include: respiratory infection (pneumonia) at 11 percent, respiratory diseases (COPD, asthma) at 9 percent, and cancer at 8 percent. India has more than 60 million people with diabetes and nearly 11 percent of the population has raised fasting blood sugar. Considering that about 50 percent of India's population is in the productive age group (16–45), this is going to be a major concern and costly over time.

In order to contend with this considerable present and future disease burden, India needs proportionate healthcare infrastructure. India has not, thus far, been able to raise public and private healthcare spending more than five percent of GDP, as compared to the Organization for Economic Cooperation and Development (OECD) average of 9.7 percent (Organization for Economic Cooperation and Development and World Health Organization 2012). India has nearly 15 beds per 10,000 people, as compared to 30 in the US. India has 355 medical colleges which annually produce over 44,000 doctors and 20,000 specialists. In addition, each year about 21,500 dentists graduate from 290 dental colleges, 120,000 nurses from 2,400 nursing schools and 1,500 colleges, 30,000 ANMs from 1,300 schools, and 70,542 pharmacists graduate from 1,211 schools or colleges. Nonetheless, India is still grappling with severe shortage of doctors, nurses, and midwives, which is presently half of the norm, 24.5 per 10,000 people.

Complying with patient safety standards across the nation is going to be a daunting task, more so when India does not have any uniform regulatory framework for the country. The introduction of NABH in 2006 was a landmark event, which provided India with a patient safety framework of global standards. During the past seven years, 200 hospitals have been able to secure NABH accreditation. However, considering that there are more than 50,000 hospitals and nursing homes, India has a long way to go.

Current Reform Activities

The Indian public financing for healthcare has been less than 1 percent of the world's total health expenditure, although it is home to over 16 percent of the world's population. Families contribute almost 70 percent of their health expenses out of their own pockets, placing disproportionate financial burden on poor households. As India contemplates a significant increase in public spending on healthcare, the World Bank has carried out the first comprehensive review of India's major Government-sponsored health insurance schemes (GSHISs). The report, "Government-Sponsored Health Insurance in India — are you covered?" found that over the last five years, Government-sponsored schemes have contributed to a significant increase in the population covered by health insurance in the country, scaling up at a pace possibly unseen elsewhere in the world (Forgia & Nagpal 2012).

The report says that the new generation of GSHISs is introducing explicit entitlements, improving accountability, and leveraging private capacity, particularly with an aim of reaching the poor. Some of the innovative features common to all these schemes include giving patients the choice to visit any public or private provider empanelled by the Government. In most schemes, transactions are fully cashless, requiring no payment to be made by the patient to the hospital. These schemes also target low-income groups, make impressive use of information and communication technology, and use pre-agreed package rates for payment.

The new generation of health financing schemes are helping India progress towards universal health coverage. According to the study, over the past five years, GSHISs have contributed to a significant increase in the population covered by health insurance in the country. Most of the growth has occurred along three lines: the National Health Insurance Plan, under the name of "RSBY," commercial insurance, and state-sponsored schemes. GSHIS coverage, the World Bank study stated, is likely to more than double to 530 million by 2015, from 243 million in 2009–2010. Over 300 million people or more than 25 percent of India's population, gained access to some form of health insurance by 2010, up from 55 million in 200304. The study added that over half of the insured are from families below the poverty line.

The study, however, recognized that coverage remains far from comprehensive, as the schemes are focused on inpatient, often surgical, care. This prompted the study to recommend increasing health insurance coverage for both outpatient and inpatient care to include all poor and near poor patients.

The Quality and Safety Landscape

India has a federal system of governance, in which the 28 provinces (states) are vested with various powers, including administration of healthcare. All states have their own regulatory framework. The regulation in most states has not been effective. The Clinical Establishments Act, 2010, has been enacted by the central Government to provide for the registration and regulation of all clinical establishments in the country, with a view to prescribing the common minimum standards of facilities and services provided by them. As health provision lies in the state domain, the Act needs to be adopted by each respective state assembly before becoming law. The Act has taken effect in eight states and in all Union Territories since March 1, 2012. The Ministry has also notified the National Council for Clinical Establishments and the Clinical Establishments (Central Government) Rules, 2012 under this Act.

Beginning in the 1980s, the private–corporate sector began to invest in healthcare. Until this time, healthcare was largely confined to the public sector and a few charitable organizations. Today, India has a sizeable number of big corporate hospitals providing tertiary level of healthcare, with indications that many of these are at par with global standards. Starting in the early 1990s, some hospitals began to adopt the ISO 9000 series of standards as a mark of quality. This was also the time when some hospitals began to receive overseas patients. Early in the twenty-first century, medical tourism established roots in India. It was during this period that the question was raised in Indian Parliament, in April 2005, through the Ministry of Tourism, about the need to have a national healthcare accreditation system in line with global standards.

The task of creating a healthcare accreditation system was taken up by Quality Council of India. An autonomous agency in the name of National Accreditation Board for Hospitals & Healthcare Providers (NABH) was established, and the first edition of accreditation standards was released in February 2006. The standards later got accredited by the International Society for Quality in Healthcare (ISQua). As of December 31, 2013, there are more than 200 hospitals accredited by NABH. This has, on one hand, created a framework for quality governance in hospitals in the country and, at the same time, provided a boost to medical tourism.

Accreditation, by design, is voluntary. It is driven by market forces and other incentives. Consumers, therefore, need to be empowered so that they demand accreditation from the hospitals. Simultaneously, we need to promote accreditation as a mark of excellence among the healthcare providers, by which they should be able to achieve greater value. Paying or empanelling agencies can play an important role in the promotion of accreditation. In most developing nations accreditation is driven by the insurance sector. Insurance companies find it convenient to rely on accreditation as it provides safeguards for minimizing risk from possible liability suits. Some of the Government-owned social schemes have adopted NABH accreditation as a basis for the empanelment of hospitals. This has begun to generate stimulate participation in NABH accreditation.

Details of the Impact of These Reform Efforts on Quality and Safety of Care

The NRHM was launched in April 2005 with the following objectives:

- reduction in IMR/MMR;
- universal access to public health services such as women's health, child health, water, sanitation and hygiene, immunization, and nutrition;
- prevention and control of communicable and non-communicable diseases;
- access to integrated comprehensive primary healthcare;
- population stabilization, gender and demographic balance;
- Revitalize revitalize local health traditions and mainstream Ayurveda Yoga & Naturopathy, Unami, Siddha and Homeopathy (AYUSH);
- promotion of healthy lifestyle.

NRHM has played a major role by strengthening health facilities to provide services, adding over 100,000 healthcare workers, improving infrastructure by increasing availability of equipment and essential supplies, and by promoting demand through community-level processes. Four major innovations have contributed to the reduction IMR/MMR. These include the *Janani Suraksha Yojana* (Mother Safety Plans) for promoting institutional delivery, the dial 108 Ambulance System to tackle the issue of emergency transport, the multi-skilling of non-specialist medical officers to address the lack of specialist skills for the provision of emergency obstetric care, and the *Janani Shishu Suraksha Karyakram* (Mother and Child Safety Program) to reduce the financial barriers of access to care.

There were some measurable indicators built in the NRHM objectives. For example IMR was envisaged to be brought down to 30 per 1,000 live births by 2012. It stands at 40 per 1,000. The MMR was envisaged to be 100 per 100,000 live births, but is 200 per 100,000. However, there has been a significant reduction in mortality due to communicable and non-communicable diseases during the period as follows:

- kala-azar mortality reduced by 21.93 percent;
- malaria mortality reduced by 45.23 percent;
- microfilaria reduced by 26.74 percent;
- dengue-related mortality reduced by 52 percent.

In terms of provision of human resources 46,690 ANMs, 8,624 MBBS doctors, 2,460 specialists and 14,490 paramedic staff were appointed under the program (Ministry of Health and Family Welfare 2011). This has significantly improved the quality and safety of healthcare services at PHCs and CHCs. This period also saw appointment of 0.8 million ASHA workers including 0.7 million equipped with drug kits.

Implementation Barriers and Solutions

India is a huge country by its sheer population size, which stands at 1,210 million. The urban population represents 31 percent of the total and is growing. Public expenditure on health is 1.2 percent of GDP which continues to be amongst the lowest in the world. Thanks to the positive in-flow from the private sector the total healthcare GDP stands at about 5 percent. Under the circumstances it is not possible to raise the expenditure and supply of healthcare services will continue to fall short at least in remote areas.

The existing public health network is in reasonably good shape but remains under-utilized. India does not have effective referral mechanisms and most patients with primary ailments end up at district hospitals. We need to strengthen the infrastructure at PHCs and CHCs so that patients gain confidence to approach these institutes for primary ailments. We similarly need to improve efficiency at district hospitals by applying quality tools such as 5S and LEAN.

In the private sector, the potential is considerable. Government can provide incentives by way of cheaper land (which is prohibitively expensive in tier-I and tier-II cities) and extend tax benefits to attract corporate companies to invest in this sector. Hospitals are presently bracketed under the commercial category in terms of payment of water, electricity, and other services. Most medical equipment is being imported and is subject to steep import duties. Lessening these restrictions can encourage small entrepreneurs to invest in healthcare. These measures will also help in opening of modern hospitals in tier-III cities, which continue to remain dependent services in tier-II and tier-I cities for serious ailments.

Quality and patient safety remain issues of concern. While accreditation has taken firm roots and is recognized universally in India, only 200 hospitals have enforced accreditation. This is largely on account of a lack of incentives for hospitals to participate in accreditation programs. In developed countries insurance companies drive participation in accreditation. In India, private insurance has very little penetration and it is left to Government subsidy or welfare schemes like the Central Government Health Scheme (CGHS), which can potentially have large-scale impacts on driving hospitals to go for accreditation. Industries on their own are not very keen, as many of them would have to invest heavily in infrastructure to comply with the requirements of the accreditation standard. Another reason for slow growth of accreditation is that hospitals have, so far, not really experienced any control, even having minimum infrastructural needs as regulation has barely been effective to date. With the advent of the Clinical Establishment Act and the launch of new social insurance schemes, demand on quality will go up and it is hoped that by 2015, things will have changed substantially.

Prospects for Success and Next Steps

India's urban population has witnessed an increase of four and a half times from 1951 to 2000, compared to a three times increase in the total population over the same period. With increased urbanization and the problems associated with modern living in urban settings, the disease profiles are shifting from infectious to lifestyle-related. It is estimated that 50 percent of beds might be occupied with patients suffering from lifestyle diseases. Government, until recently, has been focusing on NRHM. It will now need to put equal emphasis on the NUHM.

Government plans to undertake the building of six super-specialty tertiary hospitals with research and education centers across the country. This would help make high-end clinical care available to the masses. Governments need to put state-driven insurance schemes in fast track mode so as to cover the vast majority of the population. It also needs to strengthen RSBY for the workforce engaged in the un-organized sector.

Workforce shortages are a big issue. Presently, only about 22,000 specialists are graduating annually. This needs to be enhanced at least by 100 percent to match the demand of the rural population as well as urban residents. The case is similar for nursing staff. In spite of adequate numbers of nursing colleges and schools, there are few enrolling, as the perception is that there is little career progression in nursing.

Patient safety and affordability are two issues which need to be addressed simultaneously. The Government needs to prioritize a regulation framework. Equally important is the need to drive participation in accreditation. The insurance sector and payers need to come together and agree on a uniform set of standards which can ensure patient safety.

In order to make healthcare affordable, Government needs to reduce tariffs on electricity, water, and even provide subsidies for land. Similarly, there is need to reduce heavy import duties on medical equipment, as the majority of equipment is being imported. Lastly the healthcare industry needs to adopt cost competitiveness tools as adopted by engineering companies. These include 5S, Kaizen, LEAN, Six Sigma, and the Balanced Score Card.

Conclusion

India has almost the lowest international share (second to Myanmar) of public spending on health. Public expenditure is largely devoted to providing healthcare services to rural populations and to those in the below poverty segment of the urban population. The good news is that the private–corporate sector has come to the table to invest in healthcare by way of setting secondary–tertiary level hospitals in tier-I and tier-II cities. There is yet another good trend emerging, where more and more state Governments are resorting to buying healthcare services for various segments of population under their social welfare schemes. This represents a unique form of PPP, which is expected to benefit 50 percent of the population by the year 2015. This kind of PPP is also having a positive impact on quality, with state Governments, as paying agencies, able to demand high levels of quality compliance from private hospitals empanelled under their schemes. These include NABH accreditation or the patient safety criteria specified by respective state Governments.

Chapter 10

Japan

Yukihiro Matsuyama

Abstract

Health reform is a critical policy theme for the Japanese administration. The specific means of health reform have been made clear through discussion in Government councils. The Government is planning to establish a new organization to improve the quality of healthcare and patient safety through the 2014 health law amendment. As a result of the establishment of new national databases on healthcare, improvement efforts based on more detailed analysis of quality and safety data have become possible. The current healthcare delivery system is poorly organized and there is a lack of managerial governance at the regional level. This has impeded the effective formation of medical teams to deliver optimal care to patients and has had an adverse effect on the improvement of clinical practices. As a consequence, the Government is planning to grant healthcare delivery organizations a non-profit holding company status, through which large-scale healthcare entities can form core players providing comprehensive community care. The Government has coined the term "Data Health" to focus more on a healthy population achieved by prevention, a strength of Japan's, to realize longer life expectancy with lower healthcare expenditures. If it works as well as expected, Japan, already the nation with the longest healthy life expectancy in the world, may be able to further improve.

Background

The current Japanese health system was designed in the resources-rich age of high economic growth. However, Japanese economic growth rate has slowed. Even worse, nominal GDP shrank by 7.8 percent from 516 trillion Yen (US$5.16 trillion) in 1997, to 476 trillion Yen (US$4.76 trillion) in 2012. Japan's population is aging, rapidly. This has posed a problem during this deflation period. As a result, the total amount of medical care and long-term care expenditure is expected to have reached 48 trillion Yen in 2012. This suggests that by 2012 the ratio of healthcare expenditures (based on the definition of Ministry of Health, Labor and Welfare (MHLW)) to nominal GDP might have been as high as 10.1 percent, To compare this ratio to other nations, the System of Health Accounts (SHA), which is defined by the Organization for Economic Cooperation and Development (OECD), is

Table 10.1   Demographic, economic, and health information for Japan

Population (thousands)	127,000
Area (sq. km)*	364,500
Proportion of population living in urban areas (2011)	91
Gross Domestic Product (GDP US$, billions)^	5,961.1
Total expenditure on health as % of GDP	10.1
Gross national income per capita (PPP intl $)	36,300
Per capita total expenditure on health (intl $)	3,578
Proportion of health expenditure which is private	17.5
General Government expenditure on health as a percentage of total expenditure on health	82.5
Out-of-pocket expenditure as a percentage of private expenditure on health	80.6
Life expectancy at birth m/f (yrs)	80/87
Probability of dying under five (per 1,000 live births)	3
Maternal Mortality Ratio (per 100,000 live births) (2013)	6
Proportion of population using improved water and sanitation	100/100

Source: Unless otherwise stated data are for the year 2012 and taken from the World Health Organization 2014. * Area from the World Bank 2014a. ^ GDP from the World Bank 2014b.
Note: PPP is purchasing power parity, intl $ is international dollar which has the same purchasing power as US$ in the US.

used. Healthcare expenditures based on SHA are larger than that based on MHLW, because they include general over-the-counter medicines, normal delivery costs, and other items which are excluded from the definition of MHLW. The ratio based on the SHA is estimated to be around 11.0 percent in 2012. The share of people aged 65 years or older as a percentage of total population, the most influential factor affecting health system design, reached 25 percent in 2013, as shown in Table 10.2. The Government predicts that this will rise to 30.3 percent in 2025 and 38.8 percent in 2050.

According to the most recent International Monetary Fund estimate, the general Government gross debt was 1,132 trillion Yen at the end of 2012, which is 238 percent of nominal GDP. Nevertheless, the Japanese economy has not become bankrupt, because the public itself underwrites most of the debt with 1,547 trillion Yen of household financial assets. The general Government gross debt, however, will exceed the total amount of household financial assets by 2025, which is the target year of the current health reform. It will inevitably result in a period in which the Government is forced to borrow funds from abroad to meet operating budgets. As a result, interest rates on Government bonds will rise sharply, resulting

Table 10.2   The increase of elderly citizens in Japan

	2013	**2025**	**2050**
(1) Total population (thousands)	127,247	120,659	97,076
(2) Population aged 65 and over (thousands)	31,971	36,573	37,676
(2) / (1)	25.1%	30.3%	38.8%
(3) Population aged 75 and over (thousands)	15,669	21,786	23,846
(3) / (1)	12.3%	18.1 %	24.6 %

Source: National Institute of Population and Social Security Research 2012.

in a lack of financial resources for healthcare due to the burden of increasing interest payments. This inconvenient truth, along with demographic aging of the population, is the strongest driver of health reform in Japan.

The health reform has two goals: to make it sustainable and to convert the healthcare industry into an economic growth engine. Key bodies—the Social Security System Reform National Council and the Industrial Competitiveness Council and Regulatory Reform Council—have been set up to develop specific methods to achieve these aims. They recommend increasing the contributions of the wealthy, improving efficiency through increases in the scale of healthcare providers, an active commitment to advanced technology, more effective use of Information and Communication Technology (ICT), a focus on prevention, and other related measures. The draft of the 2014 Health Law Amendment includes a provision, similar to other OECD countries, for the establishment of a national organization with responsibilities to improve quality and safety.

Introduction

The current universal health insurance system (under which all citizens are obliged to enroll in one of the country's public insurance programs) was founded in 1961. The free medical care program for those 70 years or older was enacted in 1973. The health system, ranked No.1 in 2000 by the World Health Organization (WHO), was created in a time of plenty, with financial resources from high economic growth and concomitant investments in healthcare delivery systems and public health. A significant feature is its generosity. Patients can access healthcare institutions anytime and anywhere with a lower cost when compared to other countries.

The Government occasionally embarked on health reform initiatives due to worsening financial difficulties caused by falling economic growth and demographic changes. For example, Public Long-Term Care Insurance was introduced in 2000. It reflects the structural change in healthcare needs that have to be made to prompt a shift from acute care to long-term care for the older people with costly chronic illnesses. In 2008, the Medical Care System for the Advanced

Elderly began. It aims for stable acquisition by the state of healthcare financial resources for patients aged 75 and over. As Table 10.2 shows, the number of people aged 75 and over will increase sharply from 15.669 million in 2013 to 23.846 million in 2050, meaning that its ratio to the total population will rise from 12.3 percent in 2013 to 24.6 percent in 2050. The breakdown of the Medical Care System for the Advanced Elderly is: public funds 50 percent, support funds from insurers 40 percent, and premiums 10 percent. The patient premium contribution of 10 percent is much less than the 30 percent made by citizens in employment.

The health reform of the Japanese administration focuses on extending healthy life expectancy. Its policy aims are to decrease morbidity through prevention and increase quality of life. This population health initiative is the "Data Health" Project. A shared medical information system, designed to improve quality of care and safety of patients, is a prerequisite for this project. As indicated below, there are several kinds of insurers. Among them, society-managed health insurance is expected to play a leading role because of data analysis expertise.

Current Situation

A strength of Japan's health system is that it has achieved long-life expectancy for the population with relatively low healthcare expenditures by controlling medical-fee unit prices. One striking feature is that, while non-healthcare industries have produced many global companies such as Toyota, Canon, and Sony, there is no world-class healthcare delivery organization in Japan. Japan's healthcare market is ranked second in size after the United States of America (US). However, both insurers and healthcare providers are too small for the health system to keep up with technological advances. As a result, the gap between medical needs and healthcare delivery systems has been expanding without the governance of regional healthcare management resources. The management of the healthcare system as a whole has fallen behind with respect to medical technology; progress has been slow here.

The public health insurance system is classified into National Health Insurance (as of June 2012, 1,723 insurers for self-employed individuals, farmers, and unemployed 74-years-old or less), Society-managed Health Insurance (1,458 insurers for large-sized firm employees), Association-managed Health Insurance (47 insurers for small and medium-sized firm employees), Government Employees Mutual Aid Association (84 insurers), Medical Care System for the Advanced Elderly (47 insurers), and so on. There are an average of 36,400 insured people per insurer. Insurers as a whole have sustained large deficits due to the decrease of premium revenues caused by the fall in wages as a result of deflation and the increase of healthcare expenses for the elderly. Among them, a target of health reform is National Health Insurance, of which the deficit in the fiscal year 2011 was 302 billion Yen (US$3 billion). The Japanese municipalities were forced to act as guarantors for the shortfalls.

The number of medical care facilities across the country is 177,531 as of June 2013, which consists of 8,555 hospitals, 100,369 clinics, and 68,607 dental clinics. About 70 percent of the 8,555 hospitals are small and medium-sized institutions owned by individual medical doctors. These private hospitals are prohibited by medical law from paying dividends. However, a hospital owner can convert the cumulative profits into cash by selling his or her hospital. In other words, most private hospitals are for profit, with the result that their corporate tax is the same as private companies. The 274 national hospitals, 957 municipal hospitals, and 353 other public hospitals are competing, rather than cooperating with each other, in the same local medical districts. They are wasting public funds through redundant investments. In addition, the structural deficit of municipal hospitals is an especially tough barrier to healthcare delivery systems reform. The total amount of their annual patient service revenues is about 3.4 trillion Yen (US$34 billion). They cannot break even without subsidies, which amount to 760 billion Yen (US$7.6 billion), carrying forward an accumulated deficit of over two trillion Yen (US$20 billion). The information on quality and safety provided by these financially troubled hospitals is not sufficient to give an accurate picture to the Government or the population.

Detail of Current Reform Initiatives

The Government is planning to consolidate the insurers in the National Health Insurance market from 1,723 municipalities in 47 prefectures. Currently, there is a large gap in premium amounts among municipalities, even in the same prefecture. This suggests that the consolidation will generate a severe conflict of interest among residents in each prefecture. The prefectures will be given the authority to allocate financial resources. They should have responsibility for encouraging the differentiation between hospitals to reduce the gap between needs and the delivery system. They are also expected to play a key role in the Data Health Project which will be supported by national databases. One of the national databases was completed by the All Japan Federation of National Health Insurance Organizations in October 2013. The National Federation of Health Insurance Societies will also build a similar database in 2014. The Japan Health Insurance Association is expected to follow.

"Comprehensive community care" has become a key phrase of health reform. It is defined as the arrangement for providing each local resident with primary care, long-term care, health guidance, and so on, under an integrated management arrangement. The Government aims to create this for units of 10,000 people, nationally, by 2025. This should help the system to pay more attention to quality and safety in home care as well as hospital care. Acute care beyond these basic care services will be provided by large hospitals established in wider regional units.

Information sharing among medical care facilities in each region is critical to encourage the success of comprehensive community care. However, as we have seen, a significant feature of the healthcare delivery system is the disjointed state of small and medium-sized institutions. Even public hospitals do not share clinical information. Therefore, the Government has encouraged 47 prefectures to set up an information sharing program. Most prefectures started in 2013. However, it will take considerable time for this program to contribute fully to comprehensive community care, because, at this stage, participation in the program is optional rather than compulsory.

There is an area which has already implemented comprehensive community care on a large scale, providing the rest of the system for a model to emulate: Nagano Prefecture, with a population of over two million, which is located in the middle of the Japanese archipelago. Nagano is well known for having the longest life expectancy with the lowest healthcare expenditures in Japan. Nagano's healthy life expectancy of its elderly is also of the highest levels in Japan. Half a century ago, it was the worst region in terms of morbidity and healthcare costs, mainly due to cardiovascular disease and strokes caused, amongst other things, by excess salt consumption. Nagano Koseiren has provided residents with dietary guidance. It is a vertically integrated healthcare network which provides all care services needed by its residents. In Nagano Prefecture medical expenses per capita are about 12 percent less than the national average after adjusting for demographic differences. If the Nagano Koseiren system was extended to the rest of the country, this suggests that Japan can save five trillion Yen (US$50 billion) of healthcare expenses while maintaining or extending people's life expectancy. But it is not yet clear how to develop a program for disseminating the model across the country.

Status Quo of Quality of Care and Safety of Patients

While the system of healthcare financial resource management and care delivery varies from country to country, commonly both insurers and healthcare providers have a responsibility for improving quality of care and safety of local patients. As previously mentioned, the scale of each health insurer is too small to analyze data independently relating to quality and safety. Most healthcare providers are also small and lack the financial resources to acquire human resources, invest in improving quality and safety, as well as keeping up with technological advances. As a result, healthcare benchmarking programs have been premature.

National university hospitals are in a particularly serious situation, despite the fact that they should be taking the initiative in quality and safety issues. There are 45 national university hospitals. Most of them are under the control of a medical faculty, in which budget allocation is decided at faculty meetings. Those medical faculties have a tendency to focus on basic research rather than clinical or health services research. Therefore, the national university hospitals have a disadvantage in the scramble for funds between medical faculties and hospitals. The revenue from patient treatment at Tokyo University Hospital, which is the largest national university hospital in Japan, is only 42 billion Yen (US$420 million as at March 31,

2012). The total revenue of the 45 national university hospitals is 889 billion Yen (US$9 billion as at March 31, 2012), which is less than the revenue of University of Pittsburgh Medical Center (US$9.6 billion, June 30, 2012). UPMC is famous around the world as a leading healthcare industry grouping. By way of contrast, the leaders of Japanese university hospitals have no incentives to pursue world standard healthcare management.

In addition, the long working hours of Japanese hospital doctors is threatening the quality of care and safety of patients. Their working hours include not only consultation hours but also meetings, education, self-training, research, and other miscellaneous duties. According to research conducted in 2006 by The National Institute of Public Health, the average total working hours per week of a hospital doctor are 70.6. This breaks down as: consultation 39.6 hours, meeting and education related to consultation 9 hours, out of hospital activities 7.3 hours, and self-training, research, and other activities 14.7 hours. The working hours of a Japanese hospital doctor are longer than those in other countries. They bear the heavy burden of consultation work in a hospital outpatient department. This indicates a lack of proper task allocation from administrators: doctors take on non-specialized tasks which could be done by non-medical staff. According to another Government survey, 86.2 percent of doctors who ended a night shift continued on to their regular shift for the next day. In spite of such difficult working conditions, the income of hospital doctors is less than that of independent doctors. This, in turn, drives them to become independent practitioners. As a result, hospitals are caught in a vicious cycle such that the working conditions of the remaining doctors deteriorate further due to worsening medical shortages. To overcome this, Japan needs to increase the number of doctors per hospital by increasing the overall workforce supply of doctors, and doing a better job of integrating hospitals. As a way of dealing with this problem, the Government increased the enrollment capacity of medical faculties by 1,416 in 2008 up to 9,014, a record high enrollment, in 2013.

Reform Efforts of Quality and Safety

There are two sources of data regarding the quality of care and safety of patients. The first one is the Project to Collect Medical Near-miss/Adverse Event Information operated by the Japan Council for Quality Health Care. As of the end of 2012, 273 medical institutions were obliged to submit reports while 653 medical institutions participated voluntarily. As Table 10.3 shows, the number of events reported by medical institutions obliged to submit reports more than doubled from 1,114 in 2005 to 2,535 in 2012. On the other hand, although the number of voluntarily participating medical institutions has more than doubled since 2005, the number of events reported by them is only 347 in 2012, a total of 0.53 per hospital. It seems therefore that the willingness or capacity of voluntarily participating medical institutions to submit reports is poor. These facts suggest

Table 10.3   Number of reported medical adverse events

Form of participation	Year	2005	2012
Mandatory	Number of Reports	1,114	2,535
	Number of Medical Institutions	272	273
Voluntary	Number of Reports	151	347
	Number of Medical Institutions	283	653

Source: Japan Council for Quality Health Care 2011.

that there is much progress to be made. The Government intends incorporating the provisions in the 2014 health law revision to establish Medical Safety Research Committee to bolster this project.

The second data source is the National Clinical Database (NCD), which has been maintained by the Japan Surgical Society since 2011. The comparative evaluation of quality and safety is now feasible at each level of diagnosis, department, medical facility, region, and nation by collecting and analyzing surgery and treatment information across the country. However, the Government has not yet been able to provide the public with the evaluation data which they fear may prove misleading to ordinary people. It will take time for the Government to disclose them on its website as US, Canada, and Australia do, mainly because of strong resistance to information disclosure from healthcare providers. It is the responsibility of Government to disclose the evaluation data regarding national university hospitals, national hospitals, and municipality hospitals, all of which are subsidized with taxpayers' funds.

Barriers and Solutions to Reform

In order to improve the poor working environment of hospital doctors and implement world-class management systems for quality and safety, it is important to achieve business scale in healthcare, and let providers pursue a private sector-style management approach. The Regulatory Reform Council and a committee of MHLW have been discussing specific methods. One of the key phrases for healthcare management reform is a "non-profit holding company." These are vertically integrated healthcare networks. In Japan, they would provide all care services including acute care, primary care, home care, rehabilitation, long-term care, and prevention. Nagano Koseiren is an example of an organization with a similar business structure to Integrated Healthcare Networks (IHNs) in the US. It created the integration business model much earlier than American IHNs which emerged in the 1990s. The difference is that Nagano Koseiren is not allowed to own subsidiary companies as a holding company. While the annual revenues of Nagano Koseiren were 87 billion Yen (US$870 million) in 2011, there are several much larger healthcare providers such as National Hospital Organization (US$9.1 billion), Japanese Red Cross Society Hospitals (US$7.4 billion), and Social Welfare Corporation Saiseikai (US$5.5 billion). They are also non-profit organizations which do not have a holding company function. In order to help the healthcare industry contribute to economic growth, the Government needs to create healthcare providers which can expand overseas by using subsidiaries. An effective way to do this is to separate hospitals from national universities, integrate them into public hospitals in the same healthcare market and let them strive for private-style management techniques. The national university hospitals will be able to overcome the weaknesses and implement world standard quality and safety management. A holding company function is also useful to let them earn additional revenues in healthcare-related business fields. The Regulatory Reform Council is in charge of this issue.

The Japanese administration has undertaken reforms to secure additional financial resources for healthcare. The first method is an increase in the contribution of high earners. It is expected to be implemented by increasing premiums and the ratio of cost-sharing for those with higher incomes. The second method is to exclude the elderly with low care needs from Public Long-term Care Insurance. Obviously the elderly, with a strong capacity to influence elections, oppose this. In the Japanese tradition, national consensus will have to be obtained in the end.

The third method is to expand non-insured medical care in conjunction with insured medical care. This is politically the most controversial issue. Such a combination is prohibited as a general rule. If a patient receives both insured and non-insured medical care at the same medical facility simultaneously, the insured medical care becomes exempt from insurance payments so the patient is forced to pay all medical expenses. The Non-insured Associated Medical Care Program is an exemption from such prohibition. It applies mainly to new, advanced medical treatments. The market value of this is currently about ten billion Yen (US$100 million). The expansion of the program may bring some relief to public medical care financial resources, while the applicants have to pay for non-insured medical care from their own pocket. The Japan Medical Association strongly opposes this measure because of a perceived widening gap between the haves and the have-nots.

The responsibility and authority of health system management is shifting to prefectures through the healthcare reform measures. Under the new scheme, medical institutions are obliged to clarify their own functions and report to the prefecture in which they operate. The prefecture will develop a healthcare plan to tackle the gap between needs and the delivery system. The prefectures, however, lack the human resources to manage the health system at this point. The national Government should focus on developing human resources of management as well as medical doctors and nurses to make health reform successful.

Conclusion

Reform of the roles, functions, and working methods of all stakeholders in the healthcare industry including medical staff, insurers, and policymakers is critical to improve quality of care and safety of patients. It means the creation of an organizational culture which is continually pursuing world standards of quality and safety. The expansion to a business scale of both safety-net public healthcare providers and health insurers is particularly important to accomplish change in Japan. If the whole health system's management is reformed and the system uses information more strategically through the Data Health Project, Japan will be able to enhance further the levels of long, healthy life expectancy of its population. Perhaps it can also improve on its status, and become the best, most cost-effective and well-integrated health system in the world.

PART III
South Eastern Asia and Oceania

Jeffrey Braithwaite

In our journey across the world's health systems, we now move, in Part III, to South Eastern Asia and Oceania, and hear from experts in another four countries. Again, a range of income levels determine to a considerable extent the foci of health reforms and the quality and safety initiatives that are favored.

Australia and New Zealand are often grouped together as they are geopolitical neighbors, with a common system of Government based on the UK's Westminster system. However, they are different countries and have different health systems, and similarities are mostly superficial. Australia is a federation, and reform efforts are split between the states and territories on the one hand and the federal (Commonwealth) Government on the other. While there is a great deal of reform activity, most of the reforms in Australia, as Duckett shows, are structural and, from 2014, financial. The safety and quality agenda is sophisticated, has been built over many years, and seems to be in a parallel universe from the reform processes, according to this chapter.

Reorganizing structures is a feature of health reform not only in Australia, but, historically, New Zealand. Its system is more integrated—it is not a federation, but it has restructured on occasions at the meso level and, for a decade and a half, has had district health boards as a key governance mechanism. New Zealand also has embraced the quality and safety movement, according to Cummings' chapter, and now has a national agency to coordinate efforts, stimulate culture change, and make further progress.

By way of contrast, Papua New Guinea is a lower-middle income country, geographically and linguistically highly compartmentalized, with historically diverse tribalism across thousands of local, remote villages. Alongside its aid partners it has orchestrated multiple capacity-building and improvement programs, and has instituted a series of national health plans but they have often fallen short. Some commentators, according to Adu-Krow and Sikosana's chapter, have indicated the health system is in crisis. Papua New Guinea is striving to meet the Millennium Development Goals but is not likely to succeed, although it has made measurable progress in some areas. Reforms are hard to achieve in a country with its economic, social, and security challenges. Core quality and safety issues include accessibility to essential medicines, providing good facilities and equipment, having sufficient staff, and improving their skills and capacities.

Building commitment to a quality and safety agenda, and having an institutional framework for it, are important goals but are proving hard to achieve.

Indonesia is a very large country with a population of 244 million spread over 13,466 islands and faces the challenges of providing care in a middle income nation. It is in economic transition and is beginning to see more non-communicable diseases as a proportion of its total disease burden. The cornerstones of its reform measures are, according to its vision and plan for the health sector, to strive for much improved, accessible care. It has designed initiatives to revamp the workforce, making affordable medicines more widely available, and improve the health insurance system. Hermawan and Blakely note that Indonesia has made progress on a number of fronts, particularly in terms of communicable diseases and child malnutrition. Indonesia's quality and safety agenda is due to be bolstered by a new monitoring system and a range of regulatory, accreditation, and budgeting measures designed and supported particularly over the last three years. Effective implementation will be a key factor in future success, as will ongoing evaluation of the systems–strengthening initiatives.

Chapter 11
Australia

Stephen Duckett

Abstract

The last five years has seen a wave of "reform" activity in Australia, with multiple new national agencies being established, the creation of 61 new local primary care "coordinating" groups, and changes in hospital governance in many states. Although one can trace a link between this new superstructure and potential improvement in a patient's experience, it is too early to see the impact of the changes in practice.

Background

An important antecedent of health reform in Australia, at least as far as safety issues are concerned, was the recognition in the mid-1990s of significant rates of adverse events in Australian hospitals. The immediate stimulus was a report commissioned by the national Government as part of a medical indemnity review which measured adverse event rates (Wilson et al. 1995). The then Government commissioned a "task force" to recommend an appropriate response (Commonwealth Department of Health and Family Services 1996), but this reported to a new Government which dithered, reanalyzed the data, delayed, and sought further advice (National Expert Advisory Group on Safety and Quality in Australian Health Care 1999) before accepting that there was a problem. This eventually led to the establishment of a non-statutory body, the Australian Council on Quality and Safety in Health Care in 2000 to lead change (Barraclough & Birch 2006). The Council had a number of failings (Paterson 2005, Review of Future Governance Arrangements for Safety and Quality in Health Care 2005). Significant problems with care were also being disclosed in hospitals, which led to increased salience of these issues at the state level (McLean & Walsh 2003, van der Weyden 2004, van der Weyden 2005, Duckett 2009). Part of the national political response to the hospital problems and the perceived failures of the Council was to replace it with another non-statutory body, the Australian Commission on Safety and Quality in Health Care, in 2006.

Table 11.1   Demographic, economic, and health information for Australia

Population (thousands)	22,050
Area (sq. km)*	7,682,300
Proportion of population living in urban areas (2011)	89
Gross Domestic Product (GDP US$, billions)^	1,532.4
Total expenditure on health as % of GDP	9.1
Gross national income per capita (PPP intl $)	43,300
Per capita total expenditure on health (intl $)	4,068
Proportion of health expenditure which is private	33.1
General Government expenditure on health as a percentage of total expenditure on health	66.9
Out-of-pocket expenditure as a percentage of private expenditure on health	56
Life expectancy at birth m/f (yrs)	81/85
Probability of dying under five (per 1,000 live births)	5
Maternal Mortality Ratio (per 100,000 live births) (2013)	6
Proportion of population using improved water and sanitation	100/100

Source: Unless otherwise stated data are for the year 2012 and taken from the World Health Organization 2014. * Area from the World Bank 2014a. ^ GDP from the World Bank 2014b.

Note: PPP is purchasing power parity, intl $ is international dollar which has the same purchasing power as US$ in the US.

The Australian National Reform Process

Australia's health funding and delivery arrangements are shaped by its complex "marble cake" federalism where responsibility for healthcare is subject to intertwined responsibilities between the Commonwealth (national) and state Governments (Duckett 2014). The Commonwealth Government is responsible for the universal Medical Benefits Scheme and Pharmaceutical Benefits Scheme, and private health insurance. Public hospitals (which account for about 60 percent of all admissions) are a state responsibility, although about 45 percent of funding comes from the Commonwealth. The major political parties (Labor on the center-left, Liberal on the right) differ in their position on healthcare with the Liberals tending to be stronger in support of private health insurance (Duckett 2008).

The stimulus for the current wave of health reform was the election of a new Government in 2007, where the confused responsibilities between the

Commonwealth and the states had been an issue. The prospects for a renegotiation of roles were good, as at the time of its election all Governments were of the same political persuasion (Labor).

The new Government, led by Prime Minister Kevin Rudd, moved swiftly to appoint a National Health and Hospitals Reform Commission with broad-ranging terms of reference to review the health system. The media release announcing the commission identified its task as being to:

- provide a blueprint for tackling future challenges in the Australian health system including:
  - the rapidly increasing burden of chronic disease;
  - the ageing of the population;
  - rising health costs;
  - inefficiencies exacerbated by cost shifting and the blame game.

The Commission will focus on health financing, maximizing a productive relationship between public and private sectors, and improving rural health (Minister for Health and Aging 2008).

Although neglected in the media hype surrounding its appointment, the Commission's final report included recommendations relating to safety and quality (see Box) (National Health and Hospitals Reform Commission 2009).

Recommendations of National Health and Hospital Reform Commission Relating to Safety

32: To support quality improvement, we recommend that data on safety and quality should be collated, compared and provided back to hospitals, clinical units and clinicians in a timely fashion to expedite quality and quality improvement cycles. Hospitals should also be required to report on their strategies to improve safety and quality of care and actions taken in response to identified safety issues.

88: The Healthy Australia Accord would incorporate the following substantial structural reforms to the governance of the health system ... the Commonwealth, state and territory governments would agree to establish national approaches to ... patient safety and quality (including service accreditation).

110: To help embed a culture of continuous improvement, we recommend that a standard national curriculum for safety and quality is built into education and training programs as a requirement of course accreditation for all health professionals.

111. The Australian Commission for Safety and Quality in Health Care should be established as a permanent, independent national body. With a mission to measurably improve the safety and quality of healthcare, the Commission would be an authoritative knowledge-based organization responsible for:

Promoting a culture of safety and quality across the system:

- disseminating and promoting innovation, evidence and quality improvement tools;
- recommending national data sets with a focus on the measurement of safety and quality;

- identifying and recommending priorities for research and action;
- advocating for safety and quality; and
- providing advice to governments, bodies, clinicians and managers on "best practice" to drive quality improvement.

Analyzing and reporting on safety and quality across all health settings:

- reporting and public commentary on policies, progress and trends in relation to safety and quality;
- developing and conducting national patient experience surveys; and
- reporting on patient reported outcome measures.

Monitoring and assisting in regulation for safety and quality:

- recommending nationally agreed standards for safety and quality, including collection and analysis of data on compliance against these standards, the extent of such regulatory responsibilities requires further consideration of other compliance activities such as accreditation and registration processes.

112: To drive improvement and innovation across all areas of healthcare, we recommend that a nationally consistent approach is essential to the collection and comparative reporting of indicators which monitor the safety and quality of care delivery across all sectors. this process should incorporate:

- local systems of supportive feedback, including to clinicians, teams and organizations in primary health services and private and public hospitals; and
- incentive payments that reward safe and timely access, continuity of care (effective planning and communication between providers) and the quantum of improvement (compared to an evidence base, best practice target or measured outcome) to complement activity-based funding of all health services.

Following receipt of the Commission's report, the federal Government commenced an extensive consultation process led by Prime Minister Rudd, traversing the same territory as the Commission's consultations. The Government response adopted many Commission recommendations, ignored others, and changed one key recommendation in a significant way.

The Commission's recommendation for "substantial structural reform" to "establish national approaches" in a range of areas, including patient safety and quality, were largely accepted, leading to the creation of a plethora of new national bodies and a statutory basis for the Australian Commission on Safety and Quality in Health Care.

The Reform Commission identified a number of areas of new spending which were generally not picked up by the Government. The Commission proposed that this new spending could be funded by improved efficiency in public hospitals, through the national introduction of activity-based funding, building on the state of Victoria's 20 years' experience in this regard (Duckett 1995).

The Commission's proposal was that the Commonwealth Government's contribution to public hospital services should be 40 percent of the efficient cost of public hospital services, with the states continuing as the majority funder. The Rudd Government's response was to reverse this percentage, with the Commonwealth becoming the dominant funder and the increased cost to the Commonwealth to be funded by reducing the funds that flowed from the Commonwealth to the states from the national consumption tax, the Goods and Services Tax. (The Australian constitution provides that the states cannot levy excise taxes so this tax was collected by the Commonwealth and all proceeds flowed to the states). The Rudd proposal also required states to establish local governance arrangements for groups of hospitals (called "networks"). In parallel with these changes to hospitals, 61 new local organizations ("Medicare Locals") were established with very broad expectations about reforming local primary care arrangements.

Although only one state held out against this deal (Western Australia, where a newly-elected Liberal Government was in office), implementation was delayed as negotiations continued with Western Australia on the contentious issue of increased Commonwealth involvement in what as seen as a state area of responsibility (public hospitals). Shortly after this deal was announced, Rudd was replaced as Prime Minister by Julia Gillard. More importantly, Labor lost Government in the two larger states (New South Wales and Victoria), increasing the political foes arrayed against the deal.

Prime Minister Gillard renegotiated the funding deal so that the base hospital funding shares would remain unchanged, states would continue as the majority funder for the foreseeable future and were formally designated as the "system managers" for public hospitals, there would be no claw back from the Goods and Services Tax, but the Commonwealth would fund 45 percent of the cost of additional activity in public hospitals (at the efficient cost) from 2014, rising to 50 percent from 2017.

Reform Implementation: National Structures

The most obvious changes to the Australian health system have been structural. The then Liberal Opposition (now the Government) criticized many of these changes as creating a bureaucratic overlay and promised to review or abolish them.

The new national organizations include the National Health Performance Authority, charged with publishing comparative performance information on hospitals and regions. It has published a number of reports comparing hospital performance, including on safety performance, for example, levels of hospital acquired infection (National Health Performance Authority 2013). These reports compare hospitals against "peer groups," but stop short of explicitly identifying "good" or "bad" performers, despite its having the statutory authority to do so. The international literature on the effectiveness of information provision as a driver for change is quite mixed (Brien et al. 2010, Fung et al. 2008, Ryan, Nallamothu & Dimick 2012, Barker, Mengersen & Morton 2012, Gallagher & Krumholz 2011) and there is as yet no Australian study analyzing secular trends in the data being reported by the Performance Authority.

Another new national authority is the Independent Hospital Pricing Authority, charged with establishing the "National Efficient Price" for public hospital services. The Pricing Authority has so far not followed the United States, or other countries, in incorporating any safety-related aspects into price setting (Duckett 2012). This is possibly due to tension between the Pricing Authority, which is understood to be prepared to incorporate safety elements and the Australian Commission on Safety and Quality in Health Care, is unwilling to support the use of price signals.

As outlined above the antecedents of the Australian Commission on Safety and Quality in Health Care stretch back 20 years. As part of the reform initiatives it now has its own statutory foundation under legislation. It is not clear as yet whether this new found status will change its *modus operandi* or priorities.

Reform Implementation: Local Structures

The National Health Reform Agreement, the compact between the states and federal Government assigning rights and responsibilities for healthcare, described the changes as being designed to achieve "a nationally unified and *locally controlled* health system [emphasis added]" (Council of Australian Governments 2011, p. 4). The local element involved a commitment from the states to introduce local governance for "hospital networks." Most states (the notable exception being Victoria) had abolished local governance of hospitals in favor of direct accountability for regional areas or districts (similar to the England's NHS trusts and which incorporated multiple hospitals) to the state department of health. The chief executive officers of the areas and districts had performance accountability to the state Ministry of Health.

In a change not recommended by the Reform Commission, local boards of governance have been created for reshaped areas/districts with CEOs accountable to, and employed by, the boards. There is little research evidence as to the relative merits of quasi-autonomous boards compared to integrated management of hospital services (Ashton 1998), but this has not precluded periodic "restructuring" as a solution to problems with hospital systems (Dwyer 2004). The issue of center-periphery tension in organizations has long been recognized, as has the almost inevitable pendulum swings between local autonomy and centralization as the preferred form (Schön 1971), with the structural changes not necessarily leading to changes in values, norms, and ways of working (Mcfarlane 2011).

The structural changes brought no relief from ongoing financial pressures on hospitals and the new local boards of governance have not prioritized clinical governance in their processes (Bismark & Studdert 2013), nor do board members see the board as "an influential player" in determining quality.

The other change in local structures was the creation of 61 "Medicare Locals," independent organizations primarily funded by the Commonwealth Government charged with:

- improving the patient journey through developing integrated and coordinated services;

- providing support to clinicians and service providers to improve patient care;
- identification of the health needs of local areas and development of locally focused and responsive services;
- facilitation of the implementation and successful performance of primary healthcare initiatives and programs;
- being efficient and accountable with strong governance and effective management (Australian Government Department of Health and Ageing 2013).

These organizations replaced previous "Divisions of General Practice" which were dominated by GPs and aligned to their interests. The rhetoric surrounding Medicare Locals created expectations out of proportion to the funding allocated. They are expected to "coordinate" primary healthcare and improve the general practice–hospital interface, but were given no policy levers to induce either private medical practices or hospitals to change their ways. In healthcare, as in other domains, the ability to "coordinate" relies on acceptance and willingness of independent parties to change their behaviors. Coordination discourse is, in fact, a discourse of power:

> Coordination is one of the most fraudulent words of politics and administration.
> It dresses neutrally to disguise what nakedly is pure political form. Coordination
> is a political process by which the coordinated are made to change their value
> positions, their policy conceptions and their behavior to conform with the
> conceptions and expectations of the coordinator (Peres 1974, pp. 151–152).

Unfortunately, the Medicare Locals generally do not have the power to achieve the changes expected of them. The great expectations imposed on Medicare Locals were accompanied by challenges to their very existence. Even before all 61 Medicare Locals had been established, their legitimacy was questioned and they were derided as being overly bureaucratic, or at least spending funding on management which would be better allocated to "front-line" services. Twelve months out from the federal election, the then Opposition signaled it would abolish the nascent organizations, although it retreated from that as the election approached. In Government they have initiated a review of Medicare Locals.

Impact of Reforms

There are six generic levers that can be used to effect policy change: provision of new services, financial (taxes, incentives, setting up markets), regulatory and structural, information provision; rhetoric, and changing values and culture (usually by a combination of the previous five and through education) (Tuohy 1999, Hood & Margetts 2007).

The principal lever used in the Australian health reforms has been structural: new national and local organizations have been created. There have also been changes to the organizational form of the peak national quality and safety body and to public hospitals. Certainly these structural changes allow politicians to be seen to be doing something about the vexed and important issue of promoting safety and quality of care.

From 2014 the reforms will also involve financial levers, changing incentives on public hospitals through the roll out of activity-based funding for public hospital services. The pricing strategy currently does not incorporate any financial incentives to improve safety. Because the reforms mean that the Commonwealth Government will be directly exposed for the first time, to costs of increased hospital activity (previously increases in Commonwealth funding were linked to population growth), this will provide a long-term incentive on the Commonwealth to expand its investment in areas of its responsibility which might mitigate hospital activity growth such as prevention and primary care.

The creation of the National Health Performance Authority enshrines the use of information provision as a third lever for change. It is too early to assess the impact of the Performance Authority's reports.

From a safety and quality perspective, the reforms could be seen to be benign, faciliatory, and weak. The National Health and Hospitals Reform Commission identified information provision as a key national role, and this function is slowly coming to fruition. However, the Reform Commission saw information provision as stimulating local action, not public naming and shaming. The National Health Performance Authority, in contrast, was set up to report publicly on statistical performance, not on action about how hospitals are responding to identified safety issues (Duckett et al. 2008a). Policies based on public naming and shaming come from a very different paradigm than local policies of a "just and trusting culture," the dominant and best practice approach to identifying and addressing safety issues. It is unclear at this stage whether the Performance Authority's name and shame approach will have an impact either on local cultures or on improving overall safety of care.

A second key function proposed for the Safety and Quality Commission was "monitoring and assisting in regulation for safety and quality." Here, the Commission has developed and published ten "National Safety and Quality Health Service Standards" covering:

- Governance for Safety and Quality in Health Service Organisations
- Partnering with Consumers
- Preventing and Controlling Healthcare Associated Infections
- Medication Safety
- Patient Identification and Procedure Matching
- Clinical Handover
- Blood and Blood Products
- Preventing and Managing Pressure Injuries
- Recognising and Responding to Clinical Deterioration in Acute Health Care
- Preventing Falls and Harm from Falls.

Work on these standards was stimulated by the report which led to the creation of Commission (Paterson 2005) and commenced before the Commission's new statutory powers, so the real progress being made in this area cannot be attributed to the reform process.

Finally, the Reform Commission also saw a key role for the Safety and Quality Commission in "promoting a culture of safety and quality across the system." This function has not been a hallmark of the Safety and Quality Commission's activity to date, nor has the Safety and Quality Commission led a national effort to adopt evidence-based patient safety strategies (Shekelle et al. 2013).

There has been no "big bang" or national transformation to respond to safety and quality issues and no sense of urgency that the health system needs to be transformed to improve care delivery. Rather, the focus has been on new structures which have a weak and attenuated link to better outcomes. Hospitals and clinicians respond to incentives, be they financial, or reputational (Frølich et al. 2007). The new structures may lead to reputational incentives for better outcomes (naming and shaming data, results of standards reviews) but there is little evidence of this to date.

Because of this "slow and steady" approach, it is too early to tell whether the national reforms have helped or hindered progress on improving quality and safety of care in Australia.

This is not to say that there is no action occurring on improving quality and safety of care in Australia, it is just occurring outside any national framework. The scandals in public hospitals mentioned earlier stimulated state Governments to initiate a range of actions to improve safety and quality including strategies to change organizational culture (Crethar 2009), establishing new state organizations charged with improving safety and quality (Clinical Excellence Commission 2014), establishing state-based audits of surgical mortality (Retegan 2013, Azzam et al. 2013), and introducing pay-for-performance experiments (Duckett et al. 2008b). In addition, healthcare organizations have a range of quality and safety strategies in place, for example; hand hygiene, root cause analysis, critical incident reporting, and handover between shifts that are mandated or authorized by state health departments, accreditation processes, or international initiatives. These changes are evolving differently in each state, partly reflecting the different culture of each state, and the attitudes and priorities of state leadership. The state-based changes appear in some senses to be occurring in a parallel universe to the national reform agenda, neither influencing, nor influenced by, the national processes.

Lessons for Other Countries

Based on the limited evidence available, safety issues in Australia are similar to other countries in the developed world, particularly problems at the interface of systems (whether within, or between hospitals, or between primary care organizations and hospitals) and safety issues in hospitals. This account of progress in Australia in addressing these issues shows no "magic bullet" that should be immediately emulated. Rather, what the Australian experience shows is an attempt to develop national structures, somewhat peculiar to the Australian federal-state landscape, which provide a framework for safety (and quality) issues to be addressed systematically at a national level and to provide an organizational basis for improving primary care.

The likelihood of change will be impacted positively by organizational leadership, stability, resourcing (financial and in terms of human capital), and system acceptance of the legitimacy of the new organizations. Whether this new national superstructure and local structures will actually effect improvements in safety is still an emerging story.

Chapter 12

Indonesia

Sophia Hermawan and Brette Blakely

Abstract

In Indonesia, health reform initiatives related to quality and safety have been developed based upon: (1) The Health Law No. 36, 2009, (2) Vision of Ministry of Health (MOH) "Health Community with Self Motivated and Fairness" in 2010, (3) the 7 Health Development Reformation of the MOH, and (4) other related regulations. The biggest challenge in Indonesia is bedding down large-scale reform of the health system stimulated by the implementation of a National Social Insurance System (NSIS) since the beginning of 2014. This needs to be accomplished for a large population, comprising 244 million people. Meanwhile Indonesia is exposed to an epidemiological transition in which non-communicable diseases (NCDs) are increasingly becoming a considerable burden. One of the solutions for Indonesia's health problems has been the instigation of national reform initiatives to meet a health vision for quality and safety. A key feature of this is the implementing of new hospital and health center accreditation programs beginning in 2012. The intention is to integrate these reform measures with the NSIS from 2014. In this regard the MOH has implemented the NSIS, covering 63 percent of Indonesia's citizens as of 2011, with the aim of complete coverage by 2019.

Background

Indonesia is the largest archipelago country in the world, consisting of 17,466 islands, which combined have an area of 1,922,570 km^2. It lies geographically at a key strategic crossing between Asia and Australia, and between the Pacific and Indonesian Oceans. With a total population of around 244 million, Indonesia has a health expenditure of 1.8 percent of GDP, represented by public expenditure of 46.5 percent, which covers the 11.7 percent of the population who are very poor. Currently, Indonesia has an average life expectancy of 69.3 years, an obesity rate of 21.7 percent, and services its population with 2,228 hospitals (providing 0.6 beds per 1,000 people), 9,700 health centers which are staffed by approximately 0.3 doctors per 1,000 people, and approximately two nurses per 1,000 people. These are low by Organisation for Economic Cooperation and Development (OECD) standards.

Table 12.1   Demographic, economic, and health information for Indonesia

Population (thousands)	247,000
Area (sq. km)*	1,811,570
Proportion of population living in urban areas (2011)	51
Gross Domestic Product (GDP US$, billions)^	878.0
Total expenditure on health as % of GDP	3.0
Gross national income per capita (PPP intl $)	4,730
Per capita total expenditure on health (intl $)	150
Proportion of health expenditure which is private	60.4
General Government expenditure on health as a percentage of total expenditure on health	39.6
Out-of-pocket expenditure as a percentage of private expenditure on health	75.1
Life expectancy at birth m/f (yrs)	69/73
Probability of dying under five (per 1,000 live births)	31
Maternal Mortality Ratio (per 100,000 live births) (2013)	190
Proportion of population using improved water and sanitation	85/59

Source: Unless otherwise stated data are for the year 2012 and taken from the World Health Organization 2014. * Area from the World Bank 2014a. ^ GDP from the World Bank 2014b.

Note: PPP is purchasing power parity, intl $ is international dollar which has the same purchasing power as US$ in the US.

Hospitals are a mixture of private and public, with private facilities run by companies, individuals and some religious organizations (Shields & Hartati 2003). Typically, hospitals provide different levels of care at different price points with the richest patients sometimes seeking treatment overseas (Shields & Hartati 2003, Dewi et al. 2013). Some provisions have been in place for the poorest citizens to receive free basic care, notably the aid packages provided by the International Monetary Fund and World Bank through the *Jaring Pengaman Sosial bidang Kesehata* (JPSBK) scheme (Shields & Hartati 2003). During a period of decentralization combined with an increased focus on welfare in the early 2000s, many regions initiated free health insurance schemes (Aspinall 2014).

Nonetheless, due to the pay-per-service system, until recently, the largest source of funding for the health system was out-of-pocket payments. These payments represented almost half the expenditure on healthcare in Indonesia, demonstrating considerable inequities in terms of access (World Health Organization 2008). Government expenditure was low, representing only about 5 percent of an also remarkably low total expenditure per capita (only US$33 in 2004) (World Health Organization 2008).

Now, the Health Law No. 36, 2009 forms the basis of the Indonesian health system and mandates that all citizens have the right to a share of health resources, to access safe and quality healthcare, and are able to exercise levels of choice in their health treatment (Republic of Indonesia 2009a). Central to these changes was the vision of "Healthy Indonesia 2010" in 2004, which was upgraded to a "Health Community with Self Motivated and Fairness" vision in 2010. The target date for implementation of this new vision for Indonesian healthcare is 2014.

The MOH is responsible for the planning, regulation, development, and control of the operational health system in which fairness and affordability for the community is projected to be accomplished through the NSIS. In light of the data cited above in relation to health expenditure, this reform represents the most significant change to the Indonesian healthcare system in its history, and if it can be achieved, stands to increase equity and accessibility considerably. This should act to raise the standards of care and quality of services.

Controlling health system operations consists of managing human, infrastructure, and financial resources. This includes ensuring qualified health personnel are trained and available to the system, the ongoing credentialing and competency of health staff, the licensing of medical staff, oversight of ethical codes, adhering to policy requirements, reinforcing professional standards, defining standards of healthcare, determining standards of operational procedure, and allocating health staff as needed. All of these are under various strategies to induce continuous improvement of the health system.

Introduction

In 2011, the MOH launched a health development reform process based on seven principles, which consist of:

1. Revitalizing of health services.
2. Ensuring the availability, distribution, retention, and quality of human resources.
3. Promoting the availability, distribution, safety, quality, effectiveness of medicines, affordability, vaccines, and medical equipment.
4. Improving health insurance.
5. Focusing on remote areas for health problems.
6. Reforming the bureaucracy.
7. Providing world-class healthcare.

The national health system in Indonesia is based on the policy and national strategy set by Presidential Regulation No. 72, 2012. The Vision of the MOH is "Health Community with Self Motivated and Fairness." As well as promulgating this vision, Indonesia implemented a decentralization initiative which authorizes provincial and district Governments to manage health resources and services in their own areas, while following national regulations in line with the national health strategy implemented in 2008. In this system, provincial and district Governments are responsible for the output of their programs and must report the results of their programs against national indicators which demonstrate how they meet or correspond to the Indonesian health vision at a national policy level.

The Impact of Health Reform Efforts on Quality and Safety of Care

Indonesia in recent years has been focused on improving community healthcare through measures such as community empowerment, including the private sector and civil society. It is also keen to protect the public's health by ensuring the availability of health personnel, and providing comprehensive care through qualified healthcare providers as equitably as possible. This includes supporting the availability and equitable distribution of health resources and the implementation of an effective governance system. This is challenging given the size of the population and the unique geographic spread of the country.

The goals of health development 2014 include the improvement of healthcare across the community to meet the United Nation's Millennium Development Goals (MDGs). Key aims are to increase life expectancy to 72 years, decrease infant mortality rates to 24 per 1,000 live births, decrease maternal mortality rates to fewer than 118 per 100,000 live births, and decrease malnutrition prevalence in children (under five years) to less than 15 percent. These are lofty aims that, if achieved, would substantially improve the quality of life and safety of care delivered to patients and communities.

In terms of improvements to acute health services, Indonesia has implemented a quality improvement system through its hospital accreditation system, which since 1995 has been applied by a straightforward method, designed by a local independent body. At that time, Indonesia also commenced the implementation of accreditation for health centers. The basic law for hospital accreditation is stated in National Law Number 44, enacted in 2009 (Republic of Indonesia 2009b). As stipulated in this Law, all hospitals have to be accredited through the official Accreditation Body appointed by the MOH.

In accordance with Indonesia's health vision, in order to improve healthcare quality, health insurance has been mandated for all members of the community through the NSIS, including both poor and selected people who currently pay for an insurance scheme, and also civil servants. Indonesia has had health insurance arrangements since 1968, but since then the scheme has only involved parts of the community, and made a distinction between the Government and private sectors.

More recently, Indonesia has developed national reform initiatives aimed at securing its health vision for the quality and safety of healthcare by implementing hospital accreditation in line with international standards. This has been in place since 2012. The NSIS, beginning in 2014, aims to involve all the community in an integrated system.

The Current Situation

The strengths of Indonesia's health system are that it has organizational structures, levels of human resources (both managers and medical staff) in place, a new insurance system, and distributed providers in terms of health and medical facilities. However, like many countries, a major weakness is the spread of medical staff, with more in the capital and big cities than in the districts or villages. In addition, as is the case in developing countries, resources available for healthcare are limited especially when compared with OECD countries.

According to the 'Global Status Report on Noncommunicable Diseases 2010' from the World Health Organization (2011a), the greatest cause of death at any age globally is NCDs. In the last few years, Indonesia has begun to experience a double burden. Besides the long-standing problems of a high prevalence of communicable diseases in Indonesia, now, at the same time, there is the increasing burden of NCDs diseases such as stroke, hypertension, diabetes, cancer, and chronic obstructive pulmonary disease in some sections of the population. The high prevalence of NCDs are caused by accelerating changes in lifestyle which include poor choices in terms of smoking, eating an unbalanced diet, and lack of physical activity.

This situation needs to be addressed through the continuous execution of well-designed and implemented systems-level public education and health promotion strategies, and by securing resources and making available facilities and programs to address this changing disease profile. It has been estimated that such an undertaking would involve a total of 42,398 general medical practitioners, 38,095 specialist doctors, 13,114 dentists, 206,126 nurses, 136,917 midwives, 46,764 pharmacists, 125,609 other health workers, 194,272 non-medical personnel, and a total of 9,655 health centers and 2,228 hospitals (Ministry of Health Indonesia 2013).

Having a good hospital accreditation process can contribute to improving quality of care and enhancing patient safety (Greenfield & Braithwaite 2008, see also Braithwaite et al. 2012, Hinchcliff et al. 2013, and Shaw et al. 2013) but only 1,277 hospitals have accreditation to the local standards and 31 hospitals to the national standards set in 2012. Thus, not all hospitals have applied patient safety measures optimally through accreditation mechanisms, and there is room for increased take-up of accreditation and application of standards. One of the factors which should address this take-up and improve the quality of healthcare and patient safety is the MOH's directive that makes accreditation certification a requirement for hospitals. Thus, the obligation of having accreditation certification has not been implemented fully and consequently programs for patient safety in healthcare and hospitals are variable. To date, health facilities have been motivated to apply quality improvement and patient safety initiatives to the best of their abilities rather than according to national standards.

The most pressing challenge in Indonesia, however, is its large-scale reform of implementing the NSIS progressively from January 2014. If this can eventually run well, Indonesia will be the largest country to have implemented universal health coverage through a single payer (*The Economist* 2012). However, Indonesia's increasing exposure to the epidemiological transition in which NCDs are becoming a high burden, complicates the already challenging implementation of the NSIS. Management and therapy for NCDs take a long time and come at a high cost for relevant programs. This requires continuous efforts and innovation. Thus far however, the implementation of the NSIS is incomplete, and the health development budget is insufficient. Furthermore, the timeframe for implementation adds pressure to the system and its management. In 2011 the coverage of citizens by NSIS was around 63 percent and it is intended that this will be increased to 100 percent by 2019.

A key Indonesian challenge, not shared by every health system, is that its geographic area is very widespread. It is hard to reach peripheral regions, and there is reduced motivation for the health workforce to work in health facilities in remote areas. A related issue is that there is still a lack of training for those medical staff as there is a lack of expert trainers in these remote sectors.

Nevertheless, Indonesia has substantially upgraded its health profile in the last 20 years (World Health Organization 2008). Much of the improvement in health status has been attributed to Indonesia gaining control over key issues, namely communicable diseases and malnutrition in children. However, in the future, Indonesia is likely to face a variety of fresh challenges—not just the "lifestyle" challenges discussed earlier—including new emerging infectious diseases and re-emerging infectious diseases.

Indonesia has built some medical faculties, nurse schools, and midwife education programs to support the health system's development. The availability of pharmaceutical medicines and health equipment has sharply improved in the last ten years, but there remains work for Indonesia. One key is to tackle the disparity of access and poor distribution of resources between areas and social communities. For example, in 2014, in East Indonesia, there are shortages in capacity to handle NCD cases including the availability of specialist doctors.

The NSIS provides a case study example of how the Indonesian heath system's stakeholders can work collaboratively to achieve change. Establishment of the NSIS involved partnerships between Government officials, the army, the police, the private sector, professionals, businessmen, and various members of and groups representing the community (including the poorest). Quality improvement and patient safety initiatives have mainly involved the Indonesian Government, in particular the MOH, hospital managers, health centers, and health professionals. The management of NSIS is coordinated between the Government, the army, the police, and the private sector in order to reach comprehensive and general health services across whole provinces and communities. However, implementation of quality improvement and patient safety for hospitals and health centers is the responsibility of the Indonesian Commission on Accreditation of Hospitals, and local providers, with the Government only taking on a supporting role.

Current Reform Initiatives

The MOH has solved some key health problems by having a compelling vision for the future, with the aim that the system should be more focused on getting poor people quality healthcare and to increase adherence to new patient safety measures by implementing the NSIS and applying the new accreditation programs and standards. The continuity of this system will be supported by more medical staff placements in remote areas, thereby bolstering the participation of health facilities on the periphery, inducing greater levels of equity. More efforts are envisaged, including fellowships for high performance members of the health workforce or medical staff. Amongst other MOH aims, there is the intention to build more hospitals over a three year period, from 1,721 hospitals in 2012 to 2,293 hospitals by the end of 2014.

The Quality and Safety Landscape

As stated in the Health Law, the MOH is responsible for the improvement in this health system including planning, organizing, controlling, and evaluation of progress against milestones. The system involves wide-ranging and different stakeholder groups—Government, the army, the police, professionals, businessmen, and the private sector. All of them are working to support the NSIS in various ways and are participating in its management. Together, they have contributed support in the form of human resources in health services, participation as members, training in the NSIS, and are involved in studies comparing health facilities in its adoption. However, there is much work to do and the system faces many challenges.

In the pursuit of the goal to support "Quality Health Improvement and Patient Safety" measures, Indonesia has undertaken considerable work in implementing its national hospital accreditation system, dating from 2012. For the most part, the accreditation program has adopted indicators which are in line with international experience. This will serve to stimulate the raising of overall standards across Indonesian healthcare in line with best practice. Time will tell in a resource-constrained system like Indonesia's, whether, and the extent to which, this aim can be achieved.

As an initial target, the MOH has indicated that at least five Government hospitals will be accredited to international standards between 2009 and 2014 as a part of the reforms launched as "Strategic Planning, Ministry of Health in 2009—2014." Allied to this initiative is the NSIS, eventually covering all citizens of Indonesia later this decade.

NSIS is managed by a social implementation body, whose purpose is to protect the whole of the community through an insurance system whose aim is to ensure the provision of safe, credentialed, and appropriate health services. There are multiple principles on which the NSIS rests. These include that it is non-profit, and based on cooperation, openness, accountability, efficiency, and effectiveness. There are provisions for member budgeting management, mandatory membership, and portability. NSIS covers promotion, prevention, treatment, and rehabilitation, including medication and medical materials.

Although the health insurance system has been in effect now for several years, its management has been under the private sector only since the beginning of 2014. Now, with the application of the NSIS, there is the opportunity to provide an integrated system accessible to the whole community.

Synergistically with measures of quality improvement, patient safety and the NSIS, Indonesia has designed standards of accreditation for hospitals and health centers which include standards of medical care for every collegium (group of specialist doctors), standards of patient safety, standards for the NSIS (including the unit cost), and supportive standards such as those stipulated for emergency care, health technology assessment, an occupational standard, medical management utilization, and related standards.

The Impact of These Reform Efforts on Quality and Safety of Care

It is hard to measure the impact of these reform initiatives. Most of them are currently being implemented, and it is well known that it is difficult to evaluate actual impact when programs are still being rolled out. One of the reform initiatives explicitly aimed at improving quality and safety is accreditation according to international standards being applied in ten participating hospitals (three Government and seven private hospitals). It means that these facilities have applied quality improvement measures and patient safety strategies optimally, at least in theory.

Implementation: Barriers and Solutions

There are generic barriers facing all health systems intent on improving the quality of care provided, and strengthening delivery systems, not only Indonesia. These include limits to resources, the difficulty in keeping up to date, procuring the most recent technologies, and training staff for existing, and new, techniques and tasks. Some of the key implementation concerns in Indonesia's case involve the complicated process of starting the NSIS within a system which is decentralized (Hort, Djasri & Utarini 2013). The cost system in NSIS also seems rather complicated, so it could be confusing to decide the appropriate therapy and the unit cost of cases.

There are several positive indicators which suggest the system is moving in the right direction. The most successful drivers of improvement in the quality and safety of care in acute settings are hospital accreditation with international-level standards. However, not every hospital and senior staff group have demonstrated that they are engaged in the new system of accreditation and the other reform measures. Reform will take time and concerted efforts. There do seem to be signs of positive competition between hospitals stimulated by them marketing themselves to clients, which creates pressure on them to demonstrate that they provide the best healthcare quality possible, given available resources. So inevitably Indonesia's implementation model involves mixed strategies including inducing competition and cooperation between providers.

Prospects for Success and Next Steps

Indonesia has designed a very comprehensive NSIS and, importantly, created a supportive regulatory environment which involves multiple players across the sectors of the health system. This sets a promising tone against which the implementation of regulation, accreditation, and appropriate budgeting can be achieved, especially as required to support the poorer people in Indonesian society to secure health services free of charge at the point of delivery in appropriate hospitals and health centers. This represents major advances from the past. Moreover, accreditation and the implementation of associated patient safety indicators along with improved medical care under NSIS can act to support hospitals' and health centers' quality of care. The systems need to support these measures so they are as successful as possible. This means the development of a comprehensive socialization process involving training for hospital accreditation and implementation of the NSIS. Such reform initiatives will, if done well, support the system's improvement and enhance implementation measures in the future, stimulated by agreed plans with well-articulated projected timeframes and milestone targets. The MOH plans for the health system to achieve the reforms and improvement measures over the next five years, by 2019.

Conclusion

Efforts to secure health reforms and make improvements in quality of care and the safety of patients have been very important for the Indonesian MOH and other stakeholders in the last three years, perhaps especially in supporting the implementation of quality improvement through the new hospital accreditation program dating from 2012, and initial health center accreditation and the initiation of NSIS from 2014. The stage is being set for more health systems strengthening and associated improvements. Evaluation of these initiatives will be an important future step.

Chapter 13

New Zealand

Jackie Cumming

Abstract

Since 1990, the New Zealand health system has been reorganized several times, with an emphasis on improving access to services, equity of access and funding, and the overall cost-effectiveness of the system. Although major organizational reforms in the 1990s proved controversial, not achieving their desired outcomes and being overturned in 2000, they left important legacies. Organizational arrangements established in the 2000s remain in place today, such that in the 2010s the emphasis is on more collaborative working arrangements. A lack of research evidence makes it difficult to assess the impact of recent changes, however, and significant challenges lie ahead in better linking publicly and privately owned parts of the system, if the performance of the system is to be improved further.

Introduction

The key financing and organizational arrangements in the New Zealand health system go back to the late 1930s, when the New Zealand Government (1) introduced universal public funding to provide free hospital care, delivered by locally run hospitals and (2) provided partial funding for primary health care (PHC) services, delivered by a range of health professionals in private practice (Cumming et al. 2013). Since then, financing arrangements have not changed significantly, but the organizational arrangements in the health system have been reformed a number of times.

In this chapter, major reforms to the New Zealand health system since 1990 are discussed and analyzed, with a view to understanding the relationship between national reform initiatives and the quality and safety of healthcare. The focus is on system-level reforms aimed at improving the overall performance of the whole health system or key parts of the health system. The starting point for this discussion is in 1990 as, in that year, major reforms were introduced into the New Zealand health system, and, although key aspects of those reforms have been overturned, the system today continues to build on the remaining aspects of those reforms. The chapter focuses on how reforms have aimed to improve equity (of access, use, and funding), cost-effectiveness (at the system level), access, responsiveness, patient-centeredness, and safety.

Table 13.1   Demographic, economic, and health information for New Zealand

Population (thousands)	4,460
Area (sq. km)*	263,310
Proportion of population living in urban areas (2011)	86
Gross Domestic Product (GDP US$, billions)^	171.3
Total expenditure on health as % of GDP	10.3
Gross national income per capita (PPP intl $)	30,030
Per capita total expenditure on health (intl $)	3,292
Proportion of health expenditure which is private	17.3
General Government expenditure on health as a percentage of total expenditure on health	82.7
Out-of-pocket expenditure as a percentage of private expenditure on health	63.2
Life expectancy at birth m/f (yrs)	80/84
Probability of dying under five (per 1,000 live births)	6
Maternal Mortality Ratio (per 100,000 live births) (2013)	8
Proportion of population using improved water and sanitation	100/

Source: Unless otherwise stated data are for the year 2012 and taken from the World Health Organization 2014. * Area from the World Bank 2014a. ^ GDP from the World Bank 2014b.

Note: PPP is purchasing power parity, intl $ is international dollar which has the same purchasing power as US$ in the US.

The chapter firstly provides an overview of the New Zealand health system, before moving on to discuss health reforms prior to the 2000s and the current situation with respect to reforms. The chapter then discusses the strengths, weaknesses, and achievements of the current healthcare quality and safety landscape, and the prospects for future reforms. Table 13.2 summarizes the key reforms covered in this chapter; it identifies the explicit objectives of each reform and indicates successes (Ö) and failures (X), as discussed in the sections that follow.

Overview of the New Zealand Health System

New Zealand's health system is predominantly publicly financed, with Government financing currently making up 83 percent of expenditure (Ministry of Health New Zealand 2012). In recent years, expenditure on healthcare has sat just above the level expected in international comparisons given New Zealand's income (Ministry of Health New Zealand 2012), with public and total health expenditure

Table 13.2   New Zealand health reforms and summary of achievements

Goals / Reforms	Equity	Cost-effectiveness	Access	Responsiveness	Patient-centeredness	Safety
Purchaser–Provider Split 1990s		√ √ Some savings in PHC √ Some productivity improvements in hospitals X High implementation and transaction costs	√ (through improved efficiency, resulting in the freeing up of resources to reduce waiting lists and improve access) X No improvements in waiting lists	√ (for consumers) √ Māori- and Pacific-led providers X Reforms highly unpopular		
District Health Boards (DHBs) 2000s on		√ ? Reduced transaction costs compared with previous reforms X/√ Some evidence of a slow down in productivity gains, later reversed X Concerns over too many DHBs X Concerns over DHBs privileging own services		√ (to local communities) √ Stronger local focus		
Primary Health Care Strategy	√ √ Equity in funding improved ? Not always clear how changes would improve equity in health	√ √ Some evidence of reduced hospitalizations ? Better integration of services slow to being achieved	√ √ Reductions in user fees, unmet need and increases in consultation rates	√ ?	√ ?	
Targets and Financial Incentives	√ √ Improvements in rates of service use for high needs groups		√ √ Improvements in access to key services			
Elective Services Strategy 2000 on	√ √ Some evidence suggests improvements in equity of use of services	√ √ Likely given tools prioritize patients more likely to benefit	√ √ Faster access for those prioritized X Lack of information/transparency for those not prioritized			
Ministerial Advisory Group Reforms		√ (through reduced back room costs) √ Some evidence of savings	√ (services closer to home) ?	√ ? √	√ ? √	
Health Quality and Safety Commission (HQSC) (Too early to assess many achievements)	√	√				√ √ Some evidence of improvements in safety
Alliances (Too early to assess many achievements)		√	√		√	

Notes: A √ in the first row of each box shows that the reforms had the relevant goal as a key stated goal of these reforms. Subsequent √ show successes; X shows failures; ? where there is a lack of research findings.

growing faster than gross domestic product (Ministry of Health New Zealand 2012). Overall, New Zealanders have high levels of health, and the health system is generally seen as reasonably high performing, generating good levels of health relative to expenditure (Organisation for Economic Cooperation and Development 2013a). There are, however, significant inequalities, with Māori (the indigenous people of New Zealand), Pacific peoples, and those on lower incomes, having lower levels of overall health (Ministry of Health New Zealand 2013a).

New Zealand's health system covers a wide range of services, including public health, preventive, PHC, maternity, mental health, disability support, youth dental health, hospital emergency, medical and surgical, and associated community services, as well as older people's services (including home care, residential, rest home, or hospital care). Generally, adult dental health, optometry, and counseling services are the responsibility of individuals, although some social security payments are available to fund these services for lower-income New Zealanders.

A parallel "no fault" social insurance system (called ACC) sits alongside the main health system, funding services for those with injuries arising from accidents, and accounting for about 8.4 percent of expenditure (Ministry of Health New Zealand 2012). ACC-funded services are delivered by the same providers as other health services. All New Zealanders are able to purchase private health insurance, which covers PHC user charges, faster access to covered services, and a higher standard of accommodation. A third of New Zealanders are now thought to be covered (Health Fund Association of New Zealand 2013), but such insurance accounts for a very low proportion (4.9 percent) of total health expenditure (Ministry of Health New Zealand 2012).

New Zealand Governments have continually sought to get the best value-for-money from the health system, given the substantial proportion of Government expenditure spent on healthcare (21 percent of core crown expenses in 2013/14) (The Treasury 2013). Thus, many reforms have focused on dealing with the following key issues:

- New Zealanders facing difficulties in accessing PHC services, given, *inter alia*, high user charges;
- fragmented service delivery, arising from the wide range of providers delivering services to individuals/families/whānau (extended family);
- long waiting times for elective procedures;
- perceived poor performance from key agencies and perceived high overall "system" or "back-room" costs;
- perceived poor resource allocations (for example, insufficient preventive and PHC services) and decision making (for example, insufficient attention to good priority setting) resulting in poor overall value-for-money.

New Zealand's focus on these issues currently sits within a context of increasing pressures from an ageing population and growth in the numbers of people with long-term conditions, new technologies, rising expectations from consumers, and a desire to reduce unmet need and narrow inequalities in health. The recent global economic slow-down has also influenced recent reforms, although New Zealand did not suffer as much as other countries, and growth in health expenditures has now slowed down significantly (Ministry of Health New Zealand 2012).

Health Reforms Pre-2000s

Following on from the establishment of a publicly funded system in the late 1930s, early reforms focused on reducing the numbers of hospitals—to provide better value-for-money and limit unnecessary use of new technologies. Thus, during the 1980s, 14 Area Health Boards (AHBs) were established as geographically-based planning and funding bodies to encourage a focus on the health of the population as a whole and on preventive care (Cumming et al. 2013). AHBs were assigned responsibility to plan services, promote public health, and deliver hospital and related community services. Although there was a desire to integrate PHC funding into the responsibilities of AHBs, this never occurred (Cumming 2011).

Major health system reforms in the 1990s integrated all health and disability services funding into a single pool and established a "purchaser–provider split." Four geographically based purchasing authorities (Regional Health Authorities or RHAs) became responsible for the planning and purchasing/contracting of all services, and stand-alone providers (including publicly-owned hospitals) competed to win contracts to deliver services. Publicly-owned hospitals were expected to make a surplus. These reforms overturned 50 years of local governance of hospital services and hence were a major departure for the New Zealand health system.

The reforms were expensive to implement—with estimates from NZ$85 million to NZ$348 million and up to NZ$800 million (Gauld 2009)—and were criticized for their high transaction costs and focus on competition at the expense of collaboration (Ashton, Cumming & Mclean 2004); collaboration being seen to be of importance in a country with a small and geographically dispersed population. These reforms were highly unpopular with those working in the health sector and the general public, resulting in an amalgamation of the four purchasing authorities into a single, national purchasing authority, a renewed emphasis on collaboration, and removal of requirements for hospitals to make a surplus, in 1998. The model was disestablished in 2000.

These unpopular reforms did, however, leave a number of important legacies. The first was a strong emphasis on more explicit priority setting, through the establishment of the Pharmaceutical Management Agency (PHARMAC) to prioritize and manage community medicines expenditure and a National Health Committee (NHC) to consider national health and disability priorities. PHARMAC continues its work today (Cumming, Mays & Daubé 2010), having saved the health system just over NZ$1 billion to June 2006 (Pharmaceutical Management Agency 2006), and reporting savings of NZ$3.8 billion between 2002 and 2013 (Pharmaceutical Management Agency 2013). PHARMAC now has an expanded mandate including hospital medicines and devices. The NHC's work led to the implementation of a politically highly successful model for managing elective surgery (Cumming 2013), which also continues to this day. The NHC has recently had its terms of reference revised to again focus on improved priority setting (National Health Committee 2014).

The second key legacy was the voluntary establishment of meso-level PHC organizations, Independent Practitioner Associations or IPAs, by general practitioners (GPs). IPAs were the lead agencies contracting with purchasing authorities on behalf of GPs, and focused on developing and improving the quality of PHC services (Barnett 2001). It was these organizations that enabled the development of universal Primary Health Organizations (PHOs) in the 2000s (see below).

The third key legacy was the establishment and funding of many Māori and Pacific-led providers, particularly in PHC and public health service delivery, to better meet the needs of these communities (Crengle 1999, Tukuitonga 1999). These organizations continue today, playing an important role in service delivery in New Zealand.

The Current Situation

In 2000, 21 (now 20) District Health Boards (DHBs) were established, re-integrating purchasing and provision of hospital services. DHBs are responsible for planning services, delivering hospital and related community services themselves, and purchasing PHC and a range of community services from private providers. This model has been widely supported by those working in it for its local focus, but research has noted concerns over: the numbers of DHBs, resulting in duplication in functions as well as capability gaps where skills are in short supply; DHBs potentially privileging their own services rather than seeking to achieve the most cost-effective service delivery; and the more limited incentives DHBs have faced to improve hospital productivity compared to the purchaser–provider split model of the 1990s (Mays, Cumming & Tenbensel 2007).

A Primary Health Care Strategy (PHCS) was released in 2001 (King 2001). This involved: the establishment of universal, not-for-profit, meso-level PHC organizations, known as PHOs to lead and develop PHC services; formal enrolment of New Zealanders with a PHO via their usual general practice; significant new funding to reduce user charges and enhance and expand PHC services; and a change from funding GP services on a fee-for-service basis to capitation funding paid to PHOs (Cumming & Mays 2011). Within a few years, over 80 PHOs were established, user fees had reduced, reported unmet need had also reduced, and the use of PHC services had increased (Cumming & Mays 2011, Cumming, Mays & Gribben 2008, Ministry of Health New Zealand 2008a). New ways of managing user fees were also introduced, including through fees reviews processes where fee increases are seen to be too high, and through the establishment of very low-cost funding arrangements, where PHOs and practices that keep fees low (that is, below set limits) are funded at a higher capitation rate.

In spite of these positive achievements, evaluations and assessments of the PHC reforms concluded that there was a lack of clarity around the respective roles of DHBs and PHOs (Barnett, Smith & Cumming 2009); and that little had been achieved in changing the ways in which PHC services were delivered (Smith 2009). Political concerns were also expressed over a continued lack of integration of PHC services horizontally, and PHC and hospital services vertically, making services for consumers fragmented and resulting in higher than necessary costs, including unnecessary admissions to hospital (Ryall 2007).

As a result, in the last five years, PHOs have been encouraged to amalgamate (down to 36 at present), and there is a significant focus on further integrating services (Ryall 2007, DHB Shared Services 2013a), including through Integrated Family Health Centres (Ryall 2007). The latest (2013/14) developments require DHBs and PHOs to work more closely together on annual plans with clear roles and accountabilities (DHB Shared Services 2013a), and the establishment of Alliance Leadership Teams (ALTs) involving DHBs and their service providers to jointly take "whole-of-system" (DHB Shared Services 2013b) "best-for-patient, best-for-system" (DHB Shared Services 2013c) decisions.

During this time, the Government also further developed its elective services strategy to improve access to elective services. The strategy includes a formal prioritization process to determine which consumers get access, based on the consumer's ability to benefit and a DHB's ability to have the services delivered within set timeframes (Cumming 2013), now ten months in total from referral to treatment (Ministry of Health New Zealand 2013b). Punitive financial incentives are used to ensure more services are delivered and are delivered in a timely way (Cumming 2013). This has led to a highly managed electives process, and has largely removed waiting lists from the political agenda. However, there is limited transparency within the process, with no information available about how many people are turned away by DHBs at the referral stage (Cumming 2013). Associations of private health insurers and private hospitals have estimated that 170,000 people have been told they require surgery but cannot get into the electives process, about half as many people as are treated each year (TNS New Zealand 2013).

An explicit set of targets for DHBs (Ministry of Health New Zealand 2008b) and a PHO performance program with targets and financial incentives for PHOs have also been implemented in recent years (DHB Shared Services Agency 2014, District Health Boards New Zealand 2009). The PHO performance program includes some indicators that focus on higher levels of service use for higher needs populations. Performance in relation to many of the key targets has improved over recent years (Ministry of Health New Zealand 2013a).

In 2009, a Ministerial Review Group (MRG) reported on key challenges faced by the New Zealand health system and made a number of recommendations, focusing on how to slow down the rate of health expenditure growth. Its key recommendations centered on new models of care, a more seamless patient journey and care delivered "closer to home," stronger clinical and management partnerships, a sharper focus on patient safety and quality of care, a more measured and nationally uniform approach to the introduction of new technology and procedures, improving structures and processes for workforce, capital, and IT planning and funding, shifting resources to front-line services and reducing the cost and duplication of "back-office" functions, and improving hospital productivity (Ministerial Review Group 2009). The resulting changes are set out below.

In 2010, as a result of the MRG report, the Government established a national Health Quality and Safety Commission (HQSC), an independent agency that reports directly to the Minister of Health, set up in response "to concern that only modest improvements in health quality and safety had been achieved at a national level over previous years" (Health Quality and Safety Commission New Zealand 2013a). The Commission's aim is to ensure all New Zealanders receive the best health and disability care within available resources, and it is also working to achieve the New Zealand Triple Aim: specifically, improved quality, safety and experience of care, improved health and equity for all populations, and better value for public health system resources (Health Quality and Safety Commission New Zealand 2013a). Key activities include:

- initiatives to better measure and understand trends in key quality and safety markers and indicators, including an atlas of healthcare variation, mortality review committees, and serious and sentinel events reporting;
- the development of quality accounts, by which providers can assess their performance and achievements in quality of care;
- a focus on four priority areas—reducing: falls and harm from falls in care settings; healthcare associated infections; perioperative harm (that is, improving surgical safety); and medication errors;
- a national patient safety campaign (*"Open for better care"*);
- building capability in quality improvement across the country; and
- developing consumer and family/whānau engagement and partnership, with particular attention to health literacy, increased consumer participation and the development of leadership capability for providers and consumers (Health Quality and Safety Commission New Zealand 2013a).

The Commission has a focus on measuring key outcomes, and early reports do suggest there have been improvements in many key measures of safety over the past few years (Health Quality and Safety Commission New Zealand 2013b). The extent to which the Commission's work is responsible for these changes requires further teasing out, especially given that a large number of organizations are directly responsible for implementing changes to improve patient safety.

Discussion

The Quality and Safety Landscape

As a result of various reforms, the New Zealand health system currently consists of a number of key organizations, each with some responsibility for the quality and safety of health services:

- The Minister of Health (and Associate Ministers).
- A national MOH, responsible for policy, funding, regulation, and monitoring performance, as well as the purchasing of some services (for example, services for people with disabilities aged under 65, some national public health services, and midwifery services). A NHB sits within the MOH and works with DHBs, and encompasses a Health Workforce Advisory Committee and a National Health IT Board to streamline workforce and IT planning. A re-configured NHC directly advises Ministers on priorities using cost-effectiveness principles.
- Twenty DHBs—these are geographically-based, funded on a weighted capitation basis, and governed by a mix of central Government appointed and locally elected Board members. DHBs are responsible for the planning and funding of most health services in their districts, and deliver a wide range of hospital and related community (for example, district nursing, mental health) services themselves.
- Thirty-six PHOs—these are funded on a weighted capitation basis to manage and provide PHC services to their enrolled populations, contracting with general practices and other providers to deliver "first contact" services.
- A wide range of privately-owned providers delivering services, including general practices, generally owned by GPs and staffed with practice nurses and, at times, other allied health professionals: pharmacists, physiotherapists, diagnostic laboratories, midwives, nurse practitioners, and rest homes. A large number of not-for-profit providers (including Māori- and Pacific-led organizations) also deliver services such as rest home care, public health services, and mental health services.
- A wide range of advisory and regulatory bodies, including MedSafe (regulating the safety of medicines), PHARMAC (deciding which medicines and devices should be publicly funded and negotiating contracts with suppliers), the Health and Disability Commissioner (dealing with consumer complaints), a national procurement body (Health Benefits Limited) and a newly established HQSC.

Effectiveness of Reforms, Barriers and Enablers, Prospects for Success, and Next Steps

In assessing the impact of national reforms on health quality and safety in New Zealand, this chapter has begun with major reforms established in the 1990s, given that current initiatives are building on both the successes and failures of reforms back to this time. Thus, the most spectacular failure for health reforms was the 1990s reorganization, designed to bring a more "market" approach to the health system to drive improved overall cost-effectiveness. But as noted above, these reforms did leave important legacies, and this suggests reforms to a health system can make a long-term difference, even if the overall reforms themselves do not survive. Although PHARMAC and the NHC could have developed independently of the reforms, it seems unlikely that the IPAs and new Māori- and Pacific-led providers would have developed to the extent they did had the 1990s reforms not occurred. Overall, however, these reforms were costly both financially (as reported above) and politically, and it is the experiences with these reforms that have arguably resulted in few concomitant organizational reforms in recent years.

As a result, the organizational arrangements introduced in 2000 remain in place for now. This is even though there are views that there are too many DHBs for such a small country, that DHBs are too hospital-focused, and that more cost-effective service delivery requires DHBs to allocate resources not always to the DHB. Rather than reforming DHBs—perhaps through amalgamations, which are likely to be unpopular with local communities—the focus has been on getting DHBs to work together to plan and deliver services efficiently. Unfortunately, a lack of good research evidence makes it difficult to assess successes and failures with this approach.

Many of the changes brought about by the PHCS also remain in place today, and although some still view PHOs as an unnecessary layer of bureaucracy, many also see value in having high-performing organizations at this level working to improve PHC services. Early evidence suggested that not all PHOs were playing a key role and showed that change in service delivery had been slow. Recent reforms have reduced the numbers of PHOs and further encouraged change in service delivery—but again there is a lack of good research evidence on how successful these changes have been. A key recent goal has been better integration of services, and although there are frequent reports of the development of integrated family health centers (for example, Ryall & Te Heuheu 2010, Ryall 2013), there is no published information on the forms of integration occurring (Cumming 2011) and the impact, including from a consumer perspective. Again, however, there is anecdotal evidence that change is slow (Topham-Kindley 2013).

However, the more challenging and long-standing issues are in changing service delivery, where there is a particular desire to better integrate services, both horizontally within PHC services and vertically between PHC and hospital services, but where change appears to have been very slow. The reasons for this are not entirely clear, but may arise from a lack of clarity about the overall direction the system is going in and what the future might look like: overall financial pressures, multiple priorities, DHBs that continue to largely focus on their own services, few requirements for planning and reporting and few financial incentives to achieve such changes, the need for cooperation from a large number of both service delivery and professional organizations, each with their own decision-making processes and governing Board, the existence of user charges in the PHC sector alongside free care for hospital services making changes in delivery locations complex, differences in the contracts for hospital and PHC staff, and the key role that privately owned organizations need to play while they also manage their businesses as well as delivery publicly-funded services.

The Government has recently clarified planning and reporting processes (for example, with clearer roles for PHOs set out in DHB annual plans) and has sought the formal establishment of ALTs as a means of encouraging joint decision making to overcome some of these barriers. The Government is also currently working on developing a system-level performance framework to track the overall performance of the health system (Integrated Performance and Incentive Framework Expert Advisory Group 2013).

If the Government is to succeed with its further development of PHC services, however, then it must deal with one overriding issue: how to ensure there is good access to PHC services while user charges remain largely under the control of private businesses. No significant new funding has been provided to reduce user fees for all New Zealanders since 2007 and user fees are likely to have risen substantially, potentially back to the levels seen prior to the introduction of the PHCS. Evidence on changes in fees over time is lacking; however, a study using 2007 data found fees for children and young people aged 6–17 to be around NZ$12 (Raymont, Cumming & Gribben in press), while the *New Zealand Herald* recently reported fees for this group averaging NZ$22 in 2013, with some fees as high as NZ$40 and NZ$50 per visit (Johnston 2013).

There are also concerns over the viability of some general practices, particularly those working with more disadvantaged communities, which do prioritize ensuring access over user fees (practice income) (Brown & Underwood 2013). With a significant emphasis on enhancing the role of PHC in order to provide better care and keep people out of hospital, a long-term solution to this problem needs to be found.

Finally, concerns over a lack of focus on health quality and safety have led to the recent establishment of an independent agency, the HQSC, to drive culture change across the system, as set out above. The Commission is working collaboratively with a wide range of agencies at all levels of the system to improve quality and safety, although a current focus is working with DHBs, given their significant role within the system, with a particular emphasis on patient safety. Recent reports show some recent gains in key patient safety indicators (Health Quality and Safety Commission New Zealand 2013b) and a high-level evaluation of the Commission's work is underway.

Conclusion

Major reforms to the New Zealand health system in earlier years did not always succeed in achieving their overall goals, although they did leave important legacies. Reforms undertaken during the 2000s have had more longevity and successes. The focus now is on further developing the organizations established in the early 2000s, and encouraging them to increasingly make joint decisions in the best interests of both patients and the health system, but a lack of evaluation and research makes it difficult to be sure that current changes are achieving their goals.

Chapter 14

Papua New Guinea

William Adu-Krow and Paulinus Lingani Ncube Sikosana

Abstract

The Organic Law on Provincial Government and Local Level Government (OLPG and LLG) (1977) is the legal framework for decentralization of health in Papua New Guinea (PNG). The objective of the law was to improve service delivery and increase citizen participation. It also transferred public servants from national agencies and provincial Governments to districts. Subsequent reforms have been influenced by this law. Whereas in the majority of cases, the reforms and previous national health plans were not specifically designed to explicitly influence the quality of healthcare, the current National Health Plan has achieving "Quality" as part of its values. In June 2011, the National Department of Health (NDoH) launched the National Health Services Standards (NHSS) for PNG as "a blue print for providing safe, quality health services."

Background

The population of PNG (7,275,324) is considered one of the most geographically and linguistically diverse in the world—with a tendency to identify first with one's own cultural milieu leading to favoritism or nepotism, otherwise called "wantokism" (derived from "one talk" or "same language") locally. PNG is made up of 22 provinces, in four regions, with 87 percent being rural and only 10 percent serviced by roads. It has hovered between 148th and 153rd out of 187 countries on the Human Development Index from 2009 to 2011. Security has been a major concern and this has attracted the attention of both Government and development partners.

The enactment of the OLPG in 1977 (soon after independence in 1975) and its subsequent overhaul in 1995 into the OLPG and LLG brought about significant changes to power structures, roles, and responsibilities of Government at all levels. Since then, the major health reform initiatives have been largely driven by a need to either align with the Organic Law or to mitigate perceived untoward effects of decentralization. A review of the implementation of the OLPG and LLG on service delivery arrangements indicates that the delivery of basic services such as health and education "… have deteriorated and that the current system is not functioning well" (Constitutional and Law Reform Commission of Papua New Guinea 2009,

Table 14.1   Demographic, economic, and health information for Papua New Guinea

Population (thousands)	7,167
Area (sq. km)*	452,860
Proportion of population living in urban areas (2011)	12
Gross Domestic Product (GDP US$, billions)^	15.6
Total expenditure on health as % of GDP	5.2
Gross national income per capita (PPP intl $)	2,740
Per capita total expenditure on health (intl $)	151
Proportion of health expenditure which is private	17.0
General Givernment expenditure on health as a percentage of total expenditure on health	83.1
Out-of-pocket expenditure as a percentage of private expenditure on health	55.9
Life expectancy at birth m/f (yrs)	60/65
Probability of dying under five (per 1,000 live births)	63
Maternal Mortality Ratio (per 100,000 live births) (2013)	220
Proportion of population using improved water and sanitation	40/19

Source: Unless otherwise stated data are for the year 2012 and taken from the World Health Organization 2014. * Area from the World Bank 2014a. ^ GDP from the World Bank 2014b.

Note: PPP is purchasing power parity, intl $ is international dollar which has the same purchasing power as US$ in the US.

p. iv). According to many critics of the Organic Law, it has resulted in a disconnect between policy formulation at the national level and policy implementation at the sub-national level. Kase and Thomason (2009) suggest that the Organic Law has made it difficult for the NDoH to fulfill its stewardship, oversight, and regulatory role for the sector.

The country is not likely to meet most of the Millennium Development Goals (MDGs), even though there have been some gains made in various areas as in Table 14.2.

Structural health reform initiatives include the enactment of the Public Hospitals Act (1994) which transferred the management of public hospitals from provincial Governments to NDoH. The management and funding of rural health services however remained with the provincial Governments. The National Health Administration Act (1997) defined the stewardship role of NDoH in a decentralized system of service delivery.

Papua New Guinea developed a Health Reform Project (2008–2010) in line with the Government-wide Strategic Plan for Public Sector Reforms (2008–2009).

Table 14.2   Table comparing some global and PNG health indicators

	Global	PNG
<five mortality per 1,000 live births	60	63
% DPT3 immunization (% coverage among one year olds) (2012)	81	63
Maternal mortality per 100,000 live births (2013)	260	220
Skilled birth attendants (% of birth) (2012)	66	44
Contraceptive prevalence (% married women 15–45) (2012)	62	32.4
Adult HIV/AIDS prevalence (%) (2012)	0.8	0.5
Malaria mortality per 100,000 population	17	36.4
TB treatment (success rate %) (2012)	86	68
Use of improved drinking water sources (%) (2011)	87	40.2
Use of improved sanitation facilities (%) (2011)	60	18.7

Sources: National Statistical Office 2011, National Department of Health 2013, World Health Organization 2013b.

The health sector reform agenda continues to date and forms part of NDoH's successive Corporate Plans (2009–2013 and 2013–2015). The reform elements include the restructuring of NDoH, integrating the management of hospital and rural health services under one authority called the Provincial Health Authority (PHA), alternative healthcare financing options, strengthening health partnerships, and the introduction of NHSS.

In the larger scheme of things, in 2009 the Government of PNG (GoPNG) introduced a new Act to change the funding arrangements for provinces, which had been based on population and geography without regard for equal access to services or the fact that cost of service delivery is different in each province. In the same context the Government approved the "Determination" which assigns functions and responsibilities to Provincial Government and Local-level Governments (Department of Provincial and Local Government 2009a).

In 2004, the GoPNG and its development partners conceived the Health Sector Improvement Program (HSIP) as PNG's version of a Sector Wide Approach (SWAp). The HSIP SWAp arrangement was endorsed by AusAID (now Australian Government Department of Foreign Affairs and Trade—DFAT), New Zealand (DFAT), the United Nations Children's Fund (UNICEF), the United Nations Population Fund (UNFPA), the World Health Organization (WHO), and the Asian Development Bank (ADB). The Public Hospitals (Charges) Act of 1972 introduced cost sharing in the form of user fees in PNG's public hospitals. Though not provided for under any legislation, primary health facilities have been charging user fees for operational costs. As primary healthcare facilities were charging without due regard for legal provisions, in 2012 the GoPNG proclaimed a policy of "Free Primary Health Care and subsidized specialist services." This policy came into effect on February 24, 2014. A complementary policy to address bottlenecks in the flow of funds to the facility level is currently being considered for implementation. In 2005, the National Executive Council (NEC) made a decision for the NDoH to explore the feasibility of a social health insurance scheme, a decision which is yet to be implemented.

Other reform initiatives include the development of Public Private Partnership policy in 2003, the Medical Supplies Reform (Roadmap) recommended in 2008, and the Health Workforce Enhancement Plan (2013–2016). In 2008 a new structure for NDoH was approved for implementation as part of NDoH's Corporate Plan (2009–2013).

Current Situation

The national Government is the major funder and provider of health services and is complemented by grant-aided church health services that provide more than 50 percent of ambulatory services in rural areas. The private, for profit, health sector is small but growing. NDoH is responsible for setting the strategic direction for the sector through the National Health Plan, standards setting, policy development, regulation of the sector, and monitoring policy implementation. The NHSS define seven hierarchical levels of the health system, namely: Level 1 Aid Post, Level 2 Community Health Post, Level 3 Rural Health Centre/Urban Health Centre, Level 4 District Hospital, Level 5 Provincial Hospital, Level 6 Regional Hospital, and Level 7 National Referral Hospital (Government of Papua New Guinea 2011). NDoH presently funds and manages four regional hospitals, 16 provincial hospitals, and one national referral hospital. The national referral hospital is currently being considered for semi-autonomous status. Provinces manage rural health services which consist of about 736 health centers and district hospitals, and about 2,900 aid posts. Five-hundred and five of these health facilities are managed by church health services. At any one time, approximately 30 percent of aid posts are closed for various reasons, which include staff shortages and law and order problems. There are 45 urban clinics.

The PNG health system has a well-crafted and fully costed National Health Plan (2011–2020) which is a product of a broadly consultative process. The NHP Performance Assessment Framework (PAF) has 29 high-level indicators which are monitored through the routine National Health Information System (NHIS) and joint annual independent reviews.

The health system in PNG is characterized by low expenditures, poor performance, and deteriorating trends on key indicators (McKay & Lepani 2010). Access to quality health services is constrained by the rugged terrain and infrastructure which has deteriorated due to poor maintenance. The majority of health facilities do not have staff accommodation, reticulated water supply, or electricity. Funding for essential operating costs at facility level is inadequate to keep the doors open. This has reduced the ability of health staff to undertake outreach patrols on a regular basis. Shortages of essential drugs were a common feature of the system until a year and a half ago. Infrequent support supervision visits have contributed to low staff morale, absenteeism, and poor quality of healthcare. Weak capacity for policy development and analysis, weak management and leadership at the strategic level of the department, and deficient managerial skills at the subnational level (Asante & Hall 2011) are major weaknesses affecting the sector. There is a human resources crisis resulting from limited capacity for workforce planning, projection, production, deployment, management, and development (World Bank 2011) which has made it difficult for the NDoH to have accurate numbers and deployment patterns for health workers.

Health sector reforms are a result of political directives, pressure from development partners, and/or analytic studies conducted in collaboration with local and international research institutions. Over the years, the Annual Independent Monitoring Review Group (IMRG) has made a number of recommendations regarding areas for potential policy review. For example, one included the redesign of the HSIP (the health SWAp) which included the Department of Provincial and Local Level Governments, Treasury, National Department of Planning and Monitoring, Development Partners, United Nations Agencies, the Global Fund and GAVI, and non-state providers of health.

When NDoH staff, Provincial Health Advisers, Provincial Administrators, representatives from Faith-Based Organizations, Non-Government Organizations (NGOs), representatives from Central Agencies of Government, and Development Partners, convene at the annual National Health Conferences, they review progress in the implementation of Government policies and programs, and consider and agree on potential areas for policy change. The annual Medical Symposium provides another forum for stakeholders to monitor policy implementation and discuss potential areas for change in policy direction. The Monitoring, Evaluation, and Research Branch of NDoH is responsible for coordinating, monitoring, and evaluating sector performance. The Branch achieves this through the routine NHIS, coordinating the joint Independent Annual Sector Reviews (IASRG), and commissioning surveys and assessments in collaboration with the National Statistics Office and health research institutions. The Health Sector Partnership Committee (HSPC) of the health SWAp determines the thematic areas to be reviewed by the IASRG. The Provincial and Local-Level Government Services Monitoring Authority (PLLSMA) is responsible for monitoring the performance of provinces. Each of the sectors is supposed to establish PLLSMA sub-committees.

Details of Current Reform Initiatives

A new structure for the NDoH was approved in 2008 to align with the core objectives and corporate governance structure defined in the NDoH Corporate

Plan (2009–2013). A new Executive Team was established and new divisional arrangements made, regrouping branch functions within the divisions. A review of the National Health Board legislation was proposed to review its membership and establish a Secretariat. The restructuring process proved to be very slow and protracted until the end of 2012 and adversely impacted on business continuity and implementation of the reform project. A number of governance teams were established: Personnel, Project Coordination, Audit, Planning and Budgeting, and Finance Committees. The HSPC was also established under the SWAp review as a forum for high-level policy dialogue between the Government and donors.

In 2000, a baseline survey of 21 hospitals showed that an average of 42 percent of them complied with the standards set by the Minimum Standards for District Health Services of 2001 and Hospital Standards of 1997. As part of the development and implementation of its Corporate Plan (2009–2013), in 2011, NDoH published the NHSS (2011). Since then the standards have been rolled out to all four administrative regions of the country. The standards incorporate elements of the Minimum Standards for District Health Services—role delineation by service delivery level, minimum standards for essential medical and non-medical equipment, minimum health workforce requirements, clinical guidelines, health facility design, and a health service accreditation program. There are a number of initiatives currently being pursued under the NHSS: developing and/or review of treatment protocols, drug supply quality, recruitment of Clinical Specialist Chiefs as part of NDoH structure, hospital management and governance, and establishment of Community Health Posts.

The PHA reform aims to integrate the management of hospital and rural health services under one authority—the PHA, Act of 2007. An NDoH national Health Reform Team was established in 2008 to provide technical support and oversee the PHA processes. In 2011, Milne Bay, Western Highlands, and Eastern Highlands provinces were the three first phase provinces to elect to implement the provisions of the Act. The processes of establishing a PHA is detailed in the *Provincial Health Authority Act (2007) User Handbook and Arrangements (2009)* compiled by the National Department of Health. Whilst to date an additional four provinces have opted to establish PHAs, the NDoH has decided to fast track the process so that by the end of 2016 all the 22 provinces will have established PHAs.

The implementation process has focused on process issues and not the public health impact of these reforms. Challenges experienced include coordination and technical support from the NDoH Reform Team, as well as lukewarm engagement from central agencies and the majority of Provincial Administrators. The fact that the adoption of the PHA is voluntary means that national coverage is likely to be a very protracted process.

The period 2004–2007 saw the PNG health sector experience a significant decrease in health funding from both the Government and donors (Kase 2006). This necessitated the development of strategies to prioritize expenditures on health. Criteria were therefore developed to determine areas for priority spending—focusing on programs that had an impact on the greatest number of people, greatest impact on morbidity and mortality, were accessible, affordable, and cost-effective. This was the first time NDoH used priority resource allocation which is based on a health sector Medium Term Expenditure Framework (MTEF) (2004–2007). Since then, the MTEF has been refined and rolled over. The current MTEF covers the period 2014–2016 with the costs of the NHP (2011–2020) retrofitted into the MTEF and made to reflect a three-year rolling timeframe. Within the context of the current SWAp, the METF identifies resource requirements and the funding gaps and assists donors and the Government to agree on resource allocation over the three-year period.

The health SWAp in PNG was established in 1996 as the Health Sector Development Program (HSDP). This was initially to handle the ADB loan. In 2000 a "Partnership Agreement" was signed between the Government and the Australian Government DFAT to establish a HSIP Trust Account (TA) as a mechanism for handling pool funds. In 2003, New Zealand AID, WHO, UNICEF, and UNFPA joined the HSIP TA. The Global Fund for HIV/AIDS, Malaria and TB (GFATM) joined the SWAp in 2004. Donor projects continued despite the establishment of the SWAp pool fund account. Weak financial management capacity at all levels resulted in poor liquidation of funds, bottlenecks to fund flows to the sub-national level, and very low implementation rates for the HSIP TA. The significantly increased flow of funds from the GFATM and the rigorous reporting requirements simply overwhelmed the existing capacity to handle the volume of funds flowing through this account. Problems of absorptive capacity, bottlenecks in the flow of funds to the front line of service delivery, and the perception of a lack of inclusiveness in the SWAp led to the IMRG of 2009 to recommend a redesign of the SWAp.

Subsequent to the release of the World Bank report, "PNG Health Workforce Crisis: A Call to Action" in 2011, the NDoH has developed a "Health Workforce Enhancement Plan (2013–2016). This plan details a number of short-term measures which include retention strategies, increasing the retirement age to 65 years, recruitment of expatriate health workers, recruiting retired health workers, and increasing training capacity amongst others.

Quality and Safety Landscape

The main actors in the quality and safety agenda in healthcare include the NDoH which has the responsibility to set and monitor the implementation of policies and standards. Universities and professional bodies such as the Nursing Council, work with NDoH to develop curricula and to accredit training institutions. These and other training institutions collaborate with NDoH and the sub-national levels in delivering in-service training and continuing medical education programs. Health facilities at all levels are obliged to establish infection control committees, maternal mortality committees, and where appropriate to conduct regular clinical audits. In addition there are hospital medical records officers, the pharmaceutical committee in NDoH, and medical education committees—all of which are not coordinated into a common model to address the quality agenda.

Providers of health services, public, "private-for-profit," and "private-not-for-profit" have an obligation to comply with quality assurance policies and standards. The accreditation process is voluntary and mainly focuses on public health facilities. Accreditation surveys are conducted every four years. Development Partners contribute to this process by providing technical support, funding for analytic work, policy development, standards setting, and the purchase of inputs that contribute to improving the quality of healthcare. From the demand side, beneficiaries, in some cases with assistance from civil society organizations, demand what they perceive as quality care and a safe treatment environment.

Impact of Reforms on Quality and Safety of Care

All the components of the NHSS reform initiative have a direct bearing on the quality and safety of care. The medical supplies reform agenda has a direct impact on the availability of quality, safe, and affordable essential medicines. By defining the minimum standards for staffing levels, essential medicines, medical and non-medical equipment, and facility design the NHSS addresses a number of quality of care dimensions. These include assisting health staff achieve technical competencies, ensuring continuity of care through strengthening the referral system, and ensuring health facility designs include amenities such as running water and electricity. The development of treatment guidelines and training of health workers addresses the effectiveness of healthcare interventions. The PHA reform has the potential to improve the referral system and continuity of care. The abolition of user fees has the potential to improve community access to and utilization of primary health services. Increasing the quality and quantity of health workers and deploying them rationally and equitably have the potential to increase access to quality, as well as people centered healthcare services.

Under the Organic Law, provinces have significant autonomy which has resulted in a "management disconnect." Provincial authorities are not necessarily obliged to follow national directives, or policies. For example they may not allocate enough funds for the distribution of drugs, or prioritize support and supervision of district health services. The fragmented nature of service delivery has resulted in an inefficient referral system between rural health and hospital services which disrupts the continuity of care. The immediate effect of the abolition of user fees is to deprive health facilities of the revenue they relied on for their operational costs. This means that health facility staff will not be able to purchase cleaning materials and commercially available essential medicines or conduct planned outreach health patrols. The potential upsurge in health facility utilization resulting from free primary healthcare services could overwhelm the system, potentially resulting in the deterioration of the quality of healthcare provided.

The development and implementation of the NHSS and the restructuring of NDoH created an environment that is conducive for reform initiatives to improve quality of care. The PHA establishes a unitary health system at the sub-national level that makes health workers accountable to health professionals. Under the PHA arrangement the planning and budgeting framework for health services at the sub-national level is under the full control of health managers.

Barriers and Solutions to Quality and Safe Care

The health delivery system faces a number of challenges to the achievement of quality and safe care. Combined with other factors, low Government expenditures on healthcare have left the health sector struggling to meet the needs of the population which is increasing at an annual growth rate of 3.1 percent (National Statistical Office 2011). Though significant efforts have been invested in building the capacity for corporate governance within NDoH, there still exist inadequate administrative and management structures, weak supportive supervision at some levels of the system, inefficient and ineffective procurement and supply systems, currently being addressed through annual procurement planning, and weak health management information systems. Some drugs which are necessary for quality care are often not available. The critical shortage of human resources for health means that available staff is overworked, poorly motivated, and inadequately supported. In addition, facilities are dilapidated. The system focuses on technical quality issues and little on quality as perceived by consumers. There is inadequate provision of information to empower users. As a result, issues with quality of care remain constrained by the asymmetry of information between the providers and the consumers of healthcare.

There is a need to build national commitment and leadership that provides an institutional framework for quality assurance within the sector and a civil service ethos which emphasizes the accountability of staff. Current efforts in leadership and management training for executive managers and middle managers will a go a long way to strengthen this capacity. Supervision can ensure good documentation and proper management of patient data. It is crucial to ensure that available funds actually reach the front line of service delivery so as to keep the doors open. Direct Facility Funding (DFF) has the potential to increase the flow of funds at the facility level. It is also important and imperative to build the management capacity of district health managers.

Prospects for Success and Next Steps

The reforms discussed in this chapter are an integral part of the current NHP (2011–2020) and the NDoH Corporate Plan (2013–2015). The policy on "Free Primary Health Care and Subsidized Specialist Services" is one of the priorities for the ninth term of Parliament under the Alotau Accord of 2012. After the initial restructuring of NDoH, the department will be embarking on an "organizational transitional plan" during the life of its current corporate plan. This round of restructuring will facilitate the gradual transfer of non-core activities, requiring service level agreements and organizational restructuring.

Whilst the voluntary nature of the PHA adoption process was likely to constrain its roll out to all the provinces, new political directions require all provinces to be covered by 2016. In order to accelerate this process the PHA Act needs to be reviewed to make it compulsory. The first step is being the current review of the Organic Law. There will be a need to strengthen the capacity of NDoH, PHAs, and provinces to monitor the performance of contracts entered into with non-state providers.

The cost implications of rolling out the NHSS ubiquitously are yet to be estimated. It is unlikely that the Government will be able to afford the resources. A "Clinicians' Tool Kit for Health Services in Papua New Guinea: Clinical Governance: Improving Patient Care" is currently under development. As part of this roll out, it is proposed to strengthen clinical governance within health facilities, and monitor compliance through the analysis of relevant NHIS indicators and information from surveys. Success depends on the availability of adequate human resources for health, a comprehensive and well-resourced infrastructure rehabilitation program, and completion of the medical supplies reform program. This is a continuing reform that will go beyond the life of the current NHP.

A communications strategy around the free primary healthcare declaration will have to be developed. According to the current Corporate Plan, NDoH will monitor the impact of this policy on the quality and utilization of health services and programs. In view of certain specialist services continuing to attract user fees, NDoH is currently consulting relevant GoPNG Central Agencies to review options for a health insurance scheme for PNG. The evaluation of DFF recommended that it be considered as a complementary policy to the abolition of user fees, to fill the revenue gap created. The Senior Executive Management in NDoH is yet to consider the implications of the evaluation report and share these with the Department of Provincial and Local Level Government Affairs (DPLGA) and the National Economic and Fiscal Commission (NEFC). The Corporate Plan proposes further examination of DFF to determine its applicability.

Recommendations on medical supplies reform initiatives are contained in a report compiled in 2008. The medical supplies reform agenda was approved for implementation in 2013 and will remain through the life of the NHP. Proposals for outsourcing the procurement of medicines and the establishment of an independent procurement authority seem to be gaining momentum within NDoH. As long as the management information systems for the medical stores remain rudimentary, the quantification of national requirements inadequate, and procurement processes lacking transparency, the problems of essential drugs will remain—even beyond the life of the current NHP.

Future

For the future, there are plans to set up a Mental Health Directorate with 5 percent of the total budget of the health department allocated. Though this will become a pace-setter for the Pacific nations where mental health services are usually neglected, it is deemed that the percentage set aside is more than the unit can utilize and is therefore still under negotiation.

The NDoH is considering establishing a Public Health Institute which will be a prototype of the United States Centers for Disease Control and Prevention (CDC). The Government of PNG has approved a Bill to deepen decentralization to the district level. District Development Authorities (DDA) will be established "to perform service delivery functions and carry out service delivery responsibilities, to approve disbursement of district support grants," amongst other functions. This development has serious and complicated implications for the functions of and relationships with PHAs.

Conclusion

The current NHP and the various Corporate Plans acknowledge the fact that the health system is in crisis, as evidenced by a general decline in system performance, diminishing capacity, and deteriorating quality of services. The Organic Law has been largely blamed for the evolution of this crisis. The fact that PNG recently graduated into a lower-middle income country does not seem to reverse this decline; economic growth, in itself, is clearly not sufficient to lead to an improvement and the health of a country's population.

The PHA is the health sector's strategy to operate within the constraints of the Organic Law and to make the process of reform politically acceptable, legally feasible, and to deal with opposition to the reforms. There is a "principal–agent" dilemma in which the NDoH is perceived to have its own objectives which are not understood by the provinces as agents of service delivery. The PHA in particular is perceived as a threat to the power base of the provincial administrators. A locally appropriate and functioning district-based health system complemented by targeted investment in the rehabilitation of infrastructure, increased personnel deployed to the right places, practice-based and problem-oriented management capacity building, and the strengthening of information systems are essential. "To stay open health facilities require a basic level of operational funding, without which they simply cannot function" (National Economic and Fiscal Commission 2010). Funds must be available at the facility level to address the non-negotiable Minimum Priority Activities (MPAs), namely "integrated rural health outreach patrols," "the distribution of drugs" and "basic operational funding to keep the doors open." Success will only be guaranteed if the changes are an evolutionary process as opposed to "big bang" reforms.

PART IV
The Americas

Julie Johnson

We now move to Part IV and the Americas, represented by Argentina, Brazil, Chile, Mexico, and the United States (US). The countries included in Part IV represent diverse populations and diverse healthcare systems with fundamental differences, similarities, and transferrable lessons learned.

Fundamental differences can be observed in how each country finances its healthcare system, yet it is the fragmentation of financing—public and private systems—that represents some of the biggest challenges for these healthcare systems. Regardless of how a nation finances its healthcare, there are implications for quality and safety.

Arce and Elorrio report that quality and patient safety have been marginal strategies in health policy in Argentina, and that the provinces are autonomous from the nation in regards to health, as well as education. Brazil mandated universal healthcare coverage for its citizens in 1988 and has one of the largest public healthcare systems in the world, free at the point of delivery, with egalitarian mandate and provision. While quality and safety have a prominent place on the healthcare agenda in Brazil, Carvalho de Noronha and colleagues report that the vast income disparities pose tremendous challenges for the delivery of high quality care.

The central focus of healthcare reform in Chile is on the explicit guarantee of services for the 80 most prevalent diseases in the country. Potential unintended consequences of this type of reform is that people with other, non-prioritized illnesses and conditions, are at risk of neglected or delayed care. Solimano and Valdivia raise an important issue that is transferrable from Chile's experience—it is hard to fully understand the impact without a comprehensive and rigorous evaluation that runs parallel to reform effort.

If we compare total expenditures on health as a percentage of Gross Domestic Product (GDP), the US far outpaces other countries—not just the countries included in Part IV, but all other countries—with a percentage of GDP that is nearly twice the OECD average. What does the US gain from spending so much on health? Not enough, as the comparative data on health indicators show. Efforts to reduce costs have been a mainstay of health reform in the US.

What can we learn from a comparison of the counties represented in Part IV? Perhaps one important lesson is that once universal coverage is guaranteed for a population, the focus can turn to quality and safety of care. As our colleagues in

Brazil emphasize, greater public awareness coupled with providers' commitment to quality and safety will be important drivers to achieving significant gains in health outcomes. Ruelas and colleagues provide a systems level view of quality and safety and identify a basic, yet fundamental lesson from Mexico's experience. If the aim is to improve quality system wide, it is necessary to establish an explicit comprehensive strategy which includes an ethical platform for providers and patients, organizational redesign at the federal and state levels, a quality measurement system, quality improvement training, accreditation, and incentives. The final lesson from Part IV is that evaluation of health reform efforts and the effect on quality and safety of care should be prominent on everyone's future research agenda.

Chapter 15
Argentina

Hugo Arce and Ezequiel García Elorrio

Abstract

The Argentine Constitution has a federal structure, where the provinces are autonomous from the nation, in regard to the areas of health and education. Health resources (public hospitals and outpatient clinics) and several health programs are managed by the provinces, while the national Ministry of Health establishes general policies and priorities, finances strategic programs, and oversees the health system. Argentine healthcare is organized as a mixed system made up by the public, private, and social security sub-systems. Social security was fundamentally of non-governmental origin: multiple mutual insurance funds organized by immigrants became official entities and were placed under the control of trade unions from each production branch. Moreover, entities of governmental origin were set up for public employees from the provinces and for retirees. In spite of the widespread availability of public services, private services, such as social security providers, are the most dynamic. In Argentina, patient quality and safety have been marginal strategies in health policy, regardless of the intentions of health authorities in the 1990s and 2000s. Different governmental and non-governmental actors have as yet been unable to have a significant impact. To achieve such a purpose, it would be necessary to have a convergence of the provincial and the national Governments, together with professional associations, social security agencies managed by trade unions, and corporate chambers. This would enable development of transformational strategies that may reduce the gap between what happens in the country and what could be achieved, with the available resources and the quality of their scientific professionals.

Background

The Argentine Constitution has a federal structure, where the provinces are autonomous from the nation, in regard to the areas of health and education. Health resources (public hospitals and outpatient clinics) and preventive programs are managed by the provinces, while the national Ministry of Health establishes general policies and priorities, finances strategic programs, and directs the health system. The Argentine health organization—as in most Latin American countries—is basically a mixed system made up by the public, private, and social security sub-

Table 15.1   Demographic, economic, and health information for Argentina

Population (thousands)	41,087
Area (sq. km)*	2,736,690
Proportion of population living in urban areas (2011)	93
Gross Domestic Product (GDP US$, billions)^	475.5
Total expenditure on health as % of GDP	8.5
Gross national income per capita (PPP intl $) (2006)	11,730
Per capita total expenditure on health (intl $)	1,551
Proportion of health expenditure which is private	30.8
General Government expenditure on health as a percentage of total expenditure on health	69.2
Out-of-pocket expenditure as a percentage of private expenditure on health	65.3
Life expectancy at birth m/f (yrs)	73/79
Probability of dying under five (per 1,000 live births)	14
Maternal Mortality Ratio (per 100,000 live births) (2013)	69
Proportion of population using improved water and sanitation	99/97

Source: Unless otherwise stated data are for the year 2012 and taken from the World Health Organization 2014. * Area from the World Bank 2014a. ^GDP from the World Bank 2014b.

Notes: PPP is purchasing power parity, intl $ is international dollar which has the same purchasing power as US$ in the US.

systems. The country's distinctive feature is that social security originated outside the state, from multiple mutual insurance funds organized by immigrants, which in the mid-twentieth century became official entities (the so-called "Obras Sociales") and were placed under the control of trade unions from all branches of production. Today these entities number more than 300. To these Obras Sociales, others of state origin were added for the public employees of the provinces (24 entities) and for retirees (Programa de Atención Médica Integral—PAMI*[1]).

During the last 25 years, the main changes in the system have not modified its basic structure, but rather, they have attempted to establish new rules and partial regulations, seeking to solve current aspects and harmonize relationships between different actors. Overall, the system tries to evolve from a "pluralist model of decentralized regulation" to an "integrated pluralist model of regulated competition" (Arce 2010, pp. 14–22). Another important factor that needs to be emphasized is the geographic scope of the country, the diversity of climates, and

---

1   * indicates Spanish acronyms.

the difficulties in connecting certain locations to the health system in an efficient and equitable manner. Development efforts applied to quality as a health system value have been, to say the least, uncoordinated and driven by different actors; such as the national Government, provincial Governments, private financers, and institutional and professional providers without a continuity pattern, with a high presence of non-governmental initiatives. Quality has been a marginal strategy in health policy, regardless of the intentions of the health authorities in the 1990s and 2000s.

Recently, the country has been characterized by ideologically different macroeconomic policies and political orientations which determined overall aspects of the economy that partially affected the healthcare market: exchange rate, inflation, trade barriers, and social policies. Changes were accelerated by two important and institutional crises: hyperinflation in 1989 and 1990 and debt default in 2002. Similar to the rest of Latin America, in Argentina, there is a high percentage of informal workers (more than 30 percent), who do not appear in legal records and do not contribute to any social protection system. However, in the mid-term, several regulatory efforts and partial health reforms can be identified, together with social security actions aiming at redistribution, which have stimulated some changes in health system operation. The abovementioned succession of economic cycles has generated a visible inequality in the access to services and their availability. A low-income population without contribution capacity uses exclusively public services, whereas formal workers with sufficient resources are covered by social security or private health programs.

Introduction

During the 1990s health reform was mainly oriented towards the organization of social security, seeking to prevent the Obras Sociales (tied to trade unions) from retaining captive populations, to integrate the service coverage between social security and private healthcare, and to decentralize public hospital administration. During the first decade of the twenty-first century, instead, there was a greater effort towards strengthening of the first level of care, by means of community health programs for outpatients, provision of basic medication in public health centers, state coverage of pregnancy, birth and first five years of life, and different types of social benefits. Although there were isolated initiatives by the Government regarding patient quality and safety, these did not constitute a unified strategy within health policies.

The cultural characteristics of the country, which are also found in other Latin American countries, are strongly influenced by European immigration, especially of Latin origin, indigenous populations, and populations of African origin to a lesser extent (Arce 1999). Some social and cultural characteristics determine behavior regarding patient quality and safety, which may be found in most countries in the region. Among the features that describe—in our opinion—the health system, the following may be mentioned:

- Central health authorities limit their guiding function to public services, and they have a weak influence over other areas of this activity.
- There is a general fragmentation of the system, with multiple actors and decision makers, which makes their management difficult.
- In public hospitals, management budgetary models, with little autonomy in decision making by the hospital authorities, prevail (Bogue, Hall & La Forgia 2007).
- Most privately-installed capacity is based upon small local clinics, with little investment capacity and/or low-development facilities.
- Among the population of public service users there is a prevalence of an informal economy population with no contributing capacity.
- There are large disparities in public and private providers, and a coexistence of very developed facilities with others with severe structural deficiencies.
- Projects of administrative performance decentralization have stumbled in general with low management capacity of the local authorities.
- Other than professional certification, licensing, and hospital accreditation, no ongoing efforts have been made to improve quality and promote safety for patients (Arce 1998).

The Current Situation

Apart from the three sectors—public, private, and social security—there are internal divisions within each. In addition to the National Ministry of Health, there are 24 provincial ministries, which as a whole manage 55 percent of hospital beds and almost half of the outpatient care centers. The private sub-sector is made up of multiple private healthcare institutions, of different nature and size, with 45 percent of hospital beds and more than half of outpatient centers, as well as the population's out-of-pocket expenses. Social security is made up of more than 300 Obras Sociales, 24 for public employees of the provinces and one for retirees (PAMI*). This configuration hinders the system's capacity for coordination and articulation, preventing the organization of a "formal" health system and conspires against the efficient use of resources and the achievement of acceptable levels of equality in coverage (Bisang & Centrángolo 1997). In the case of the public sub-sector, there is an agency for the coordination of health ministries, the Federal Health Council (Consejo Federal de Salud—CoFeSa*), which has no management functions and simply allows the sharing of information and the coordination of technical programs. In turn, insurance entities (Obras Sociales and private healthcare) are linked to private providers, as they refer all their patients to that sector. Such behavior occurs because the covered population prefers to receive care at private facilities, although in some cases public hospitals have greater technical capabilities than private ones.

So far as the administrative relationship between insurers and healthcare service providers is concerned, medical, hospital, dental, and biochemical associations have an important role as middlemen in the invoicing and payment of the delivered care. Such institutions are organized by each province and are signatories on the agreements with insurance entities, although in some cases there is direct hiring, especially in big cities. This healthcare management model, as it adds administrative steps to contractual mechanisms, increases inequalities in accessibility to the care provided and deepens its regional heterogeneity. In spite of such circumstances, although the public sub-sector has the largest share in installed capacity, in economic terms approximately 60 percent of the system's financial resources circulate through the administrative connections between insurers and private providers. Therefore, these sectors have an important role in decision making and in the configuration of the health system overall (Abuelafia 2002).

This complex matrix of actors and healthcare financing exposes what is probably the biggest weakness of the system, which is fragmentation, with its concomitant consequences such as inefficiency, lack of continuity in health policies, and inequality among the different sectors. Although Argentina is placed among the countries with better health indicators in the region, trends show that improvements achieved in past decades have halted and in some cases, have even deteriorated (Departamento de Estadísticas e Información de Salud 2012). The prevalence of adverse events and patient harm in the region was also estimated by the Latin American Study of Adverse Events, sponsored by the Pan-American Health Organization (PAHO) (Aranaz-Andres et al. 2011). This situation led the national Government to seek the development of centralized efforts to ensure basic health services, such as mother–child care and primary care.

Detail of Current Reform Initiatives

Between 1960 and 1992 almost all the existing public hospitals in the national jurisdiction were transferred to provincial jurisdictions. Just a few hospitals remain within the national scope, with a shared regime between the two jurisdictions. University hospitals and the hospitals that provide care to the Armed Forces and Law Enforcement personnel remain within the national jurisdiction. During the 1990s as well, a decentralized hospital model was pursued, with the intention to have services billed to social security; however, such efforts were unable to modify the traditional culture of public hospitals, which still depend mostly on the state budget for resources. During that decade, a process developed under the name of "deregulation of Obras Sociales," based upon the concept that workers of one production area should not be captive to their corresponding Obra Social and that they should be able to choose another. Likewise, higher-income workers could access—through their Obra Social—programs managed by private healthcare organizations. On the other hand, a basic benefit package was established under the Mandatory Medical Program (Programa Médico Obligatorio—PMO*). These actions were influenced by the general trend to introduce pro-competition reforms and to ensure the sustainability of the social security system.

During the 2000s, most actions were aimed at the strengthening of the first level of care and to facilitate the access to healthcare for important sectors of the population that were excluded after the 2001–2002 crisis. These efforts were supported by loans from the World Bank and the Inter-American Development Bank (IDB), which contributed to the financing of: (1) the Remediar Program, to provide basic medication (as defined by PAHO) to outpatient clinics, (2) the Community Doctors Program, seeking to train professionals with social vocation and community orientation, (3) the Nacer Plan for the coverage of pregnancy, birth and first year of life, and (4) the Sumar Plan for the coverage of teen care and influence in other stages of life. During this stage, progress was made in the implementation of the Categorizing Authorization program, in order to unify the different oversight regimes of the provinces, including public hospitals, as an object of oversight. In the social security sub-sector, it is during this period that the freedom of Obra Social choice got a foothold. There was an increase in coverage, outsourcing to private healthcare for higher-income members and new legislation was enacted specifically regarding private healthcare.

The Quality and Safety Landscape

Since the mid-1980s a group of public health specialists, encouraged by the social security regulating entity, started several pilots of standards elaboration and assessments in the field. These initiatives led to the decision by the PAHO, by means of an agreement with the Latin American Hospital Federation (FLH*), to commission the Argentine group for a working document for an Accreditation program with standards adequate for the Latin American scenario. This made possible, after consolidation during a few consensus meetings, the publication of the *Hospital Accreditation Handbook for Latin America and the Caribbean* (Pan-American Health Organization—Latin American Hospital Federation 1992). In 1992 the Ministry of Health created the National Program of Quality Assurance in Health Care (Programa Nacional de Garantía de Calidad de la Atención—PNGCAM*), especially focused on the elaboration of technical standards by specialty, with the collaboration of multiple scientific societies. However, this Ministry could not support the distribution of that handbook. This hindered its application in the rest of the countries of the region. Among the aims of the authorities at that time, priority was given to the unification of the Licensing and Categorization standards across the country, as each province had different conditions to authorize services and to determine their resolution capacity.

A decade later, in 2004, CoFeSa subscribed a general agreement of Health Ministers, under the name, Federal Health Plan 2004–2007. The plan explicitly included a unified model of Categorizing Authorization, as well as the promotion of accreditation for health facilities. However, most of the development of the quality and patient safety drive occurred outside Government, with a great diversity of initiatives. In 1994 activities started at the Technical Institute for the Accreditation of Health Facilities (Instituto Técnico para la Acreditación de Establecimientos de Salud—ITAES*), which operates to this date. This was followed by the Biochemical Foundation (Fundación Bioquímica—FABA*) for clinical test laboratories in 1996 and by the Specialized Center for Health Standardization and Accreditation (Centro Especializado para la Normalización y Acreditación en Salud—CENAS*) in 1998, all of them devoted to developing and implementing accreditation programs (Paganini 1999).

Similar measures are seen with entities devoted to clinical quality: the Institute for Clinical Effectiveness and Health Policy (Instituto de Efectividad Clínica y Sanitaria—IECS*) is in charge of activities related to care training, research programs, clinical care guidelines, and technology assessment, and the National Medicine Academy's Institute of Epidemiological Research (Instituto de Investigaciones Epidemiológicas de la Academia Nacional de Medicina) which publicized the focus on care practice, developed research on medical errors, clinical care guidelines and clinical epidemiology training. Also, four scientific societies were organized: the Argentine Society for Medical Audits (Sociedad Argentina de Auditoría Médica—SADAM*) which initiated the quality drive since the 1980s, the Argentine Society for Quality in Health Care (Sociedad Argentina para la Calidad en Atención de la Salud—SACAS*) which was the organizer of the 18th International Society for Quality in Healthcare Conference in Buenos Aires in 2001, the Association for Audits and Medical Quality of Córdoba (Asociación de Auditoría y Calidad Médica de Córdoba—ASACAM*), and the Avedis Donabedian Foundation (Fundación Avedis Donabedian—FAD*). There are at present two quality awards: the Quality Award of the Government of the City of Buenos Aires, specific for hospital services, and the National Quality Award, which evaluates the performance of Total Quality Management guidelines, along with other similar awards, such as Japan's Deming, Europe's European Foundation for Quality Management and Baldridge in the United States of America (US). Finally, there are at least seven training programs focused on quality and safety, offered in different cities, which have operated on an ongoing fashion for the last two decades. All these initiatives seek to raise awareness among the different stakeholders, but their impact is nevertheless limited due to low demand, either because of the scarce statutory regulation in force, or because the eventual quality improvement and error prevention are not later reflected in tangible benefits for the system actors.

These initiatives have had two aspects in common: they were initiated with a high degree of personal or institutional voluntarism, without sustained support actions by the state. With the exception of the particular circumstances of PNGCAM and the national advisory committee for patient safety in 2007, promoted from the national Government, they have been focal points of non-governmental guidance for the health system, regarding how to approach quality and safety programs. On the other hand, they diversified and supplemented international influences, from PAHO, the World Health Organization (WHO), and Joint Commission and Accreditation Canada, which since the early 1980s drew the attention of the physicians who visited the US, impressed by the improvements introduced by hospital accreditation (Sánchez Zinny 1979, Canitrot 1980). Global initiatives such as the hand hygiene campaign, the surgical checklist, and the Patients for Patient Safety initiatives promoted by WHO, were actively endorsed by the national Government and were pilots for models of collaboration between the different actors (World Health Organization 2007)

The Impact of These Reform Efforts on Quality and Safety of Care

Due to the institutional fragmentation of the organization model of Argentina there are no consistent data that allow a global outlook of the impact of actions taken on quality and safety, other than the indicators elaborated by each institution or program as a result of their own activities. There are statistical data on benefits and coverage provided by different national state agencies within the framework of different programs (Remediar, Community Doctors, Nacer Plan, Sumar Plan), but still there are no consistent findings on their impact besides program reports with promising results. Regarding this, it is useful to explain that the events that make up the vital statistics of the country (child mortality rates, general mortality rates, births, maternal mortality rates, fecundity), come mostly from legal entities instead of specific health records. Frequently, primary and secondary causes of deaths are recorded for administrative reasons and do not represent the actual clinical causes. In geographically isolated areas and in socially vulnerable populations, frequently such events are underreported.

On the other hand, morbidity data come from the National Program of Hospital Statistics for morbidity and mortality, which is based upon the WHO's diagnostic classification, with the inclusion of child, maternal, and general mortality data with more reliable diagnostics. However, these are not cross-referenced with births and deaths data in legal records. These data are only collected in public hospitals and are published by the Ministry of Health. However, public hospitals represent 40 percent of care activity and private facilities in general do not keep any statistical records. Taking into account these limiting factors, it is difficult to assess the actual impact and scope of the quality and safety programs. In the case of infection control, better records have been kept, as there are two programs in place, one public (VIHDA) and another private (VIGILAR), which have acted consistently for years to help reduce the impact of healthcare associated infections, but with mixed results. These are well-developed clinical initiatives, although their impact and scope has not been as expected, but they may be a model for other similar programs.

Implementation: Barriers and Solutions

Some of the weak points in the Argentine patient quality and safety efforts are most likely influenced, as mentioned, by the population's origin. Typical behavior includes a general unwillingness to obey rules, with a tendency to react after the fact, rather than proactively preventing problems. In hospitals there is a generalized tendency to conceal mistakes, in implicit "silence pacts," which could be part of the main obstacles for the incorporation of improvement programs based upon the analysis and prevention of adverse events, although no formal Argentinean research findings yet support this statement. Apart from these cultural characteristics, there are other barriers that, in our judgment, may have a significant impact:

- There is, in general, a latent resistance against the application of procedure standards (for example, surgical checklists), both between the professional and the technical personnel, even though it has been endorsed by the central Government.
- Whenever there is an adverse event, there is, most of the time, a tendency to conceal the medical error, perhaps due to a lack of organizational conscience. Most of the time, therefore, there is a tendency to react after the fact, rather than plan proactively.
- Lack of data that may otherwise help to identify the magnitude of failures and damage caused by bad care quality. This prevents an adequate awareness by the population and health professionals.
- Nursing personnel are less skilled than they should be, they are badly paid and they work mainly as assistants, without making autonomous decisions based on the professional role.
- Among hospital personnel it is common to find condescending and superior attitudes whenever relating to patients and families.
- Little presence of personnel skilled in issues related to quality of care and patient safety.
- Poor participation of the public in decision making on health issues and lack of interest in receiving information about system performance in order to exercise rights of choice based upon quality.
- Regarding quality improvement, external assessments (licensing, professional certification, accreditation) have received more attention and funding than improvements in everyday management and the prevention of events that may harm patients (Arce 2001).

On the other hand, regarding strengths, it may be said that the health system and its professionals have been historically well-regarded within the region, and even in industrialized countries where they migrate for residences or rotations. The level of training is also respected (although these are exceptional cases, three Medicine Nobel Prizes have been awarded to Argentinean professionals), because of a well-developed scientific environment and a long tradition in teaching and research. As potential facilitating features for improvement initiatives, we may refer to, among others:

- Highly developed technical and scientific human capital regarding healthcare, research and teaching at a regional level.
- More than 20 years of experience in hospital external assessment programs, as well as a great diversity in non-governmental initiatives related to patient quality and safety.
- A long tradition of civil society organizations that has influenced the field of health, by means of non-profit associations, scientific societies, private universities, and a great number of undergraduate and graduate education programs.
- A vigorous trade union organization and associations of professionals in the health field, that may be an anchor for the dissemination and eventual standardization of initiatives related to care quality.
- The existence of successful initiatives in other countries in the region, that may be effectively adapted to our country, in the same way as the Argentine experience in external assessment programs has been usefully applied in other countries.

Prospects for Success and Next Steps

The exercise of federal management in Argentina has been particularly disorganized, due to an ill-defined distribution of health responsibilities among the provinces and the central Government. This fact has endangered most the described quality and safety initiatives in the country. Unlike in Brazil, Uruguay, and Chile it has not been possible to consolidate public and social security funding sources under a centralized management, impacting on the planning and execution of quality and safety programs (Andrés Bello University 2011). Change may come from the central Government, provinces acting on their own will, or disease-specific national programs that may incorporate quality of care as a main goal beyond coverage.

A priority strategy to ensure quality of care and to reduce adverse events should at least take into account the experiences of Colombia and Mexico (Ruelas & Poblano 2007, Kerguelén 2008), as examples to be considered. However, in these countries there has been a long tradition of health reform, statutorily implemented, a path that has met difficulties in Argentina due to the fact that transit through Congress usually neutralizes core aspects of the reforms. In these reforms, adequate quality goals should be defined (Committee on Quality of Health Care in America,

Institute of Medicine 2001), there should be a promotion of the patient´s rights in the care received, and the results of care performance should be publicized. Quality incentives should be implemented and the population should be allowed to participate in decisions regarding their health.

Conclusion

In Argentina, quality and safety has been, unfortunately, a marginal strategy in health policy, regardless of the intentions of health authorities in the 1990s and 2000s. It is evident that there is still much to be done in terms of regulation, and likewise, it is necessary to continue to develop initiatives for the benefit of vulnerable sectors of the population, whose health indicators should be improved. The diversity and lack of synergy of the actors has not facilitated the intended results, for which reason it is considered necessary that the national Government and the provincial Governments should approach professional associations like Obras Sociales, provider chambers, and the academic sector, in order to achieve a consensus about the way forward. The purpose would be to develop consensual strategies that may narrow the gap between the current situation in the country and what should be, with regard to the history of the health system, the development of its human capital and available resources.

Chapter 16

Brazil

José Carvalho de Noronha, Victor Grabois, and
Adelia Quadros Farias Gomes

Abstract

Brazil initiated major healthcare reforms just after the restoration of a democratic Government in 1985 and the promulgation of a New Constitution in 1988. Provisions for universal and egalitarian health services were mandated and quality of care and patient safety increasingly became prevalent on the healthcare agenda. From the 1990s on, major regulatory legislation has been passed and a growing number of programs and initiatives have been developed both in the public and private sectors. There is still significant fragmentation between the sectors but indications of greater coordination may be observed. Current reform efforts are being redirected to the delivery of integrated services through regional healthcare networks. Greater public awareness and providers' commitment to quality and safety are important driving forces although, overall, appropriate financing of the system and persistent inequities and challenges to access remain significant constraints.

Introduction

Major healthcare reforms in Brazil have the dispositions of the 1988 Federal Constitution (Brasil 2010) as their pivotal landmark. The Constitution was promulgated after the country had lived under 20 years of military rule, and following three years of intense debate on the future of political, economic, cultural, and social institutions under the reborn democracy. The shaping of the health policy fundamentals engaged citizen's organizations, labor unions, health professionals, healthcare providers, industry, political parties, patient's organizations, media, and academics mobilized with their specific agendas. The results of this political momentum were translated in the Constitution into a full Chapter on health within the broad scope of the provisions of the organization of the social security.

The Constitution article that summarizes the Brazilian healthcare reform desiderata states that:

> Health is a right of all and a duty of the state and shall be guaranteed by means of social and economic policies aimed at reducing the risk of illness and other hazards and at the universal and equal access to actions and services for its promotion, protection and recovery. (Article 196, Brazilian Constitution)

**Table 16.1	Demographic, economic, and health information for Brazil**

Population (thousands)	199,000
Area (sq. km)*	8,459,420
Proportion of population living in urban areas (2011)	85
Gross Domestic Product (GDP US$, billions)^	2,252.7
Total expenditure on health as % of GDP	9.3
Gross national income per capita (PPP intl $)	11,530
Per capita total expenditure on health (intl $)	1,109
Proportion of health expenditure which is private	53.6
General Government expenditure on health as a percentage of total expenditure on health	46.4
Out-of-pocket expenditure as a percentage of private expenditure on health	57.8
Life expectancy at birth m/f (yrs)	70/77
Probability of dying under five (per 1,000 live births)	14
Maternal Mortality Ratio (per 100,000 live births) (2013)	69
Proportion of population using improved water and sanitation	98/81

Source: Unless otherwise stated data are for the year 2012 and taken from the World Health Organization 2014. * Area from the World Bank 2014a. ^GDP from the World Bank 2014b.
Note: PPP is purchasing power parity, intl $ is international dollar which has the same purchasing power as US$ in the US.

Provisions for the reorganization of the public health system were established which mandated the creation of a unified health system (SUS), integrating under a single command the healthcare activities that were divided between the Ministry of Health and Social Security, and similarly at the state and municipal levels. The healthcare system was to be financed by general taxation at the three tiers of Government and specific social contributions associated with social security.[1]

The healthcare landscape in Brazil has been almost entirely reorganized since 1988, both as much as a consequence resulting from the health reform processes as from the deep changes in Brazilian economic and social changes over a quarter of a century. Quality of care and patient safety issues slowly entered the healthcare agenda in the private and public sectors. By the 2010s, many problems have not been solved, but quality and safety considerations have a clear place on that agenda.

1	A good review of the Brazilian healthcare system can be found in an article published by Paim et al. in the 2011, Health in Brazil series of *The Lancet*.

The Current Situation

One may say that Brazil has a dual-level, but interconnected, healthcare system. Twenty-five percent of the population, the upper strata of people's income distribution, despite being entitled to the publicly financed unified health system, is also covered by private health plans and insurance. About 80 percent of this coverage is contracted by employers with varied degrees of employee participation. Almost all health plans and insurers contract services on a fee for service basis, but most choose fixed reimbursement rates and lists of preferred providers.

The other three-quarters of the population have no other entitlements beyond those services provided under the arrangements of the SUS. The SUS is a three-tiered system with defined roles and processes played by the Union, the 26 States and the Federal District, and the 5,562 municipalities.

Brazil has one of the largest public healthcare systems in the world, free at the point of delivery with egalitarian mandate and provisions. However, the middle level of development of the country and its historically very high wealth disparities pose tremendous challenges for the delivery of high-quality care.

In short, there is a wide differential in the quality of the care provided which is strongly influenced by the amount of and mechanisms available for its financing. The public share of total healthcare spending (43 percent) (Instituto Brasileiro de Geografia e Estatística 2012) is still very low such that it cannot fully assure the rights established in the Constitution. There is a large range of reimbursement for the services provided among the private plans and as compared to the SUS. As an example, the average payment for a single admission to inpatient care by the highest premium health insurances in 2012 (US$9,818) was almost 18 times greater than the payment by the public system (US$550).[2] How to leverage the quality of care so all benefit is thus a major challenge. Some health services are likely to be exposing patients to significant hazards and damages.

Healthcare reform in Brazil celebrated its quarter of a century anniversary in 2013. The major processes and changes have therefore had a reasonable time span to mature, even more so within a country facing the challenges to overcome the huge historical handicaps both in social and economic development. More recently Brazil is embarking on more progressive changes in its pathways toward greater development and social and economic equality.

Access to healthcare has expanded following an important set of laws and regulations passed after the 1988 Constitution. A few of them can be noted as having particular impact in the quality of care beyond financial arrangements. In 1990, a key structure of social participation and control was passed, determining the organization of health councils at the three levels of Government: Federal, State, and Municipal (Law 8142/1990). The composition of these councils is

---

2 Derived from data available for the private plans (Agência Nacional de Saúde Suplementar 2013) and calculated for the SUS with data obtained from the Ministry of Health (DATASUS n.d.).

designed to reflect the major stakeholders in the healthcare arena. Fifty percent of their members must be users, including labor representatives, neighborhood associations, and patient interest groups. A further quarter are represented by health professionals and academics and the remaining quarter by healthcare providers' representatives, public and private. These councils, besides their legal responsibilities of overseeing the healthcare provisions in their respective tier, play an important role in raising quality of care issues. In 2012 their roles and obligations were further regulated, requiring health plans and budgets to be formally approved and monitored by them (Complementary Law 141/2012).

The Quality and Safety Landscape

Regulatory Agencies

The first major move in the quality field was in the regulatory domain. In 1999 a law was passed completely restructuring the health surveillance system (Law 9872/1999). The law determined the organization of a national system, with roles defined for the three levels of Government under the coordination of a federal agency then created under the Ministry of Health—the National Agency of Health Surveillance (ANVISA). The ANVISA's scope of activities includes, besides norms concerning licensing and auditing of health services, a full range of roles in food, drug, and border regulations. Typically, standards are federal and surveillance is delegated to states and municipalities, although these levels may produce additional norms to address local conditions and issues.

In the mid 1990s quality improvement awareness emerged and entered the healthcare leadership agenda, both in the public and private sector. Aligned with other countries in implementing strategies to improve the quality of care and safety of the patient, Brazil has been developing initiatives which, albeit fragmented, seek to improve the quality of healthcare in both the public and the private sectors. These initiatives have been implemented at different levels of the management system, in various areas of care, and with different types of emphases, including monitoring, evaluation, the introduction of new practices, and the dissemination of scientific information, amongst others.

In 2000, a national agency was created by law to oversee and monitor health plan insurers, called National Agency of Supplementary Health (Law 9661/2000). All health plans and insurers are required to register with the agency and comply with a series of requisites varying from providing data on their beneficiaries, to financial sustainability, and quality of care offered by their contracted care providers.

Quality Improvement Approaches

In 1995, the Ministry of Health launched a program aimed at improving quality based on five main points: the use of performance indicators (institutional and population), the adoption of a hospital accreditation system conducted by non-governmental agencies, the use of tools to improve quality, the establishment of clinical guidelines, and the strengthening of community/consumer control over healthcare (Noronha & Rosa 1999).

In the area of hospital accreditation, several initiatives are worth mentioning. In 1986, the Brazilian College of Surgeons created the Standing Committee for the Qualification of Hospitals. The Sao Paulo association of medicine and the regional council of medicine of Sao Paulo set up the Hospital Quality Control Program (CQH) in 1990.

At the end of the 1990s, the Ministry of Health produced a standards manual focused on the health system's structure. It had a list of chapters covering the organization of care, diagnostic and therapeutic support, logistics and administrative services.

In 1994, the National Academy of Medicine, the Brazilian College of Surgeons and the State University of Rio de Janeiro got together to create a Committee of Evaluation and Quality Improvement of Health Services. In 1998, these institutions created the Brazilian Consortium of Accreditation of Systems and Health Services (CBA) which partnered with Joint Commission International (JCI) and developed international accreditation processes.

Federal Government[3]

ANVISA

Although national ANVISA requirements are for licensing of services, in the mid-1990s ANVISA expanded its activities towards a broader approach:

• In 1997, ANVISA launched the National Program to Control Hospital Infections, aspiring to reduce the rate of infections within health services by 30 percent, in addition to ensuring guidance for basic healthcare measures. It also aimed to prevent the indiscriminate use of antibiotics and hospital germicides, attempting to prevent resistance and contributing to a marked decrease in overall hospital costs.

• Launched in 2001, the Rede Sentinela de Hospitais (Sentinel Hospitals Network) project acts as an active observer of the performance and safety of regularly used health products, encouraging the organization of health risk management teams within hospitals, and implementation of improvement plans focused on the rational use of medicines and technology. In addition, it sought information about adverse events and technical complaints related

---

3 The following paragraphs containing an inventory of Brazilian initiatives were extracted from a part of the technical report "Qualidade dos Serviços de Saúde no SUS" (Quality of Health Services in the SUS) commissioned to the Oswaldo Cruz Foundation by the Federal Ministry of Health, co-authored by this chapter's authors, delivered in December 2013 (Unpublished to date).

to health products and subsequently notified ANVISA about these issues using the online Health Surveillance Notification system (NOTIVISA).

- Established in 2004, the National Network for the Investigation of Outbreaks and Adverse Events in Health Services (RENISS) aimed to train a multidisciplinary team to work to reduce the severity of cases and the number of people affected by investigating possible risk factors and the sources and causes of outbreaks. Thus, this would help to better understand the dynamic of the occurrence of these types of events and guide changes in care practices and regulations.

- The National Network for Monitoring Microbial Resistance in Health Services (RedeRM) was set up in 2004 to increase the effectiveness of healthcare through timely detection and the rational use of antimicrobial agents as well as to prevent and control the emergence and spread of antimicrobial resistance in health services in the country.

- In 2007, the Hand Hygiene in Health Services Program was launched, aligned with Organizzazione Mondiale della Sanità's "Clean Care is Safe Care" program. Its aim was to reduce the spread of infections and multi-resistant microorganisms as well as reduce the number of patients who contract preventable infections related to their healthcare.

- The NOTIVISA was developed in 2009. The main objective of the system is to strengthen the post-use/post-marketing surveillance of products by monitoring adverse events and technical defects related to them. This service provides an information system which notifies of adverse events and technical defects related to the following products under health surveillance: drugs, vaccines and immunoglobulins, medical articles, medical and hospital equipment, in vitro diagnostic products, use of blood or components, cosmetics, toiletries and perfume, disinfectants, and pesticides.

- In 2012 Patients for Patient Safety in Healthcare Program was initiated which is based on the World Health Organization (WHO) program of the same title. The main objective is to provide the general public with tools and information about health hazards and answer questions about the healthcare process to enhance the quality of care in clinics, during surgical procedures, hospitalizations, and clinical examinations. Patients and their families become active participants in decisions about the quality and safety of their care.

Federal Ministry of Health

- Launched in 2001, the National Humanization Policy (HumanizaSUS) aimed to put the SUS principles into practice in the daily routine of the health services, bringing about changes in management and care methods, involving health professionals, managers and users.

- The Safe Surgery Program was launched in 2009 in line with the WHO's "Safe Surgery Saves Lives" Program. The aim was to improve quality and ensure safety of surgical interventions, which would gradually result in more lives being saved and more disabilities being prevented. It also intends to raise the desired standards in health services. These include: (1) prevention of surgical infections, (2) safe anesthesia, (3) safe surgical teams, and (4) surgical care indicators.
- The Improving Quality and Access to Primary Care Program (PMAQ-AB) was launched in 2011. It sought to increase access to and improve the quality of primary care, with a comparable guaranteed standard of quality at national, regional, and local level, so as to enable greater transparency and effectiveness of Government measures aimed at primary healthcare throughout Brazil. The program targets family health teams and state and municipal managers. It involves the external assessment of the conditions of access and the quality of all of the municipalities and teams taking part in the program which takes place after the teams have been trained. In conjunction with educational and research institutions, the Ministry of Health carries out visits to the teams to assess a number of aspects, from infrastructure and inputs to issues related to the work process.
- Formalized in 2011, the Training and Quality Improvement in the Health Care Network Program (QualiSUS-Rede) includes a strategic systems intervention component focused on national priorities and supporting the implementation of care networks and a definition of healthcare whose scope includes: support for the organization and quality of healthcare management, management and classification of healthcare, quality in healthcare, technology and innovation in health, funding mechanisms and allocation of resources, and monitoring and evaluation of sub-projects.
- The 2011 Evidence-Based Health Portal is a joint initiative between the Ministry of Health and Coordination for the Improvement of Higher Education Personnel (Capes/MEC) which aims to provide rapid access to scientific knowledge by means of current and systematically reviewed publications. It is targeted to professionals in the fields of biology, biomedicine, physical education, nursing, pharmacy, physiotherapy, and occupational therapy, speech therapy, medicine, veterinary medicine, nursing, dentistry, psychology, and social work.
- The latest Ministry of Health initiative is the National Patient Safety Program (PNSP), launched in April 2013. The PNSP has the overall objective of contributing to the quality of healthcare in all health facilities nationwide.

Overarchingly, the main strategies are to promote and support the implementation of initiatives focused on patient safety in different areas of care, organization, and management of health services through the implantation of risk management and patient safety nuclei in health facilities, involve the patient and their families in patient safety measures, increase the general public's access to information on patient safety, produce, systematize, and disseminate information on patient safety, and promote the inclusion of the subject of patient safety in technical, undergraduate, and post-graduate courses in the area of health.

A National Patient Safety Program Committee (CIPNSP) has been established and it has developed proposals for strategies to implement the program. Protocols were developed and distributed relating to: Patient Identification, Safety in Surgery, Safety in the Prescription, Use, and Management of Medicines, the Practice of Hand Hygiene in Health Services, Fall Prevention, and Pressure Ulcer Prevention. A host site was created to access all the information and documents relating to the Program.

In addition, all health services in the country are asked to appoint a center for patient safety to manage all actions related to risk management and patient safety in healthcare processes.

Oswaldo Cruz Foundation—Fiocruz

The Collaborating Center for Quality of Care and Patient Safety (PROQUALIS), based in the Oswaldo Cruz Foundation Fiocruz, was created in 2009 to contribute to the improvement of health practices, in order to make them more safe and effective. The main activities of PROQUALIS are related to the portal available on the website www.proqualis.net.

The center works on identifying, selecting, and editing scientific literature for publication on the portal, production of content such as lessons, videos, reviews, and other; translation and adaptation of relevant content from WHO and other leading institutions; the creation and utilization of profiles and channels on social network sites; and the identification and publication of initiatives to implement safety practices in hospitals of excellence in hospital management.

Allied to these national measures, a significant number of initiatives and programs have been established at state and municipal levels of Government. Many have beneficial effects on the quality of care provided.

Initiatives of Private Institutions

The CQH developed by the Sao Paulo Medical Association in conjunction with the Sao Paulo Regional Council of Medicine aims to contribute to the continuing improvement of the quality of hospital organizations. It encourages participation and self-assessment, as well as containing a very important educational component, which is an incentive to change attitudes and behaviors.

The "National Quality Award" has been conferred by the Foundation for the National Quality (FNQ) Award since 1991 and is aimed at encouraging improvement in the quality of management and increased competitiveness between organizations. Companies who enter themselves for the award then have their management performance evaluated by trained FNQ examiners. At the end of the process, the companies are given a broad assessment report. The winning companies are considered models of competent organizations.

The Accreditation of Health Services is carried out according to the decisions of the institutions, using national and/or international methodology, the latter of which is based on Canadian and North American models.

The accreditation program, using the methodology of the National Accreditation Organisation (ONA), has been in use since 1999 and aims to promote the implementation of ongoing assessment and certification of quality in health services. It is aimed at continually improving care in institutions providing health services. Accrediting institutions, themselves accredited by the ONA, and applying the standards of the Brazilian Accreditation System and the Brazilian Accreditation Manual—(ONA specific), are responsible for the accreditation evaluation process.

The International Accreditation of Health Services, using the methodology of the JCI has been carried out by the Consortium for Brazilian Accreditation (CBA) since 1998. The objective is to help to improve the quality of services provided to the patient through a process of accreditation of organizations of health service providers who apply to the process employing the methodology and standards of the JCI.

The International Accreditation of Health Services, using the methodology of Accreditation Canada has been carried out by the Qualisa Management Institute since 2006, adopting Canadian methodology.

The Guidelines Project was developed in 2000 by the Brazilian Medical Association in conjunction with the Federal Council of Medicine. It has developed clinical guidelines for a significant number of clinical conditions.

The Brazilian Association of Private Hospitals (ANAHP) developed two initiatives for associated hospitals: the 2002 Integrated System of Hospital Indicators (SINHA) project and the 2004 Better Practices Assistance project. The SINHA Project aims to provide members with ongoing and periodic indicators to encourage processes for improvement in the provision of medical and hospital services as well as in the human resources and financial sectors. The strategies used to implement the project were, the definition of indicators, the forming of the Information Board, Analysis and Quality (CIAQ), and the publication of an annual journal of the SINHA project's annual indicators. Each hospital receives the indicators, always protecting the identity of the hospitals. The process of data collection is carried out via the internet and indicators are periodically measured and presented in tables and graphs to participating hospitals. The indicators are published in the *Obervatorio* magazine.

The "Better Care Practices" Project, aims to generate subsidies for continuous improvement in the quality of healthcare and excellence in patient care, monitoring the indicators of participating hospitals. The implementation strategies are as follows: 1) Hospitals were provided with the list of 100 medical guidelines developed by the Brazilian Medical Association and the Federal Council of

Medicine, so that those of interest could be implemented in each hospital institution and 2) together with its team of doctors and clinical staff, established its performance line, including the development of clinical and managerial indicators, so that through the measuring of results, it was possible to make an objective analysis of the work.

Implementation: Barriers and Solutions

It becomes evident when analyzing the spectrum of initiatives currently in place in the country and the historical timeline of implementation, that quality of care and patient safety concerns have acquired a priority status in Brazil. However, it must be said that the most effective and widespread measures have occurred in the regulatory domains.

Unfortunately there is a strong punitive approach associated with rigid regulatory prescriptive norms that often impedes the development of a blameless culture, promoting a defensive attitude among healthcare providers, be they health professionals or organizations. An important segment of the media strongly contributes to the search for someone or something to blame, quickly identifying and exposing persons, organizations, or Governments to be guilty of any mishap.

In spite of current progress, the medical profession in general remains reluctant to both admit to the occurrence of errors or adverse events, and to accept shared knowledge or strategies to promote inter-professional collaboration. Public institutions are very much vulnerable to political point-scoring by opponents or by the media. Private groups fear losing their market share.

On the other hand, the growing engagement of informed users demanding—and wanting to help provide—good quality of care has helped to disseminate among providers a culture of demonstrating that they are engaged in an ethos of improving the quality of their care. And the occasional "safety scandals" exposed in the media can put Governments on notice, stimulating them to advance safety policies.

The Future

How to actually achieve the Constitutional desiderata of providing egalitarian access to quality healthcare for all citizens irrespective of their ability to pay for is the greatest challenge lying ahead for Brazil. This means that the country faces a long journey in order to overcome its social and economic development constraints and increase the overall wealth to be shared in an equitable way. The public healthcare system, SUS, is very much underfinanced and this must be corrected. Many facilities are underequipped and understaffed. Poor areas still struggle to have a permanent medical doctor to serve their population.

Health professionals must constantly renew their commitment to safe and good quality care. Medical and other professional schools should introduce concepts and approaches on quality and safety of care in their curricula. As the epidemiological profile of the population evolves and there is a growing burden of non-communicable diseases, the delivery of healthcare needs to be profoundly reshaped. The blurring between health and social care, the multi-morbidity patterns presented by an ageing population increasingly require the implementation of networks of integrated care. Stronger coordination among providers is required and the fragmentation of care observed in competing private organizations needs to be reversed.

Currently Brazilian healthcare reform movements are very much oriented toward these goals. In 2011, a Presidential Decree (Decree 7508/2011) was passed mandating the reorganization of the SUS along the lines of regional healthcare networks of integrated care. This implies a redefinition of the roles of the three levels of Government. Public and private partnerships for the delivery of care are being strengthened. In the private sector, health plans and insurers are increasingly restructuring their networks of providers in a similar direction.

In the domain of quality of care it is expected that the patient safety program initiated in 2013 will progressively augment its reach and scope. More structured quality bodies or agencies are expected to come into existence in forthcoming years.

Brazil has an identifiable, acquired maturity in demonstrating that the burdens of underdevelopment and inequity can be overcome with political will and people's engagement and participation. The scarcity of resources has not been an insurmountable impediment to move towards safer and better care more equitably provided to Brazil's citizens.

Chapter 17
Chile

Giorgio Solimano and Leonel Valdivia[1]

Abstract

Over the past decade, Chile has implemented several significant health reform initiatives, including "Universal Access with Explicit Guarantees" (Acceso Universal con Garantías Explícitas—AUGE), which guarantees opportune, quality, and financially protected treatment for 80 priority health conditions. While these reforms have achieved considerable improvements in access to healthcare, even for the most disadvantaged groups, the impact of the policies is not yet sufficiently felt in the quality and safety of healthcare, particularly in the public system. Several mechanisms have been established to provide quality assurance and safety of care, and an institutional framework is in place for its enforcement at both national and regional levels. Full and successful implementation of the reforms, however, has faced obstacles in terms of the availability of expert human resources, the resolutive capacity of the primary care centers, and the timeliness of attention. It is expected that the administration of the New Majority will address these pressing issues and continue to thoroughly evaluate and improve the healthcare system's quality and effectiveness for the entire Chilean population.

Background

Current healthcare reform initiatives in Chile date back to the early 2000s, during the administration of President Ricardo Lagos (Bastias & Valdivia 2007, Erazo 2011). These reforms, beginning with the passage of Law 19.996 in 2004, focus on health promotion, protection, and recovery (República de Chile 2008). The aforementioned law expanded coverage of medical services through a system of legally binding, explicit care guarantees for the most prevalent pathologies in the country, AUGE. A group of experts meet annually to decide which pathologies should be included based on several criteria, including burden of disease, socioeconomic and gender inequality, societal (population) preferences, associated costs, and cost-effectiveness (Ministerio de Salud 2002). At present, 80

1 Acknowledgement: The authors gratefully acknowledge Sara Schilling, MPH student at the University of Chile, School of Public Health, for her invaluable assistance with data collection and processing, and extensive text editing.

Table 17.1   Demographic, economic, and health information for Chile

Population (thousands)	17,465
Area (sq. km)*	743,532
Proportion of population living in urban areas (2011)	89
Gross Domestic Product (GDP US$, billions)^	269.9
Total expenditure on health as % of GDP	7.2
Gross national income per capita (PPP intl $)	21,310
Per capita total expenditure on health (intl $)	1,606
Proportion of health expenditure which is private	51.4
General Government expenditure on health as a percentage of total expenditure on health	48.6
Out-of-pocket expenditure as a percentage of private expenditure on health	62.5
Life expectancy at birth m/f (yrs)	77/83
Probability of dying under five (per 1,000 live births)	9
Maternal Mortality Ratio (per 100,000 live births) (2013)	22
Proportion of population using improved water and sanitation	99/99

Source: Unless otherwise stated data are for the year 2012 and taken from the World Health Organization 2014. * Area from the World Bank 2014a. ^GDP from the World Bank 2014b.

Note: PPP is purchasing power parity, intl $ is international dollar which has the same purchasing power as US$ in the US.

pathologies are covered by AUGE (see Table 17.2 for included conditions, listed by their year of incorporation) (Ministerio de Salud 2013).

There has been limited evaluation of the effects of AUGE to date, but available evidence indicate that while medical care coverage expansion has been relatively successful, quality, safety, and equity of healthcare offerings has not met expectations (Erazo 2011, Paraje & Vásquez 2012, Luis Vera Benavides 2012, Unger et al. 2008). The most important efforts to improve healthcare include expanding availability of medical specialists, producing clinical protocols for AUGE pathologies, strengthening partnership with private providers, and improving quality standards for accreditation.

In Chile, attempts at health reforms in the 1990s came at a time when the country was emerging from a 17-year military dictatorship, characterized by the imposition of a neoliberal ideology affecting all aspects of the Chilean society and particularly social policies and programs (Erazo 2011). For over 20 years, Chile lived with the inheritance of the dictatorship with a superficially reformed Constitution, and a mixed (public and private) health system based on a market approach to healthcare provision. At present, the country, with a center-left New Majority ("Nueva Mayoria") administration, led by the re-elected President Michelle Bachelet, is on the threshold of major political reforms, such as an authentically democratic constitution and social reform strengthening public services and limiting private sector profit in health, social security, and education. We are entering an exciting era, and there is much progress to be made.

Introduction

Chile has a long history of healthcare and public health reforms, with improvement efforts dating back to 1924 with the Workers Insurance Act, followed by the Preventive Medicine Act of 1938, and culminating with the creation of the National Health Service in 1952. All these reform efforts focused on protecting the disadvantaged population, such as reducing the prevailing high infant mortality rate due to infectious diseases and malnutrition, and maternal mortality rates mainly due to obstetric risks related to lack of access to contraceptives leading to unsafe abortions. In the mid-seventies, under the military Government, drastic changes were made in the provision of healthcare services, including the weakening of the public system and the imposition of a market approach to health financing through the establishment of individual private health insurance.

This chapter presents a case study of Chile, a country achieving considerable progress in the expansion of service coverage but still weak in improving quality and safety. Such weakness is inherent to unresolved health equity issues.

The Current Situation

From an organizational point of view, the original National Health Service was transformed into the National Health System in 1980, which remains in place to date. This system consists of a network of 29 autonomous territorial healthcare services, that are responsible for hospital care—both inpatient and ambulatory—and supervise over 300 urban and rural primary care centers, which are managed by municipal authorities.

The Chilean healthcare system has succeeded in numerous areas: expansion and strengthening of the primary healthcare (PHC) network, the eradication or control of major infectious diseases, significant improvement in health status indicators, a well-established health authority and supervision system, a consistent increase in budgetary allocation, and extension of the country's healthcare infrastructure.

On the other hand, the system also has various weaknesses: the prevailing inequities in healthcare quality and safety associated with user's income level, the high level of centralization and concentration of health resources in the Capital of Santiago and a few other large cities, and a shortage of professional health human resources necessary to provide adequate care to the majority of the population.

The overarching challenge facing Chilean healthcare, as mentioned above, is the need to ensure better quality and safety of care for users of both the public and private systems, in order to diminish the evident disparities. An urgent task the new administration must take on is the ongoing evaluation and improvement of health services and their administrative and clinical procedures, in order to provide better quality care.

Reform Initiatives

The responsibility for initiating and monitoring reform efforts lies chiefly with the Ministry of Health and, to a lesser extent, with the health authorities of the 15 regions of the country, while the implementation of these reforms is the responsibility of the healthcare service network. In addition, there is a Health Superintendent Office responsible for supervising both public and private providers.

Noteworthy among Chilean healthcare indicators is the low rate of general mortality, which has remained stable since the early 1990s at 5.5 per 1,000. Infant mortality in 1992 was 15.1 per 1,000 and decreased to 10 per 1,000 in 2011 (Departamento de Estadísticas e Información de Salud n.d.). During the past decade, there has been a marked increase in the number of beneficiaries in the public sector, with coverage reaching 76.2 percent in 2011, alongside a concomitant decrease in the number of private system users.

The Quality and Safety Landscape

Although responsibility for healthcare monitoring tasks has been delegated, as described above, quality and safety standards still tend to be fairly basic in the public system, and there is unfortunately little to no supervision and evaluation of existing practices. Thus, private providers use their superior quality and safety as a publicity mechanism to attract clientele.

Other relevant stakeholders include the private-for-profit sector, civil society, and the judicial system. Firstly, private sector entities are entrenched in the defense of corporate interests and often significantly increase premium costs of insurance, limit plans' benefits, protect pharmaceutical patents to block access to generic medications, and lobby on behalf of tobacco, alcohol, and other drug and food industries, in an effort to limit regulatory legislation. Civil society stakeholders—citizens involved in community councils, user groups, and Non-Government Organizations (NGOs)—serve as decision makers in a few, limited instances, but they are decidedly not yet as active in health matters as they are in other issues, such as public education and environmental protection. The judicial system is gradually facing increased demands to prosecute denial of services and unjustified increases in the costs of premiums of healthcare plans. However, no institutionalized judicial mechanisms exist to deal with these demands; legal remedies are in the purview of the Labor Tribunals and the Environmental Public Prosecutor.

The Impact of These Reform Efforts on Quality and Safety of Care

Healthcare reform initiatives in letter and spirit are aimed at improving and safeguarding the quality and safety of care offered by both institutional and individual professional providers. Three specific mechanisms for quality and safety assurance have been established within the AUGE framework: accreditation of institutional providers (such as public hospitals, clinics, and centers); specialty and sub-specialty certification for individual providers; and a national registration system for medical and paramedical personnel. The responsibility for enforcing the standards contained in these instruments lies with the Office of the Health Superintendent within the Ministry of Health. The Health Superintendent is in charge of supervising both the public and private health insurance companies and the institutional and individual care providers, ensuring adherence to published accreditation standards and procedures.

The initiative aimed at improving quality and safety of care—the 2012 Patient Rights and Responsibility Law—is quite recent. While it is early to fully ascertain the impact of this law, it appears to already be having an effect on the behavior of providers, and enhancing the awareness of patients and families about their rights as users of the system. Measures such as informed consent for clinical procedures, as well protection of privacy regulations, are becoming routine at most public and private care establishments.

Additionally, in recent years, there have been efforts to increase regulation of the accreditation of public, as well as private, healthcare institutions, in light of user complaints, some of which reached the judicial system. The Ministry of Health has strengthened the National Accreditation System for Quality Healthcare, and assurance of safe and effective quality care has been incorporated in the national health goals for the 2011–2020 decade (Velasquez 2012, Escobar 2013, Concha 2007). Various instruments and procedures for provider certification and accreditation are in place, and institutions are increasingly going through this process.

The Chilean healthcare reforms, initiated a decade ago, have been, necessarily, a gradual process. Implementation still requires additional measures to fine-tune progress and management of the system, and it is therefore difficult to clearly identify the successful drivers of improvement in quality and safety. We will nevertheless venture to mention a few. The selection of a number of pathologies as priority for treatment through AUGE has tackled the most pressing problems affecting vulnerable groups. An important dimension of the AUGE system is its emphasis on timely, opportune treatment. If expedited care cannot be offered, providers are required to direct patients to any available service, either private or public. This policy has had an important effect on reducing the age-old problem of waiting lists in the public sector: 380,000 people were waiting for treatment of an AUGE condition in 2010, and in June 2013, that number lowered to around 8,000, although with incorporation of new pathologies in July 2013, the waiting list rose to nearly 11,000 in August of 2013 (Sandoval, Fernandez & Perez 2013). The current state of the AUGE waiting lists is being reviewed by the new administration.

Just as it is not yet possible to completely pinpoint the various factors associated with healthcare improvements, it is also difficult to single out reform measures, which have had a negative impact on quality and safety of care. Concerns, however, are being expressed, from various sources, on certain risks derived from some of the basic tenets of the reforms (Erazo 2011, Unger et al. 2008, Missoni & Solimano 2010). As mentioned, the central focus of the reform is the system of explicit guarantees of services (AUGE), which at present prioritizes and, ultimately, guarantees services for 80 selected pathologies (see Table 17.2). While this prioritization makes sense in terms of the country's burden of disease, it bears risk—the danger of neglecting or delaying care for non-prioritized illnesses and conditions. Legally mandated assurance of timeliness of service often forces public hospitals to transfer patients to private providers. While this measure assures timeliness of service, it considerably increases the costs of such services and expands the presence of the private, profit-making sector to the detriment of the public health institutions. In response, the current Ministry of Health administration has declared that new pathologies will not be added to the AUGE list until the situation can be properly assessed, in terms of the clinical solutions and the waiting lists for the 80 pathologies currently guaranteed under AUGE.

Another concern being expressed relates to the danger of excessive judicial litigation in healthcare (Sánchez Rodríguez & Nancuante Almonacid 2013). While the new legislation on patients' rights is considered necessary, and a potentially powerful instrument to improve quality and safety of care, it may herald the danger of over vigilance on the part of providers, which may in turn delay treatment. From the patients' perspective, there may also be excessive appeals to judicial procedures, adding to the cost and administrative burden.

Implementation: Barriers and Solutions

There should be no doubt that the Chilean healthcare reform process underway has achieved progress in increased access to healthcare service, and preliminary work has been done to improve quality and safety (Bastias & Valdivia 2007, Unger et al. 2008). However, there are a number of barriers, related to the availability and deployment of healthcare personnel, infrastructure utilization, and resolutive capacity at the primary care level.

One of the most significant barriers to quality and safety improvement is the shortage and the inadequate distribution of health professionals. The personnel shortage is particularly acute in establishments serving the urban poor and in locations far from the capital or other large cities, especially in small, isolated

2005	2006	2007	2009	2013
Chronic terminal kidney failure	Cholecystectomy (symptomatic 35—49 years)	Medical treatment for mild and moderate hip and/or knee arthosis (≥55 years)	Retinopathy of prematurity	Colorectal cáncer (>15 years)
Operable congenital cardiopathy	Stomach cancer	Subarachnoidalhaemorrhage secondary to rupture of cerebral aneurysms	Pulmonary dysplasia premature	Epithelial ovarian cancer
Cervical cancer	Prostate cancer	Primary central nervous system tumors needing surgery	Bilateral sensorineural hearing loss of prematurity	Bladder Cancer in persons (≥15 years)
Palliative care and pain relief for terminal cancer	Vision impairment (≥65 years)	Herniated lumbar nucleus pulposus needing surgery	Non-refractory epilepsy in persons (≥15 years)	Osteosarcoma in persons (≥15 years)
Acute myocardial infarction	Strabismus (<9 years)	Leukaemia	Bronchial asthma (≥15 years)	Surgical treatment of aortic valve lesions in persons (≥15 years)
Type 1 Diabetes	Diabetic retinopathy	Dental emergencies (ambulatory)	Parkinson's disease	Bipolar disorder in persons (≥15 years)
Type 2 Diabetes	Non-traumatic retinal detachment	Integral dental care (60-year-old adults)	Juvenile idiopathic arthritis	Hypothyroidism in persons (≥15 years)
Breast cancer	Haemophilia	Severe multiple trauma	Secondary prevention of ESRD	Treatment of moderate hearing loss (children <2 years)
Spinal dysraphias	Depression (≥15 years)	Moderate or severe cranial trauma (emergency care)	Laxative hip dysplasia	Lupus Erythematosus
Scoliosis needing surgery (<25 years)	Prostate hyperplasia needing surgery	Severe ocular trauma	Comprehensive oral health of pregnant women	Surgical treatment of lesions of the mitral and tricuspid valves in persons (≥15 years)
Cataracts	Othesis and technical aids (≥65 years)	Cystic fibrosis	Remitting multiple sclerosis recurrent	Eradication therapy for Helicobacter Pylori
Hip replacement for arthosis with severe functional limitation (≥ 65 years)	Stroke (≥15 years)	Rheumatoide arthritis	Hepatitis B	
Cleft palate (born after July 1, 2005)	Chronic obstructive pulmonary disease (ambulatory treatment)	Harmful use and dependence on alcohol and drugs (<20 years)	Hepatitis C	
Childhood cancer (<15)	Moderate and severe asthma (<15 years)	Labor analgesia		
Schizophrenia (fist symptoms after July 1, 2005)	Neonatal respiratory distress syndrome	Major burns		
Testicular cancer		Bilateral hearing loss needing a hearing aid (≥65 years)		
Lymphoma				
HIV/AIDS				
Upper and lower respiratory infection (<5 years)				
Community-acquired pneumonia susceptible to ambulatory care (≥65 years)				
Primary arterial hypertension (≥15)				
Epilepsy susceptible to treatment in primary care (<15 years)				
Integral dental care (6-year-old children)				
Prematurity				
Alterations of impulse generation and conduction that require pacemaker				

Table 17.2   AUGE included conditions, listed by their year of incorporation

communities. Moreover, the current health workforce has historically been neglected in terms of pay and working conditions, creating frequent labor unrest and strikes, which greatly affects the quality of care. Low pay in the public sector often means that health professionals, particularly physicians, tend to hold jobs at both public and private establishments, in addition to maintaining their own private practices.

Physicians with several jobs normally attend to their public sector responsibilities for only a few hours a day, and see many patients within those short periods. In turn, limited time availability of physicians results in over scheduled healthcare services, extremely rushed care of patients, and underutilization of the healthcare infrastructure. This problem is compounded by the fact that most healthcare teams lack coordination and communication, which are much needed to provide comprehensive and high-quality care to patients.

The healthcare reform process has not been able to reduce the historically heavy dependence on tertiary care institutions. Overcrowded public hospitals remain a permanent feature of the healthcare system, which hampers the quality of the care provided. Although Chile has an extensive PHC network, its limited resolutive capacity does not motivate patients to stop going directly to hospitals to resolve their medical needs, however minor, and only exacerbates their dependence on tertiary care.

Several enablers and implementation opportunities for quality and safety improvement can be elicited. First among them is the profound need to strengthen the diagnostic and treatment capabilities of the PHC network, which implies the availability of basic instruments, lab facilities, and other diagnostic tools, as well as trained personnel. Partial deployment of specialists to the PHC units will strengthen their resolutive capacities and reduce dependency on hospitals. Second, referral and counter-referral processes in the healthcare network should be expedited. Third, the healthcare team approach should be revamped, with physicians playing a leading, but not monopolizing, role, to improve trust, collaboration, and communication among the professionals in the PHCs. Fourth, quality of healthcare would be improved by resolving the historical debt with the public health workforce, in terms of their salaries, contracts, and working conditions. Finally, the Chilean health reform would be greatly strengthened with the formulation of an explicit healthcare human resource policy, which strategically anticipates the medium- and long-term needs of the population, in line with the evolution of the epidemiological and demographic profile of the country.

Prospects for Success and Next Steps

Chile's extensive experience in health reform shows that no quick fixes are possible. Prospects for success are dependent on a number of factors, many of them outside the sphere of influence of the health sector, such as improvement in the public education system, overcoming social and economic disparities, empowerment and participation of the civil society, sustainable economic growth, and social development. In addition, healthcare reform requires a long-term, strategic perspective, and avoidance of the current emphasis on short-term results that, although very visible through public announcements by health authorities, do not radically modify the root causes of the problems. The success of such reforms will require an active role of the state in terms of supervision, enforcement, and evaluation of the implemented policies and programs.

In addition to healthcare reform legislation, a judicial framework must be developed that will enable courts to adequately prosecute the infringement of health laws and any other unlawful behavior of health providers, pharmaceutical companies, and health insurance companies, among others.

A necessary next step is the elevation and enhancement of the role of universities and research centers in educating and training the required human resources, as well as expanding research to generate scientific evidence in support of policy formulation, strategy development, and program evaluation, responsive to the priority needs of the country. Furthermore, the sharing of ideas among academic institutions and their integration with public service providers are important pre-requisites for healthcare quality improvement.

A positive development that favors the prospects of success is the increasingly active participation, in recent years, of civil society. Several interest groups have emerged, rallying around specific diseases, such as cancer, diabetes, lupus, and multiple sclerosis. These organizations act as pressure groups vis-à-vis the Government and its policies. Citizens are increasingly present in the decision-making process at the Executive Councils of public hospitals, and their participation and vigilance of resource allocation is expected to be a factor in ensuring improved quality of service.

Ultimately, health reform initiatives are closely linked to and dependent on long-term, cultural changes in society. In Chile, one clear example of a needed radical cultural change is overcoming the notion of healthcare as a market commodity and adopting the notion of healthcare as a human right. Undoubtedly, this type of cultural change will take time, but it is a fundamental pre-condition for a successful health reform, guaranteeing quality and safety of service for all.

Chapter 18
Mexico

Enrique Ruelas, Octavio Gómez-Danté, and Walverly Morales

Abstract

A major, comprehensive, system-wide quality improvement strategy for healthcare was launched in Mexico in January, 2001, for a six-year period. This strategy was one of the key components of a health reform initiated by a new Government that took office in December, 2000. This strategy, called the National Crusade for Quality in Healthcare, encompassed several interventions aimed at improving technical and interpersonal quality. This chapter summarizes each of these interventions and reflects on some lessons learned. The main messages are that the sum of quality improvements of individual healthcare providers, processes or even units, is not necessarily equal to the quality of the whole system, that in order to improve quality system-wide it is necessary to design a comprehensive strategy, and that this is possible in a middle-income country.

Introduction

On December 1, 2000, a new administration took office in Mexico for a six-year term. A month and a half later, a comprehensive system-wide quality improvement strategy was launched by the President of Mexico, Vicente Fox, in a ceremony that gathered all the key actors within the healthcare system: public and private healthcare provider organizations, union leaders from all major public provider institutions, heads of the associations of schools of medicine and nursing, leaders of healthcare professional associations, representatives of the National Academies of Medicine and Surgery, and the National College of Nurses, as well as representatives of the pharmaceutical industry and the unions of the main healthcare provider institutions, among others. The strategy was called the National Crusade for Quality in Healthcare, and was a central component of a healthcare reform initiative that was implemented during that period. The main objective of this strategy was to promote the necessary changes to establish quality of care as a core value in the culture of healthcare organizations, both public and private, and improve the technical and interpersonal quality of healthcare services system-wide.

The purpose of this chapter is to describe this strategy which included: the establishment of an explicit ethical platform for healthcare providers and

Table 18.1   Demographic, economic, and health information for Mexico

Population (thousands)	121,000
Area (sq. km)*	1,943,950
Proportion of population living in urban areas (2011)	78
Gross Domestic Product (GDP US$, billions)^	1,178.1
Total expenditure on health as % of GDP	6.2
Gross national income per capita (PPP intl $)	16,450
Per capita total expenditure on health (intl $)	1,062
Proportion of health expenditure which is private	48.2
General Government expenditure on health as a percentage of total expenditure on health	51.8
Out-of-pocket expenditure as a percentage of private expenditure on health	91.5
Life expectancy at birth m/f (yrs)	73/79
Probability of dying under five (per 1,000 live births)	16
Maternal Mortality Ratio (per 100,000 live births) (2013)	49
Proportion of population using improved water and sanitation	95/85

Source: Unless otherwise stated data are for the year 2012 and taken from the World Health Organization 2014. * Area from the World Bank 2014a. ^GDP from the World Bank 2014b.
Notes: PPP is purchasing power parity, intl $ is international dollar which has the same purchasing power as US$ in the US.

patients, an organizational redesign of the federal Ministry of Health (MoH) and state ministries of health to support this strategy, the development of a quality measurement system, a major training component for healthcare professionals on quality improvement tools (QIT), the implementation of specific quality improvement actions, and the reinforcement of the accreditation system for healthcare facilities. The strategy also included financial incentives for healthcare organizations to implement quality improvement initiatives, the creation of a national quality award for healthcare organizations, and the participation of service users and citizens in monitoring the quality of care of health facilities. Even though the administration that launched this Crusade left office in 2006, the strategy was adopted, with some changes, by the next Government which was in term till 2012 and by the current administration which has been in charge since 2012 and will continue to be until 2018.

The three main messages of this chapter are, first, the sum of quality improvements of individual healthcare providers, processes, or even healthcare units is not necessarily equal to the quality of a whole system. The second is that in order to improve quality system-wide it is necessary to design a comprehensive strategy. Lastly, in the third instance, that it is possible to design and implement a system-wide quality improvement strategy in a middle-income country. The first part describes the comprehensive reform approved by the Mexican Congress in 2003. Part two discusses the conditions that demanded the implementation of a quality improvement strategy for the Mexican health system. Part three is devoted to a discussion of the various components of the strategy and its results, many of which were identified and measured through formal evaluations. The chapter ends with the basic lessons of this initiative, which are of particular relevance for middle-income countries.

Quality and Healthcare Reform

Mexico is a middle-income country with 117 million inhabitants, most of them Spanish speaking. Therefore, it is considered a Latin American country, although it is located in North America along with the United States of America (US) and Canada. It has 33 states and a federal district where the President and most Federal Government offices are located. Even though Mexico was the eleventh largest economy in the world, by 2000, the GDP devoted to healthcare was 5.8 percent, one of the lowest in the Continent. It has a mixed healthcare system with public and private providers. As an example of the proportion of this public–private mix and of the size of the system, there are around 4,000 hospitals in the country, out of which, 3,000 are private and have 25 percent of all beds, whereas 1,000 public hospitals have the remaining 75 percent. In general, most public hospitals are larger and have better trained healthcare professionals and medical equipment. Yet, many people tend to prefer private hospitals, although they have to pay out-of-pocket, because they avoid waiting times and receive friendlier care. Before 2003, there were two major social insurance schemes that covered around 50 percent of the population. The rest had no formal public healthcare coverage. Private insurance has been traditionally scarce since no more than 6 percent of the population is covered by private policies.

A major legislative reform establishing a system of social health protection was approved by a large majority of the Mexican Congress in 2003 (Frenk 2006, Frenk et al. 2006). This system required reorganizing and increasing public funding by a full percentage point of GDP over eight years in order to provide universal health coverage. The vehicle for achieving this aim was a third public insurance scheme called *Seguro Popular* (Popular Insurance), which now guarantees legislated access to a package of 275 essential health interventions and a package of 57 specialized and costly interventions, including neonatal intensive care, treatment for cancer in children and teenagers, cervical and breast cancer, and HIV/AIDS. The program has elicited an enthusiastic response from the population, such that by December of 2011, 52 million people had enrolled (Gobierno Federal Estados Unidos Mexicanos 2011).

The financial reform has been complemented by a management reform which is strengthening the delivery of services through efficient schemes for drug supply, outcome-oriented information systems, comprehensive planning of new health facilities, technology assessment, and a comprehensive evaluation system. One of the central programs of this managerial reform was the National Crusade for Quality in Healthcare, the purpose of which was to improve patient safety, responsiveness and assure effective healthcare.

Need for a System-Wide Strategy

The initial concerns for quality improvement in the Mexican healthcare system and the first initiatives to achieve it date back to the 1980s, when the first "quality circles" where organized in an acute care public teaching hospital (Ruelas et al. 1990). Other quality improvement initiatives followed this initial experience, but, overall, these were isolated efforts with poor documented evidence of improvement.

In 1994, the Mexican Health Foundation implemented the first National Satisfaction Survey of the Mexican Health System (Fundación Mexicana para la Salud 1994, Ruelas & Querol 1994). The main problem identified by this survey was the low quality of healthcare perceived by the population, followed by insufficient resources and low access to health services. In 1997 the MoH made an assessment of the levels of technical quality in 288 public hospitals. The level of quality was poor on average, with significant variations among hospitals (Secretaría de Salud 2001a). Within one state in Mexico, for example, the assessment found the second best and the worst of all hospitals in the country. In 2000, a second National Satisfaction Survey was implemented with similar results as the previous one. The need was clear: to enhance the public perception on quality of care and improve the technical quality as well as lower, as much as possible, the enormous variations.

With this information at hand, in January of 2001, the new administration of the MoH launched a national quality strategy that was directly supported by the incoming President of Mexico. There was a clear awareness about the possibility of implementing a strategy to address not only specific quality problems in particular organizations and institutions, but a set of interventions to create a wide platform to improve the quality of healthcare at the individual, organizational, and system levels.

National Crusade for Quality in Healthcare

The new President of Mexico, Vicente Fox, was elected in July 2000 and he immediately appointed several transition teams to develop action plans for a Government that was to take office on December 1, 2000. Between August and December of that year, the health transition team designed a system-wide quality improvement strategy that was embedded in a National Health Program that promised to address the problems of equity, quality, and financial protection of the Mexican health system (Secretaría de Salud 2001b). The name for the strategy was "National Crusade for Quality in Healthcare" and was chosen in order to create a sense of urgency and a common aim, since the word "crusade" is defined as "a remedial enterprise undertaken with zeal and enthusiasm" (Merriam-Webster. com n.d.).

Within the health transition team, a group of five people chaired by the future Deputy Minister for Innovation and Quality at the MoH was established to design the strategy. A conceptual model was developed considering, among other factors, the following: values, key processes to be improved, indicators, information system, training, incentives, expected outcomes, change management, organizational culture, and leadership. A framework for the strategy was also designed and it included a vision towards 2006 and 2025, a visual image, challenges to be overcome, objectives, operational strategies, and specific actions.

Feasibility Assessment

Three different assessments examining the feasibility of implementing a system-wide strategy were made. The first was conducted during the design stage and the other two during the first 100 days of the new Government.

For the first assessment, two external groups of around 20 experts from a wide variety of backgrounds in healthcare were formed. These two groups were gathered separately to make an assessment of the proposed strategy with the following criteria: integrity, internal consistency, clarity, potential to motivate, feasibility of implementation within a six-year period, and risk of failure. The results of both groups were compared and the coincidence in the marks given by both gave an indication that the strategy might have a high potential of success (Secretaría de Salud 2001a).

During the first 100 days of the new Government, two surveys were made, one to healthcare providers and the other to users of healthcare facilities. The purpose was to identify their perception of the need to improve the quality of care and implement a specific strategy to do so. It was encouraging to learn that both groups agreed in their perceptions.

Framework

The vision of the Crusade towards 2006 was that by the end of the period, quality should be explicitly recognized as an important value within the culture of healthcare organizations, and that improvement would be evident throughout the system and able to be perceived by patients and the general population.

The visual image included a logo and a single word. The logo for the strategy was a smiling face using a stethoscope ending in a heart shape, which encapsulated the two dimensions of quality, the technical and the interpersonal. The word *sonríe* (smile), was proposed as an acrostic which proved to be very useful to convey not only a target but an operational definition of quality to healthcare providers since the Spanish word "sonríe" allows to build the following words with the first three letters: safety (*seguridad*), opportunity (*oportunidad*), and met needs (*necesidades satisfechas*). The following three letters were split in two branches, one for technical quality—outcomes (*resultados*), indicators (*indicadores*), and effectiveness (*efectividad*)—and the other branch for the interpersonal dimension—respect (*respeto*), information (*información*), and empathy (*empatía*).

The main challenges to be overcome were to improve quality, reduce variation, and improve public perceptions on quality of healthcare. Overall, the main objective was to increase the quality of healthcare and the level of satisfaction with the healthcare system. In order to achieve this objective, 70 actions were defined and grouped in the following ten categories:

Ethical platform
During 2001, different ethically-oriented documents were developed by groups of nurses and doctors with the endorsement of key academic organizations. These documents, and their summarized contents in posters, were widely distributed in healthcare facilities: patient's rights, code of ethics for health professionals, and physician's and nurses' rights.

Education on quality and about quality
Three main actions can be mentioned in this regard: first, the implementation of training programs on quality improvement for health professionals; second, the implementation of a National Quality in Health Care Forum as a gathering of all those interested in learning and sharing experiences on quality improvement in all kinds of settings; and third, the creation of an incentive to increase the number of accredited schools of medicine. The first action reached over 58,000 healthcare professionals from all over the country across a five-year period. The Forum started in 2003. By 2006 the number of attendants on site was 2,000, and virtually (through the internet), 11,000. The third action consisted of a regulation issued by the MoH which blocked access to healthcare facilities to students from non-accredited schools of medicine.

Indicators
A set of 50 indicators was established to be monitored. The plan was to implement them gradually through the six-year period. By the end of the term only 17 were measured regularly, among them: waiting times (in primary care units and in hospitals), fully filled-in prescriptions in public healthcare facilities, satisfaction with the information provided to patients on their diagnosis and treatments, care of pregnant women, care of children with diarrhea, care of diabetic patients, care of hypertensive patients, rate of cesarean sections, and hospital infection rates.

Monitoring

Several mechanisms for monitoring the indicators were designed and implemented. The first was the "Quality Indicators" (INDICA) system. This is an electronic database that, by the end of 2006, was providing information on the 17 indicators from over 7,000 healthcare facilities. The second was a monthly survey implemented by the Office of the President of Mexico to monitor the satisfaction levels of users of healthcare units all over the country. Even though the trend in the level of satisfaction was very stable during the first five years of the Administration, a slight improvement was demonstrated towards the sixth year. The third mechanism was called "Calidatel," a toll-free telephone number to address complaints and suggestions to healthcare organizations. The fourth was an annual publication called the *Observatory of Hospital Performance* with a benchmarking format that allowed comparison of the performance of public hospitals from different institutions and states.

Specific quality improvement actions

Hundreds of specific quality improvement actions were documented throughout the six-year period to improve clinical and administrative processes as well as patient satisfaction, both in hospitals and primary healthcare units.

Recognition

Three actions were implemented in this regard: the National Quality in Health Care Award, performance agreements, and citizen endorsement groups. The award was granted for the first time in 2003 to one hospital and one primary healthcare center among 87 participating facilities. By 2006 the number of participating facilities reached 1,929. Performance agreements were designed to provide financial incentives to those healthcare units that justified the need for financial resources to implement simple but effective quality improvement actions. Between 2002 and 2006, 512 primary healthcare centers and 219 hospitals benefited from around US$10 million. The "citizen-endorsement groups" initiative is described in the following section.

Citizen Participation

The purpose of the "citizen-endorsement groups" was to train groups of volunteers from the community to assess the responsiveness of healthcare facilities through pre-designed checklists (Ruelas 2006). Once an assessment was made, the group would make recommendations to the executive team of the facility and agree on the improvements to be made and the timeframe to achieve the suggested improvements. If the unit met the agreements it was "endorsed" by the group. In 2006, there were 1764 active citizen groups, one per hospital or primary healthcare center; 1,210 were groups formed by people living in the surroundings of a particular healthcare facility and the rest were non-governmental organizations, universities, and even employees of business companies that attended a nearby unit. That same year, 1,153 units were endorsed. Due to this initiative, the Federal

MoH was granted the 2005 "Transparency Award" by the National Institute of Public Administration of Mexico, which rates all governmental efforts to provide good services to the population.

Processes standardization
Several processes were standardized in public facilities, including the care in emergency units and the care of pregnant women, children with diarrhea, diabetic patients, and patients with hypertension. This action evolved in the following administration to the development of more than 300 clinical guidelines which are now in place.

Accreditation of healthcare organizations
From 1999, a voluntary accreditation system of hospitals was established under the responsibility of the General Health Council of Mexico. In 2001 the standards and survey methods were updated to include standards for patient safety and new standards for different types of healthcare facilities. In the following administration (2006–2012), the whole system was harmonized to meet international accreditation standards. In addition, according to the law that created the System for Social Health Protection, a specific, basic, and compulsory accreditation was established for all units providing services to those affiliated with *Seguro Popular*, a first step towards the more comprehensive accreditation provided by the General Health Council.

Organizational redesign
The reform also included organizational redesign of the federal MoH and the state ministries. One of the Deputy Ministries was renamed Deputy Ministry for Innovation and Quality, the second position in command at the federal MoH. This Deputy Ministry was comprehensively redesigned to include the following general directorates: Health Information, Performance Evaluation, Planning and Development, Quality and Education, and the newly created National Center for Technology Excellence in charge of technology assessment. In addition, 32 local committees in charge of quality-oriented activities were established in each state of the country. Each committee was comprised of representatives from all public healthcare institutions and private providers, and was chaired by the state Minister of Health. In the present administration, around 1,600 quality promoters have been appointed all over the country and quality and safety committees have been established in hospitals and primary healthcare units.

Execution

The execution of the strategy was under the responsibility of a Steering Committee chaired by the Deputy Minister for Innovation and Quality, with the participation of the top medical officers of the main public healthcare institutions. In addition, all state Ministers of Health were given feedback every three months on the performance of their states in a session devoted to the National Crusade within the regular meeting of the National Health Council, the organization that gathers all state Ministers of Health under the chairmanship of the Federal Minister of Health. A key component of the implementation strategy was a set of lectures and conferences dictated by top officers of the MoH in many professional association meetings as well as in hospitals and other healthcare facilities. These lectures were devoted to the discussion of the National Crusade recognizing not only the successes, but also the shortcomings in order to maintain the momentum created from the beginning of the strategy.

Evaluation

Annual external evaluations of the Crusade were requested until 2006. These evaluations provided crucial inputs for the adjustment of this initiative and were critical for the accountability mechanism established by law.

Lessons Learned

The National Crusade for Quality in Healthcare implemented in Mexico offers several lessons for developing countries wishing to develop a system-wide quality improvement culture:

1. A system-wide approach provides high visibility to quality in healthcare in a short period and can therefore influence the whole organizational culture.
2. Implementing a system-wide strategy generates a trade-off between the capacity to create a strong national momentum in a short period of time and a weak control of processes and outcomes.
3. The Crusade indicated that the more interventions are implemented, the higher the impact on many aspects of care. However, the increasing number of interventions also adds complexity to the execution of the strategy. For example, at the beginning, there were 50 indicators proposed to be measured, however it was impossible to monitor all of them appropriately. At the end, only 17 were monitored reliably.
4. A large number of healthcare facilities and providers included within this strategy facilitated the momentum for change, however it was also a major obstacle for the adequate control of processes and outcomes because of, among other things, the amount of variables to be monitored, the number of professionals to be coached on quality improvement interventions, and the number of facilities to be supervised.
5. A strategic approach built on focused actions on specific geographic areas, facilities, and indicators evolving in a cascade fashion could have rendered similar results, but stronger efforts would have been needed to grant

      visibility to the strategy and create the necessary momentum to influence the whole system

6. Patient satisfaction can be improved and the general perception of healthcare services, influenced with systems-level activities such as these.
7. In health systems of low- and middle-income countries where there is not enough managerial capacity, attention should be paid to the training of managers, who can complement the work of healthcare providers in the execution of a quality strategy.
8. Even though middle-income countries like Mexico do not have the resources available in high-income nations as it was mentioned before, quality improvements can be achieved with limited additional resources.
9. Periodic external assessment of quality strategies are needed to adjust their implementation and contribute to transparency and accountability.
10. Turnover of local leaders, such as Governors and State Ministers of Health, need to be considered in the design of the strategy to cope with the instability created by these changes.

Chapter 19

United States of America

Julie K Johnson and Arlene S Bierman

Abstract

The United States of America (US) is the only developed nation that does not have a universal system of healthcare coverage, and there has been a long-standing debate about how to structure the healthcare system to provide access to care. In 2010, despite fierce opposition, the US Congress passed the Patient Protection and Affordable Care Act (ACA) (US Congress 2010) and President Barack Obama signed the Act into law. While this law represented a sweeping reform of the US healthcare system with provisions to expand coverage and to control costs, it also included provisions to improve the quality of healthcare and foster innovation in research and design of the healthcare delivery system. The ACA has encountered many political and logistical barriers to implementation, but has also sparked many health system reforms and innovation aimed at improving the quality and efficiency of healthcare delivery. It is too early to judge the ultimate impact of this landmark legislation.

Background

Although the US has the highest per capita health expenditures in the world, it lags behind many developed nations in important measures of health (Schroeder 2007). For decades, the rise in healthcare costs in the US outpaced growth in the economy as a whole. Yet despite the unprecedented levels of spending, it is clear that Americans are not gaining benefits commensurate with higher expenditures: the quality of care received in the US is not what it should be. Dozens of countries boast superior life expectancy and lower infant mortality, harmful medical errors abound, and there are pervasive disparities associated with race, ethnicity, and socioeconomic status (Institute of Medicine 1999, National Research Council & Institute of Medicine 2013).

It is within this context that the US enacted the ACA in 2010. The ACA established fundamental health insurance reforms implemented over a span of four years, 2010–2014 (US Department of Health and Human Services 2014). At the time of its enactment, the ACA was expected to extend health insurance coverage to 32 million uninsured US citizens and permanent residents by 2016 (Congressional Budget Office 2011), thus reducing the proportion of uninsured legal residents from 17 percent to 5 percent (Kominski 2014). Attaining this goal

Table 19.1   Demographic, economic, and health information for the United States of America

Population (thousands)	318,000
Area (sq. km)*	9,147,420
Proportion of population living in urban areas (2011)	82
Gross Domestic Product (GDP US$, billions)^	16,244.6
Total expenditure on health as % of GDP	17.9
Gross national income per capita (PPP intl $)	52.610
Per capita total expenditure on health (intl $)	8,895
Proportion of health expenditure which is private	53.6
General Government expenditure on health as a percentage of total expenditure on health	46.4
Out-of-pocket expenditure as a percentage of private expenditure on health	20.7
Life expectancy at birth m/f (yrs)	76/81
Probability of dying under five (per 1,000 live births)	7
Maternal Mortality Ratio (per 100,000 live births) (2013)	28
Proportion of population using improved water and sanitation	99/100

Source: Unless otherwise stated data are for the year 2012 and taken from the World Health Organization 2014. * Area from the World Bank 2014a. ^GDP from the World Bank 2014b.

Notes: PPP is purchasing power parity, intl $ is international dollar which has the same purchasing power as US$ in the US.

is unlikely, given the Supreme Court decision on the expansion of Medicaid, the safety net program for low-income families and individuals, delayed and flawed implementation, and Congressional opposition.

Our aim is to examine the relationship between the US national reform initiatives and the quality and safety of healthcare. We provide a brief history of healthcare reform initiatives and outline the current status of healthcare quality in the US that underscores the imperative for change driving current reform efforts. Then we turn to a discussion of specific aspects of the ACA that promote innovation around quality and safety, the significant barriers that challenge reform efforts in the US, and lessons learned.

Brief History of Healthcare Reform in the US

The US has a rich history of healthcare reform spanning more than a century. In the early twentieth century, progressive reformers proposed a system of compulsory health insurance initiatives to protect workers in the industrial sector against both wage loss and medical costs during sickness—the American Association for Labor Legislation. The proposal was introduced as legislation in many states. The characteristics of the reform—proposed by academics without input from the people their proposal would cover—had important (but largely disregarded) lessons for future reform efforts (Hoffman 2003).

Healthcare reform has been part of the political platform for a number of US presidents, of both major political persuasions, who attempted to implement some type of national health insurance: Theodore Roosevelt in the 1910s, Franklin D Roosevelt in the 1930s, Harry Truman in the 1940s, John Kennedy and Lyndon Johnson in the 1960s, Richard Nixon in the 1970s, and Bill Clinton in the 1990s.

In 1912, Theodore Roosevelt was the first presidential candidate to include a healthcare insurance plan as part of his presidential campaign platform. In the 1930s, as part of the famous New Deal, Franklin D Roosevelt proposed a more expansive concept of reform to create a national health insurance system that would insure everyone in the US. The legislation was designed so that healthcare reform would be part of a larger program that introduced a social security program for retirement. The American Medical Association (AMA) vehemently opposed the idea of a national health insurance scheme on the grounds of protecting physician autonomy and preventing Government from intruding into the practice of medicine. Also, at this time in US history, the perceived "threat of socialism" was high, so the AMA framed the debate as a battle against "socialized medicine." In an effort to avoid derailing legislation for a retirement security program, Congress removed the section on healthcare reform. Roosevelt's plan to introduce a national health insurance scheme fell to his successor, Harry S Truman. Although health reform was President Truman's number one campaign issues, he was unable to secure a majority of votes in Congress to pass the legislation. Healthcare reform became the Holy Grail for Democrats and Liberals, who continued to argue for a Government-run, national health insurance program (Quince 2009). In 1952 the incumbent Republican Party put forth private health insurance as the alternative to a Government-sponsored "socialist" plan. The era of employer-based health insurance was born, and by 1960 many employees had private health insurance. However, other non-unionized, low-wage workers, and those with part-time employment, remained uninsured.

John F Kennedy made healthcare a major campaign issue, but as president he was unable to get a plan for the elderly through Congress. Lyndon Johnson was successful in pushing for national health insurance for two population groups—people over 65 years old, which became the Medicare program and Medicaid (a means-tested national health insurance program for people of low income). Medicare and Medicaid were signed into law in 1965. Richard Nixon put forth a proposal for a national insurance plan that required employers to cover their employees, kept Medicare and Medicaid in place, and provided a national health insurance plan for all others who weren't covered. Before this plan went through, Nixon was impeached and the issue of a national insurance plan didn't emerge again until the Clinton administration in the 1990s. Clinton's proposed expansive reform to guarantee coverage for all Americans, control costs, and make the healthcare system more efficient failed to pass Congress, but Clinton's efforts did result in the Children's Health Insurance Program (CHIP) (Medicaid. gov 2014). CHIP was signed into law in 1997 and provides health coverage for children of low-income families with incomes too high to qualify for Medicaid, but who cannot afford private insurance.

Moving to the current era of health reform efforts, the Obama Administration had a legacy of lessons learned from political failures for a comprehensive national health insurance plan coupled with examples of successful efforts in "gap filling" reform. The political odds were stacked against Obama and his campaign promise to provide all Americans quality, affordable health insurance. Furthermore, the stakes were high, because it is not just a political battle to be fought and won, but also a battle about the health outcomes of a nation.

Current Status of Quality and Safety of Care in the US

The US has an opportunity to benefit from an abundance of research that highlights the shortcomings of its healthcare system. In 1999, the Institute of Medicine of the National Academies published its seminal report, *To Err is Human*, which highlighted the problem of medical errors and set the stage for national and international attention on quality and safety. The landmark report estimated that preventable medical errors led to between 44,000–98,000 deaths per year (Institute of Medicine 1999). A more recent study suggests that adverse events occur in one-third of all hospital admissions (Classen et al. 2011). Medical errors don't stop at the hospital doors. McGlynn and colleagues showed that people, on average, only receive about half of all recommended ambulatory care treatments (McGlynn et al. 2003, Mangione-Smith et al. 2007). Data from the Organisation for Economic Cooperation and Development (OECD), 2011, reveals that the US ranks 27 out of 34 OECD countries in terms of life expectancy at birth—with an average that is more than one year below the OECD average. In the US, the reduction in infant mortality has been slower than most other OECD countries and is currently well above the OECD average. The US has more obese adults than any other OECD country and ranks fifth in obesity among children. US citizens, however, are an optimistic lot, and rank as number one in their perceived health status (Organisation for Economic Cooperation and Development 2013a).

In a country with such an abundance of resources, how did this happen? Without oversimplifying the complexities of the issues, Paul Batalden's observation, "Every system is perfectly designed to get the results it gets," seems to have particular relevance (Carr 2008). All indicators of health outcomes show that Americans are "leaving life years on the table," with disadvantages beginning at birth—the US has the highest rate of infant mortality and the highest rate of child poverty among high-income countries (Detsky 2014). The social determinants of health—education, income, early childhood development, living and working conditions, and social and economic status—leads to America performing poorly in international comparisons of health status, and the gap is widening despite increased spending on healthcare. The US ranks first among OECD countries in healthcare expenditures and 25 in spending on social services (National Research Council & Institute of Medicine 2013, Detsky 2014).

The healthcare system in the US is a patchwork quilt of private health insurance either provided by employers as a fringe benefit or purchased by individuals and Government-provided insurance for those who serve or have served in the military, the elderly, and those who are below a certain level of poverty as determined by each state. There are overlaps in the coverage, as well as gaps that have left many people uninsured. In 2010, when the ACA legislation passed, 18.4 percent of non-elderly Americans (people not covered by Medicare) did not have health insurance (Assistant Secretary for Planning and Evaluation 2011). Many more have periods of un-insurance over the course of a year. The number one reason that people lack coverage is cost. Indeed, healthcare accounts for a remarkably large portion of the US economy. In 2010, the US spent US$2.6 trillion on healthcare, an average of more than US$8,000 per person (up from US$1,110 in 1980). The percentage of the GDP devoted to healthcare increased from 7.2 percent in 1970 to 17.9 percent in 2010 (Kaiser Family Foundation 2012).

Rising healthcare costs over the past decade have had systemic effects, leading to a decrease in the number of employers offering health insurance and the number of employees who can afford the premiums when health insurance is offered (Committee on Health Insurance Status and Its Consequences, Institute of Medicine 2009). In addition, rising costs have led to cost-shifting to patients, with higher deductibles and copayments and limited physician networks, leading to more who are underinsured, have access barriers, or discontinuity of care. The implications of being uninsured sets off a predictable cascade of events: people who lack insurance find it difficult to afford necessary care, healthcare becomes a luxury, and the lack of preventive care and ongoing care for chronic conditions adversely affects health outcomes. As a result, people who are uninsured have a greater likelihood than people with insurance of being diagnosed with severe health conditions (such as cancer that could have been diagnosed at an earlier stage), being hospitalized for preventable health problems, or dying prematurely (Committee on Health Insurance Status and Its Consequences, Institute of Medicine 2009).

The Affordable Care Act (ACA)

The ACA is the most significant piece of healthcare legislation in the US since the enactment of Medicare and Medicaid in 1965. When the United States House of Representatives passed the legislation with a 219 to 212 vote, Obama said, "What this day represents is another stone firmly laid in the foundation of the American dream …. We answered the call of history as so many generations of Americans have before us. When faced with crisis, we did not shrink from our challenge—we overcame it. We did not avoid our responsibility—we embraced it. We did not fear our future—we shaped it" (Connolly 2010).

The ACA aims to address fundamental problems with the current healthcare system. It phases in, over a period of four years, expanded access and coverage, an increased emphasis on quality measurement and reporting, controls for healthcare costs, a focus on prevention to improve population health, and enhancements to the delivery system.

Expansion of Access and Coverage

To expand coverage to the uninsured, the ACA builds on the extant system–employer-based insurance, individual private insurance, and public (Medicare and Medicaid) insurance. For those ineligible for group insurance through an employer or an association, private premiums are very high and unaffordable for many. Most people are required to have health insurance by 2014 or to pay a penalty. States maintain a certain level of control in this process. For example, each state is required to have a Health Benefits Exchange to help individuals who do not have access to affordable employer-based coverage. If a state chooses not to create an Exchange, the federal Government will do so. Qualified health plans offered through the Exchange are required to provide specified essential health benefits.

The ACA additionally called for a nationwide expansion of Medicaid eligibility. As the law was written, nearly all US citizens under 65 with family incomes up to 138 percent of the federal poverty level would qualify for Medicaid under the expansion. The Medicaid expansion was a provision at stake in the ACA cases decided by the Supreme Court in June 2012. The Court upheld the Medicaid expansion, but limited the federal Government's ability to penalize states that don't comply. Therefore, what was originally essentially mandatory—for states to expand Medicaid—is now effectively optional.

Performance Measurement and Reporting

The ACA includes provisions to improve quality of care and health system performance such as a requirement for the Secretary of the US Department of Health and Human Services to develop quality measures. These measures are intended to be used to assess healthcare outcomes, functional status, transitions of care, consumer decision making, meaningful use of health information technology, safety, efficiency, equity, and health disparities, and patient experience. Healthcare professionals and providers will be required to report data on these new measures to the Centers for Medicare and Medicaid Services (CMS). Ultimately, these data will be made available to the public. In addition, the ACA changes the Medicare (and in some cases, Medicaid) reimbursement structures to reward providers and healthcare professionals, in part, on the quality of services provided.

Payment Reform

The ACA created new Accountable Care Organizations (ACOs) that incentivize doctors and other providers to work together to provide more coordinated care to their patients. Over 250 organizations are participating in Medicare ACOs, giving more than four million Medicare beneficiaries access to high-quality coordinated care. ACOs are estimated to save the Medicare program up to US$940 million in the first four years.

The Hospital Readmissions Reduction Program decreases Medicare payments to hospitals with relatively high rates of potentially preventable readmissions to encourage them to focus on this key indicator of patient safety and care quality. In 2015, physician payment will be tied to the quality of care they provide. Those providing higher value will receive higher payments.

Public Health Initiatives

With a focus on prevention and population health, the ACA requires hospitals to conduct a community health needs assessment and take steps toward addressing those health needs. The ACA includes new funding to invest in prevention, wellness, and public health infrastructure. The ACA includes US$500 million in 2010, US$750 million in 2011, and US$1 billion in 2012 for a new Prevention and Public Health fund to invest in prevention, wellness, and public health infrastructure.

Innovations in Improving Quality and Health System Performance

Several initiatives were funded as part of the ACA, specifically to address innovation for quality and safety. The CMS Innovation Center was established as part of the ACA for the purpose of testing "innovative payment and service delivery models to reduce program expenditures ... while preserving or enhancing the quality of care" for those individuals who receive Medicare, Medicaid, or CHIP benefits (CMS.gov 2014). The Innovation Center, funded with US$10 billion over a decade, is currently focused on testing new payment and delivery system models, evaluating results and advancing best practices, engaging a broad range of stakeholders to develop additional models for testing. The Innovation Center has come under scrutiny and criticism because of its reliance on demonstration projects to test ideas in practice, instead of using randomized controlled trials (Kolata 2014).

The Patient Centered Outcomes Research Institute (PCORI) was established as part of the ACA to conduct research and provide information about the best available evidence in order to help patients, and their healthcare providers, make more informed decisions. PCORI's research is intended to give patients a better understanding of the prevention, treatment, and care options available, and the science that supports those options. To date, PCORI has funded almost US$500 million to advance patient centered, comparative clinical effectiveness research projects. National priorities for research include evaluating prevention, diagnosis and treatment options, improving health systems, enhancing communication and disseminating evidence, addressing disparities in health and healthcare, and improving comparative effectiveness research methods and data infrastructure (Selby & Lipstein 2014). Patient centeredness, engagement, and likelihood of changing practice—not explicit in National Institutes of Health or Agency for Healthcare Research and Quality funding—are fundamental to the research PCORI funds.

The ACA designated that Patient Safety Organizations (PSOs) help hospitals with high readmission rates improve their performance. The ACA also called for the Department of Health and Human Services to provide a program to support PSOs in this work.

Implementation: Barriers and Solutions

Economist Victor Fuchs, quoting Niccolo Machiavelli from 1553, writes that the Law of Reform suggests that "There is nothing more difficult to manage, more dubious to accomplish, nor more doubtful of success … than to initiate a new order of things. The reformer has enemies in all those who profit from the old order and only lukewarm defenders in all those who would profit from the new order" (Fuchs 2009).

Small-scale improvements—the incremental changes proposed by the ACA—can be seen as a barrier to large-scale system change. They detract attention from what needs to be accomplished. The "new order of things" of the ACA has met opposition and challenges since it was enacted into law.

There are several reasons why health reform efforts in the US have met such resistance. Many individuals (people who are satisfied with their healthcare and political conservatives who are ideologically opposed to big Government) and organizations (drug companies, insurance companies, and manufacturers of equipment and devices) prefer the status quo (Fuchs 2009). The majority of Americans were (and still are) well-insured and were generally satisfied with their coverage, and in particular with their doctor. Opponents to large-scale health reform played on people's fears that radical change would jeopardize what people valued in their current healthcare system. ACA was crafted to leave in place as much as possible of the pre-existing system of health insurance, but the result was that the reform was built on the most complex, clunky, and costly healthcare system in the world (Aaron 2014).

The US is historically a country of social movements, characterized by "change from below"—grassroots participation of the people, organizing and demanding change on their own behalf. These grassroots efforts played out across the population, effecting change intermittently such as in equal rights for women, Civil rights, and workers rights. However, there has never been such a movement for universal healthcare and compared to other industrialized countries, healthcare in the US is not considered a right (Hoffman 2003).

The ultimate success of the ACA will depend on how elected officials respond to the challenges that emerge (Aaron 2014)—and how the reforms are accepted in communities and across the population. It is too early to understand the implications of the ACA provisions on quality and safety, and at this juncture it is easier to measure the effects of healthcare reform on the levels of uninsured Americans. As of March 31, 2014, ACA had reached its targets for open enrolment. The percentage of uninsured adults has dropped to from 18.4 percent to 15.8 percent. Among those gaining coverage, most are enrolled through employer—sponsored coverage and Medicaid (Carman & Eibner 2014). Expanding insurance coverage is certainly an important goal of the ACA and the early results are positive.

Conclusions

The reform landscape in the US continues to evolve but there are lessons learned as we review past and current reform efforts. Repeal of the ACA is not likely but amendments and further changes are almost guaranteed.

While the ACA was enacted to address the fundamental problems with the current healthcare system, most features of the ACA were built on one binding constraint—healthcare reform in the US had to be incremental. A single payer system that covered all Americans was never a viable option for the US, yet many individual states, for example Vermont with its Green Mountain Care, have moved closer to universal access. Without a doubt we can conclude that the ACA suffered from flawed implementation. The task facing Obama and future legislators is determining what parts work best, which parts should be jettisoned, and which parts need further revision.

There are objectives that should be cornerstones of health reform: (1) universal coverage for basic and essential healthcare that meets societal needs, not unlimited individual wants; (2) a defined budget for federal healthcare expenditures that sets limits on spending; (3) the establishment of national evidence-based standards for the practice of medicine and the issuance of prescription drugs in order to improve consistency, enhance quality, reduce costs, and dramatically reduce litigation; and (4) enhanced personal responsibility and accountability for health and wellness.

The ACA offers opportunities to improve healthcare in the US by expanding coverage and reducing healthcare costs. Simultaneously, the ACA will create new challenges as the legislation is implemented and experienced at different levels of the healthcare system—the individual patient and consumer level, the micro-system level and the macro-system level. There is a need to rigorously test and evaluate new models of care that emerge from the legislation.

PART V
Europe

Russell Mannion

Part V continues by now common themes, this time, in relation to Europe, with representation from seven countries: Denmark, England, Scotland, Sweden, Norway, Germany, and Italy. All are high-income countries with well-established and advanced healthcare systems that have been developed within a broader set of arrangements which, in addition to covering primary and secondary care, also embrace public health services, and a range of community care and social care agencies. In terms of the total size of population they can be split into two broad groups, with Denmark, Scotland, Sweden, and Norway all having relatively small populations of around five to nine million people and those with much larger populations—England, Italy, and Germany having 53 million, 61 million, and 82 million respectively. All of the health systems, apart from Germany, are, to a greater or lesser extent, based on the Beveridge model whereby healthcare services are funded through general taxation, with universal access and coverage with services that are free at the point of use. In contrast, the German health system is based on the Bismarckian model which is financed by private insurance plans funded jointly by employers and employees through payroll deductions.

Although the nature and trajectory of health policy in each country is intimately tied to each nation's unique history, intrinsic cultural values, legal and political institutions, and traditions, a number of convergent trends across these countries can be discerned in relation to emergent approaches towards healthcare quality and patient safety. First, there has been a shift from healthcare quality being viewed as a predominantly medical concern and preoccupation to the development of more managerial and organizational approaches towards promoting high-quality care. In all countries there have been national initiatives to promote quality and in many countries these are being linked with local and more "bottom up" approaches to safeguarding care. Second, there has been an increased emphasis on the use of published comparative data on provider quality and performance as a means to stimulate improvement, although in many countries data quality and coverage remains poor, lacks credibility among clinicians, and is rarely used by patients to select providers. Third, there has been a growing emphasis on involving patients and engaging the general public in quality improvement activities and evaluations. This ranges from developing more, individualized approaches, to patient involvement and empowerment such as "personalized" care in England, to broader approaches to engaging citizens and the third sector in policy debates about the nature of health reform, particularly in Germany and Scotland. Fourth, in some countries, particularly England, Sweden and Norway, there has been an increase in the use of financial payment for performance schemes to reward and incentivize providers for improving quality and performance. Finally, in some countries, most notably England and Sweden, there has been a focus on the creation of pro-market mechanisms and the use of competition and choice to stimulate quality improvement, although in some countries, most notably Scotland, such pro-market approaches have been resisted strongly.

Chapter 20

Denmark

Janne Lehmann Knudsen, Carsten Engel, and Jesper Eriksen

Abstract

Over the years the Danish health system has seen significant reformed in relation to rationalizing its governance structure. Alongside reforms in the distribution of responsibilities for the provision of services, the central and regional Governments have embarked on major hospital reforms. The reforms have driven hospitals towards centralization, specialization, standardization, and higher efficiency. At the same time, healthcare has moved from hospitals into the primary sector, resulting in changed expectations and roles for family physicians, and there has been a major expansion of municipality-based healthcare responsibilities. General practice, however, has not been correspondingly reorganized

The effort during the past 20 years towards increased quality has transformed the agenda and management of quality improvement and patient safety. It has increasingly become a matter of central regulation, thus moving from local responsibility and private ownership to becoming an obligation for healthcare leaders based on standards defined at a national level. Transparency has increased as well as public access to data. The agenda has changed from ensuring high professional standards and efficiency, to include patient safety and a patient engagement agenda, aimed at enhancing patient-centered care. Quality improvement has also steadily become more data-driven.

The health reforms have been politically driven. The perspective on quality has mainly been towards achieving higher specialized care. In the latest reform it was also a main objective to ensure coherence, mainly between primary and secondary healthcare. Improvements in quality of care have been pushed by health professionals, patient organizations, and public demands expressed through the media. Technology has, only to a minor degree, influenced the reforms and efforts.

Introduction

Healthcare reforms with profound political, structural, and financial implications were carried out in 1970 and 2007, rationalizing the governance structure at the regional and local levels. The latest reform also introduced a new quality agenda by shifting power and clarifying responsibilities between the governance levels.

Table 20.1   Demographic, economic, and health information for Denmark

Population (thousands)	5,598
Area (sq. km)*	42,430
Proportion of population living in urban areas (2011)	87
Gross Domestic Product (GDP US$, billions)^	315.2
Total expenditure on health as % of GDP	11.2
Gross national income per capita (PPP intl $)	43,430
Per capita total expenditure on health (intl $)	4,720
Proportion of health expenditure which is private	14.5
General Government expenditure on health as a percentage of total expenditure on health	85.5
Out-of-pocket expenditure as a percentage of private expenditure on health	87.2
Life expectancy at birth m/f (yrs)	78/82
Probability of dying under five (per 1,000 live births)	4
Maternal Mortality Ratio (per 100,000 live births) (2013)	5
Proportion of population using improved water and sanitation	100/100

Source: Unless otherwise stated data are for the year 2012 and taken from the World Health Organization 2014. * Area from the World Bank 2014a. ^GDP from the World Bank 2014b.

Notes: PPP is purchasing power parity, intl $ is international dollar which has the same purchasing power as US$ in the US.

The evolution of quality improvement began 20 years earlier and was initially pushed by the medical societies and later on this altered, due to increasing public and political demands as well as the professional engagement. Within the changing structural frameworks, a number of plans and strategies have been vehicles to reform quality and safety, including ad hoc legislation and economic contracts between the Government and, primarily, the regional health authorities. These efforts were integrated and became formalized by the comprehensive Act on Health Care, which framed the health reform in 2007. Since then other political initiatives have followed, changing the quality landscape. Accreditation is now an integrated part of the quality development framework and based on a mutual agreement between the national and regional health authorities.

The aim of this chapter is to describe the relationship between the national Danish health reform carried out in 2007 and supplementary national key efforts reforming quality and safety during the last two decades and to explore the relationship between this and the subsequent transformation of quality and improvement.

The Current Situation

The Danish population of 5.6 million people is serviced by a public healthcare system, with equal access for all citizens, financed through taxes. Less than 2 percent of hospital services are delivered by private providers. The services are generally free of charge, but there are consumer fees, mainly on medications and dentistry, accounting for about 20 percent of total healthcare expenses. Any resident is entitled to be enlisted to a general practitioner (GP) who, apart from delivering family medicine, acts as gatekeeper to specialized care.

Governance is three-tiered, with each tier headed by elected political bodies:

- The Government, mainly the Ministry of Health, including agencies and the Ministry of Finance, is responsible for the overall regulatory, supervisory, and fiscal functions, including the expenditure framework for regional and local services. The Danish Health and Medicines Authority is an agency with the task of supervising and regulating healthcare, and authorization and supervision of healthcare professionals including the governance of pharmaceuticals, drugs, and medical equipment. The National Serum Institute controls infections, attends to biological threats, and monitors activity, cost-effectiveness, and quality. It has the responsibility of IT development at the national level, monitors the health status of the population, and operates the national bio bank.
- Five regions are responsible for hospital care, mental health services, general practice, and practicing specialists. Hospitals are owned by the regions. In contrast, the 3,600 GPs practicing in Denmark are, in principle, independent, but are almost exclusively financed by a mixture of per-capita and fee-for-service payments.
- Ninety-eight municipalities are responsible for the promotion of health, home care and long-term care, rehabilitation, and substance abuse.

A recently published Organisation for Economic Cooperation and Development (OECD) report emphasized the comparatively high degree of equity in Danish healthcare and the far-reaching reforms in the hospital sector as the primary strengths (Organisation for Economic Cooperation and Development 2013c). The system is judged as efficient, with an overall high level of public trust and satisfaction. The report highlights impressive quality monitoring and improvement initiatives with a commitment at the national, institutional, and individual levels to monitor and improve quality. But when it comes to quality management, the OECD report identified a need for consolidation—to create coherence across the many initiatives, with a special focus on measuring and maximizing the contribution made by primary care.

The management model today is based on economic, rather than quality-based incentives, and evaluation of reforms is not systematic. The three-tiered governance structure adds stability to the system, but creates opportunities for power struggles and turf protection.

In spite of the level of public health service and free access to care, life expectancy has not increased as much as in other comparable countries. One of the main reasons is that cancer incidence and mortality are high compared to other developed countries. On the other hand, when it comes to providing the best treatment and outcome of heart disease, Denmark is a world leader. The reasons for these differences are not well understood or studied. Health equity is a stated priority but until recently few policies and interventions have been carried out. Lately, a gap of about 20 years in life expectancy between psychiatric patients and the general population has attracted much attention (Nordentoft et al. 2013).

The primary weakness concerning quality seems to be the lack of coherence across the health system, creating discontinuity of care and safety hazards when responsibility for patients is handed over between institutions. The OECD report identified primary care as a specific area of concern and highlighted a need for a different, stronger, and more modernized sector. The report also addresses that formal continuing professional education is not in place, but ought to be.

Detail of Current Reform Initiatives

The two major healthcare reforms in 1970 and 2007 changed the system politically, financially, and structurally. The reform in 2007 also changed the quality landscape.

The purpose of the 2007 healthcare reform was to further develop a democratically-controlled public sector as a basis for the Danish welfare society. The reform drew up a new public sector, where 98 municipalities (previously 298), five regions (previously 14 counties), and the state have their own task-related identity. The number of taxation levels was reduced from three to two, as the regions, in contrast to the former counties, cannot levy taxes. Before the reform the counties—as those responsible of medical care—had tax-raising power. After the reform the regions—as the new custodians—are financed out of the state budget and paid by the municipalities according to the services they offer.

As a consequence of the reform, the responsibility for healthcare at the operational level was split. The major responsibility for healthcare was left with the regional level, while the local level (municipalities) took over new responsibilities within primary care, in addition to their well-established role in social care. As a consequence, it became mandatory for the two political systems to establish joint Health-coordination Councils at the regional level, to enter into health contracts within specific geographic areas, specifying which tasks should be carried out by whom, and to develop care pathways as a platform for managing specific patient groups across the sectors. The main aim is to ensure better coordination of care.

Overall, the healthcare reform established a new operational agenda for the health system, but without the involvement of general practice. A comprehensive Act on Health Care consolidated the regulation of healthcare by defining the responsibilities and tasks within the system. It also increased the power of the central health authorities to regulate clinical care and the organization supporting this.

The Danish Health and Medicines Authority became empowered to further regulate the specialized hospital-based care. The organization of the specialized services has to be based on considerations of ensuring the highest quality but also an efficient use of resources. Planning is carried out in cooperation with the Associations of Medical Society as well as the regions, but with the Danish Health and Medicines Authority as the lead agency. Over the years highly specialized care has been concentrated into fewer hospitals: in 2005 surgery of ovarian cancer was carried out at 30 hospitals, today there are five. Colorectal cancer surgery was handled at 38 units in 2003, this was reduced to 19 in 2012.

The health reform in 2007 reinforced an overall centralization trend of hospital care as illustrated below (Table 20.2).

The number of acute care hospitals will be further reduced to 21. The Government has pushed the development by deciding to finance highly specialized so called "Super Hospitals" in each of the five regions, which has triggered a major construction program.

The reform has had substantial implications for the municipalities. They became formal healthcare providers and had to build up competences and infrastructure to support their task. They are obliged to manage the provision of social care as well as healthcare.

Table 20.2   Numbers of public hospitals in Denmark

Year	1945	1955	1965	1975	1995	2005	2013
Number of hospitals	166	156	148	132	95	59	31

The Quality and Safety Landscape

The responsibility for quality and safety is divided among formal stakeholders. The reform in 2007 changed the quality landscape and pushed forward a stronger commitment; the Health Care Act more specifically defined the responsibility of management to promote and control quality. Quality improvement was defined as an obligation for leadership at all levels, and included the municipalities as new healthcare providers. The mandate of the Danish Health and Medicine Authority was expanded to include a clear obligation to supervise institutions as well as individual professionals, which included an expanded role in planning the specialized services. The responsibility of the National Safety Database was moved away from the Danish Health and Medicine Authority to a new organization named Patientombuddet, which also was given the task to investigate patient complaints. The aim was to emphasize that reporting of adverse events and disciplinary actions are two distinct systems.

Health professionals have an obligation to report clinical data to approximately 60 national quality registries, and to meet professional standards. National clinical guidelines are developed in collaboration with professional associations and The Danish Health and Medicine Authority. Hospital-based doctors are employees working under direction by leaders, while GPs are not. Formal re-certification via a Continuing Medical Education (CME) program is not an obligation in any healthcare professions.

The Danish Health and Medicine Authority carries out the central regulation of the professionals and health institutions—public as well as private providers. The regions and the municipalities have operational responsibility and a wide range of powers to organize services for their citizens, as well as determining the level of quality. The National Serum Institute is building an extensive analytic capacity on a national level.

Rigsrevisionen, the Danish National Audit Office, is an independent public institution reviewing public governance on behalf of the Parliament. As a consequence of the health reform in 2007, the institution was given the task of auditing the hospitals, and in 2012 a critical revision of quality improvement was published (Rigsrevisionen 2012). Rigsrevisionen concluded that there is a substantial lack of formal evaluation, follow-up and leadership engagement, and its recommendations highlighted a clear need for improvement. This institution has also carried out an external audit of the governance of cancer care, which has resulted in a better ongoing monitoring of quality and a stronger leadership.

Other stakeholders who have a notable impact on the quality and safety agenda include the Danish Medical Association (DMA), as well as the specific medical societies and the Nurse Association, who are engaged in promoting quality and safety, mainly focusing on clinical care. They promote quality improvement and transparency based on non-punitive principles. They partner to a high degree with the national health authority. Maintaining the independent status and autonomy of GPs is high on the agenda of the Organization of General Practitioners. This can make it challenging to integrate the GPs into national strategies. Only recently have GPs been obliged to report a minimum dataset on quality, and there is no transparency in the quality of individual practitioners or practices.

The power of patient organizations has increased—not formally, but indirectly though lobbying and the publishing of data based on research and patient experiences, addressing the need for improving quality in healthcare. In 2008 the majority of patient organizations cooperated to establish Danish Patients—an umbrella organization working from a joint agenda. Efforts towards achieving better care and outcome are central. Danish Patients has become an accepted partner, and its influence is increasing. Danish Patients acts as the patients' voice on generic themes, as well as partnering in improvement efforts. The Danish Cancer Society is the biggest and politically most powerful single patient organization.

The Impact of These Reform Efforts on Quality and Safety of Care

The specific reform efforts explicitly aimed at quality improvement and patient safety have mainly been generic, in the sense of not being targeted at specific patient groups. But more recently, specific tools have been developed as a consequence of insufficient quality of care for specific diseases, primarily chronic diseases such as cancer.

The first National Strategy for Quality published by the Health and Medicine Authority in 1993 had a profound influence on quality improvement in the following decade. The strategy was developed in cooperation with all principal stakeholders. It was responsive and compliant and addressed the need for data-driven improvement. It combined both a bottom-up and a top-down approach by addressing the responsibility of leaders, as well as health professionals. It was, for instance, followed by a specific strategy focusing on national quality registries. Revised strategies followed, but the national strategy has not been updated since 2007, when the Act on Health Care was launched.

Patient-centered care has only recently become an expressed aim in Danish healthcare, although Denmark was one of the first countries globally to pass an Act on Patients' Rights. Legislation was passed in 1998, which focused on patients' rights to be informed before treatment, and defined a patient's right to access information in their medical record. As a consequence of the financial agreement in 2000, national surveys on patient experiences of hospital care have been carried out annually. Due to pressure from quality officers and clinical leaders, this has changed from only being a political tool to benchmark hospitals, to also serve as an improvement tool for individual clinical units.

Patient engagement is mainly understood by providers as the empowerment of patients to handle their own situation and care. The full concept of patient centeredness, meaning partnering with patients to ensure that the care is organized to fulfill patient preferences and needs, has not been consolidated. Patient organizations advocate for a broader understanding. At this time a national working group, established by the Ministry of Health, is developing a national strategy focusing on patient engagement.

There has, however, been some success, as there seems to be a drive in healthcare towards a more patient-centered approach. A number of initiatives have been aimed at changing the traditional physician centered structure of hospitals into departments corresponding to medical specialties towards a more patient-centered organizational structure. An example is the establishment of common units for emergency admission. These are not merely traditional emergency units, triaging and providing urgent treatment, but short stay hospitals within the hospital, with care provided by a cross-specialty care team. A related approach is to cluster resources and competencies needed for a specific patient pathway, rather than using professional competence types as the basic unit of organization, in order to achieve high-quality care for patients with comorbidities.

Results from the patient surveys have again and again confirmed that there is a lack of continuity in care. A financial agreement between the Government and the counties in 2001, determined that each individual patient receiving hospital care should have a dedicated point-of-contact health professional. With the Act on Heath care in 2007 this became a patient right, but was nonetheless a struggle to implement. The financial agreement in 2011 launched a supplemental "coordination officer" with the task of handling logistics in the trajectories of cancer patients and patients with heart disease, when care is handed over. Whether these efforts have had any positive impacts on patient satisfaction has not been documented.

A national mandatory accreditation program for publicly-funded hospitals was decided as part of the financial agreement in 2002. The aim is to improve quality and to ensure continuity of care as well as a more uniform level of basic care across the providers. Municipal and private healthcare providers joined the agreement. A freestanding organization, the Danish Institute for Quality and Accreditation in Healthcare (IKAS), with Board representatives from the parties to the agreement, was established in 2005 to develop and manage the accreditation programs, the Danish Healthcare Quality Program (DDKM). The first organizations were accredited in 2009; organizations will be reassessed in a three-year cycle. The program now includes public and private hospitals, community pharmacies, ambulance services, and some municipal healthcare services. Programs for GPs and office-based healthcare practitioners are being developed.

Accreditation has obtained wide acceptance among healthcare managers; it has also been embraced by many professionals, but there remain levels of resistance. The arguments behind this resistance are mainly related to the perceived burden of documentation, but also that it does not sufficiently grasp the clinical aspect of quality. The perceived lack of evidence is brought into play. Rigsrevisionen states, "The Danish Healthcare Quality Program is the most important quality program in the healthcare sector."

The patient safety agenda seems to supersede broader clinical improvement when it comes to leadership attention. The safety agenda was initiated by the Act on patient safety passed in 2004. It became mandatory for health professionals at hospitals to report adverse events to a National Safety Database through a non-punitive reporting system. The regions are obligated to act when safety hazards have been identified. Today, the Act also embraces the primary sector, and it gives patients and relatives the opportunity to report concerns. In all regions and at all hospitals, organizations supporting the reporting system have been established and are following up events. It is, however, uncertain whether the reporting system has had any real impact on outcomes. Nonetheless, work continues in this area. The Danish Society for Patient Safety, in cooperation with healthcare providers, runs big improvement projects, mainly by inspiration from the Institute of Health Care Improvement, including a Safer Hospital Program implemented at five hospitals. The safety agenda now involves the municipalities too.

Over the past ten years cancer care has received special political attention due to poorer outcomes compared with the other Nordic countries. Three national cancer plans, the establishment of an organization of multidisciplinary cancer groups, national cancer pathways, and national monitoring of waiting time have been established, and it has been estimated that around €1 billion has been dedicated by the Government to this area. Cancer care initiatives are seen as a forerunner for other clinical areas.

Implementation: Barriers and Solutions

Some of the main findings in the 2012 report from Rigsrevisionen on the quality programs at Danish hospitals were:

- The aggregate number of programs is considerable and the efforts to integrate the programs should continue.
- The programs would benefit from improved IT support.
- There is a need for evaluation of the programs to determine if the objectives have been achieved.
- The total amount of resources dedicated by the Government to the hospitals for improving care is not known.

By their very nature, national reform initiatives tend to be top-down. Consequently, resistance on the ground is to be expected. When reform efforts change structure, power issues are evoked. Physicians argue in many cases that they are detrimental to the teaching and maintenance of professional expertise. The admission units provide an example. Redistribution of resources to the units is difficult; this can result in a situation where the traditional departments complain about cutbacks, whereas the admission units are still perceived as under resourced by their staff and management. Compounding this problem, as emergency medicine is not an independent specialty in Denmark, it has been difficult to recruit and retain physicians to these departments. Also, allocation of physician time from other departments to participation in admission unit teams can be a matter of conflict.

Other reform initiatives, such as the accreditation program DDKM and The Danish Safer Hospital Program, are largely indifferent to structure but aim at improving critical work processes and monitoring quality and safety. However, not all processes in a complex system like healthcare can be pre-specified in detail. The experience, in particular from DDKM, is that perceptions of over-regulation or over-monitoring will evoke resistance. Exaggerated monitoring of compliance with procedures will lead to demotivation and gaming. The case of the Danish Safer Hospital Program shows the potential of campaigns, but also highlights the difficulties in spreading change outside the sites directly involved.

Data availability is in principle a force driving reform, but it is not enough to improve care. Delay in availability to clinicians and lack of management is often mentioned as a barrier to progress. Denmark has not yet achieved the goal of providing real-time quality data widely to close the quality improvement loop.

The regulatory efforts focusing on cancer care seem finally to have had an impact on outcomes. It has been a long journey, and it has to continue due to the increasing cancer incidence. It has been crucial for the positive results to date, that alliances have been created between the clinical cancer specialists and the Cancer Society, in turn including the policymakers, and that reliable data exists to monitor quality and progress.

Prospects for Success and Next Steps

Looking back, the regulation of quality has changed:

- from voluntary to mandatory;
- from professional responsibility to leadership responsibility;
- from local standards to national standards;
- from beliefs to data-driven improvement;
- from private data ownership to transparency with public ownership;
- from focusing on hospital care to include municipality-based care.

In view of the challenges and the state of affairs described above, how can we move on? One of the shifts that is needed is a change from viewing quality as a purely technical aspect of care, to include a keen commitment towards ensuring quality through the entire patient journey. To achieve this, the patient perspective must be taken far beyond merely being about informing patients and carrying out patient surveys. It also implies that GPs have to become integrated as equal professional partners in the health system, with reduced autonomy as a consequence. Also the municipalities must come fully on board.

The professional culture is an issue. A consequence of specialization is the tendency for the fragmentation of care. This can lead to a non-holistic attitude of "Is this a problem that belongs to me, or can I pass it on to someone else?" What has aptly been called "an episode physician." This is not only a consequence of specialization, but also of changed attitudes, due to working agreements in favor of reduced working hours for doctors, as well as the tendency among doctors to see themselves as employees. The trend is reinforced by the pressure for productivity, that will be enhanced by the resource gap facing Denmark, as well as other OECD countries, and by IT support that is, as yet, far from optimal.

It is tempting to see structure as the first choice of lever. In the case of Denmark, it seems obvious that healthcare should be united under one management. However, there are important political interests that would counter such an attempt—a lot of energy would go into struggles for power. Furthermore, altering structure does not necessarily provide a solution for what really needs to change. In the opinion of the authors, one important lever would be finding ways to shift a number of paradigms:

- From a focus on productivity to a focus on creating value for patients and realizing partnerships with patients in the care given as well as at the organizational level.
- From monitoring technical effectiveness of treatment to including quality of the entire patient pathway and ensuring that economic incentives support this.
- Promoting accountability and a holistic view among healthcare professionals by relying less on management for detailed regulation of processes, without sacrificing the need for attention to processes at the micro level.
- From everyone doing his or her best, to a realization of the importance of seeing oneself, and acting, as part of a team—on the micro, meso, and macro levels, supported by the pre and postgraduate system.

Conclusion

The case of Denmark illustrates that the quality and safety agenda can be changed profoundly by a mix of structural reforms, legislation, and national strategies, embracing bottom-up movements among professionals and patients, and using campaigns to promote attention and to demonstrate the possibility of success. The efforts can lead to improved quality of care provided, but needs to be followed by changing professional attitudes and organizational culture. It also illustrates that structural boundaries can be important barriers, and highlights the need for further collaboration based on a holistic view of patients, patient pathways, and the whole healthcare system.

Chapter 21

England

Martin Powell and Russell Mannion

Abstract

This chapter focuses on the impact of the major reforms of the New Labour (1997–2010) and Conservative–Liberal Democrat (2010–) Governments on quality and safety of care delivered in the English National Health Service (NHS). We first briefly outline the position before 1997, before setting out the main reforms of the Labour and Coalition Governments. We then briefly set out the current quality and safety landscape, linking—where possible—changes in quality and safety with recent reforms, and discuss current quality and safety issues. We find that despite scandals such as "Mid Staffordshire," most of the evidence points to improvements in quality and safety over time. However, there is an element of "Groundhog Day" as "quality" is periodically rediscovered as a major theme in the NHS and recommendations of previous inquiries being recycled after high-profile and tragic events. At times the NHS appears to be an organization without a memory. "Sorry" may be the hardest word, but learning and implementation appear to be the hardest activities.

Introduction

Established in 1948, the NHS is the oldest single payer health system in the world. It is funded directly through the general taxation system. The budget for 2012/13 was around GBP£109 billion (or about 9.8 percent of GDP, up from 6.6 percent in 1997) and health services are largely free at the point of use. The NHS is administered centrally, and is formally accountable to Parliament through the Secretary of State for Health, who is a member of the majority political party (Labour—broadly left; Conservative—right; Liberal Democrats—center). Health services in Scotland and Wales were part of the same structure as the English system until 1999, when powers were devolved to the Scottish and Welsh Governments.

Since its inception the NHS has undergone a process of continual reform, change, and adaption. This chapter focuses on the impact on quality and safety of care delivered in the NHS by the major reforms of the New Labour (1997–2010) and Conservative–Liberal Democrat (2010–) Governments. First, we first briefly discuss the position before 1997. Next we examine the main reforms of the Labour and Coalition Governments, and explore the current quality and safety landscape.

**Table 21.1   Demographic, economic, and health information for United
Kingdom (*England alone data not available*)**

Population (thousands)	62,783
Area (sq. km)*	241,930
Proportion of population living in urban areas (2011)	80
Gross Domestic Product (GDP US$, billions)^	2,475.7
Total expenditure on health as % of GDP	9.4
Gross national income per capita (PPP intl $)	37,340
Per capita total expenditure on health (intl $)	3,495
Proportion of health expenditure which is private	17.5
General Government expenditure on health as a percentage of total expenditure on health	82.5
Out-of-pocket expenditure as a percentage of private expenditure on health	56.8
Life expectancy at birth m/f (yrs)	79/83
Probability of dying under five (per 1,000 live births)	5
Maternal Mortality Ratio (per 100,000 live births) (2013)	8
Proportion of population using improved water and sanitation	100/100

Source: Unless otherwise stated data are for the year 2012 and taken from the World Health Organization 2014. * Area from the World Bank 2014a. ^GDP from the World Bank 2014b.
Notes: PPP is purchasing power parity, intl $ is international dollar which has the same purchasing power as US$ in the US.

We then attempt to link changes in quality and safety with recent reforms, before finally discussing current quality and safety issues.

Historical Background: Quality in the National Health Service (NHS) 1948–1997

Quality is defined in different ways by different commentators and agencies. However quality is defined, it was rarely discussed until the 1990s (see below; also see Thorlby & Maybin 2010). It was largely assumed not to be an issue in the NHS context, with politician's mantra being that the NHS was the "best in the world," it was largely implicit, and was defined and assessed by providers.

Nonetheless, there were occasional concerns over quality. For example, in 1969 Labour Secretary of State Richard Crossman seized the opportunity provided by a report revealing "scandalous conditions" at Ely hospital, to set up the Hospital

Advisory Service, an inspectorate in all but name (Klein 2013, p. 59). Over time, concerns of quality shifted to a new agenda: from the individual clinician to a collective clinical responsibility towards the consumer (Powell 1997). Vincent, Burnett, and Carthey (2013) write that patient safety really emerged as a high-profile issue in the late 1990s from a confluence of factors, with a series of high-profile events contributing to the heightened importance of patient safety.

Recent Reform Initiatives

Reforms Under the New Labour Government, 1997–2010

In this period, quality and safety issues were driven by a broad policy agenda together with a more specific safety agenda that was shaped more by "events." In opposition, the 1997 Labour Manifesto promised to treat an extra 100,000 patients, to end waiting for cancer surgery, and to set "tough quality standards" for hospitals (Klein 2013, p. 191). The White Paper "The New NHS" (Department of Health 1997) argued that quality was best determined by collaboration rather than competition. It introduced clinical governance (developed from a medical audit introduced during the 1990s) as a framework through which NHS organizations are accountable for continuously improving the quality of their services (Scally & Donaldson 1998). It also introduced a new wider performance measurement system, backed by threats of central intervention for miscreants, and National Service Frameworks (NSF) to reflect best practice. The National Institute of Clinical Excellence (NICE) would produce evidence about cost-effectiveness of interventions, and reduce the level of geographical inequity ("postcode lottery"). The Commission for Health Improvement (CHI) was set up as a new regulator for quality. The White Paper "A First Class Service" (Department of Health 1998) placed quality at the center of the NHS, at least theoretically. This quality agenda set up the National Clinical Assessment Authority, a body to which NHS employers could refer doctors whose performance was seen as problematic for review, and the National Patient Safety Agency, responsible for operating a national system of reporting and analyzing adverse events and "near misses." A statutory "duty of quality" shared by all providers of NHS services was established in the Health Acts of 1999 and 2003, with provider Chief Executive Officers accountable for quality as well as financial matters.

"An Organisation with a Memory" (OWAM) (Department of Health 2000b), an influential policy paper, provided data on the scope and magnitude of safety issues in the NHS. It reported an estimated 850,000 adverse events, representing 10 percent of admissions, occur annually, costing hospitals approximately GBP£2 billion. It stated that the NHS needed to develop: unified mechanisms for reporting and analysis when things go wrong; a more open culture, in which errors or service failures can be reported and discussed; mechanisms for ensuring that, where lessons are identified, the necessary changes are put into practice; and a much wider appreciation of the value of the system approach in preventing, analyzing, and learning from errors

The more specific events included a "litany of scandals, matched in NHS history only by those in the mental hospitals in the 1960s and 1970s" (Timmins 2001, p. 578). The most notable was at the Bristol Royal Infirmary (Kennedy 2001). In October 1997, the Professional Conduct Committee of the General Medical Council (GMC) began the hearing of a case "that transformed the policy landscape as far as relations between the state and the medical profession were concerned" (Klein 2013, p. 197). This resulted from the deaths of 15 children while, or after, undergoing cardiac surgery at the Bristol Royal Infirmary and, in effect, placed the medical profession on trial. It was not simply a matter of individual competence, but also the failure of medical audit and professional self-regulation, as well as ignoring the concerns of a "whistle-blower" (Klein 2013, p. 197).

The NHS Plan (Department of Health 2000a) revolved around "investment and reform." In return for a significant increase in NHS funding, the NHS would have to change its way of working. This document set the NHS back on the road towards "market-based reforms" (Dixon, Mays & Jones 2011) or reinventing competition, but a complex policy mix that blended competition with continuing top-down control (Powell et al. 2011).

A new performance measurement system initially consisted of "traffic lights" (red, amber, and green) that were later replaced with star ratings for hospitals. The ministerial assumption was that good clinical governance could be equated with good quality of care, but this was a "highly questionable assumption" as "process did not equate outcome" (Klein 2013, p. 227). The CHI changed its name to the Health Care Commission (HCC) in 2004, and reported new annual health checks.

A Quality and Outcomes Framework (QOF) was introduced in 2003 as part of the general medical services contract between the NHS and general practitioners (GPs). The QOF established standards (indicators) in five major domains including clinical standards and patient experience, and determined about 25 percent of GP payment each year. It represented an alignment between financial incentives and the standards of good medical care (Propper & Venables 2013).

A 2005 document (Department of Health 2005) regarded reform as composed of four mutually interacting streams (Dixon, Mays & Jones 2011, Powell et al. 2011): demand (choice, commissioning), supply (diversity—Foundation Trusts (FT), private providers), transactional (Payment by Results (PbR)), and system management and regulation ("targets and terror") which would result in better quality, better patient experience, better value for money, and reduced inequality.

Although there were further documents on quality and safety (for example, Department of Health 2001, 2006, and National Audit Office 2005), the Darzi Report (Department of Health 2008) signaled "a revivalist burst of enthusiasm for change in the name of quality" (Klein 2013, p. 253). It stated that the NHS must have "quality of care at its heart," and raised to importance three dimensions of quality: clinical effectiveness, safety, and patient experience. It set out the "National Quality Board," regional "Quality Observatory" and local "Quality Accounts" (selected from a menu of 400 measures), and Patient Reported Outcome Measures (PROMs). It outlined "best practice tariffs" (where a significant proportion of provider income would be linked to patient experience and satisfaction) and "Never Events" (where payment can be withheld when care does not meet the minimum standards patients can expect; see Department of Health 2009). In a "Groundhog Day" rerun of 1997–1998, quality was to be the "organizing principle" of the NHS.

Two further elements were thrown into the policy melting pot. First, the financial crisis of 2008 changed feast to famine. The "quality and productivity challenge," or so-called "Nicholson challenge," set out the need to make "efficiency savings" of GBP£15–20 billion over the three-year period from April 2011 (Department of Health 2009).

Second, events—yet again—shaped policy. A spur to action at hospital Board-level came from two further hospital "scandals" involving patient deaths from healthcare acquired infections (HCAIs), one at Stoke Mandeville Hospital in 2005 and another at Maidstone and Tunbridge Wells in 2007 (Vincent, Burnett & Carthey 2013). However, the largest spur came from a HCC Inquiry in 2009 that found "a catalogue of appalling management and failures at every level" at the Mid Staffordshire NHS FT which was estimated to result in up to 1,200 excess deaths between 2004 and 2009 (Klein 2013).

Reforms under the Coalition Government, 2010–2014

The Health Secretary of the Conservative–Liberal Democrat Government of 2010 quickly produced the White Paper "Equity and Excellence: Liberating the NHS" (Department of Health 2010), which was seen as the largest reorganization in the history of the NHS. The Parliamentary Bill was 550 pages long, with 280 clauses, and formed the basis of the Health and Social Care Act 2012, with many of the changes effective from April 1, 2013 (Timmins 2012). The main changes were the establishment of a central commissioning board (now NHS England), new local Clinical Commissioning Groups, elected local authorities to take over responsibility for public health, new Health and Wellbeing Boards, and a new consumer body set up called Health Watch to represent patients' interests.

The Coalition wished to move from the measurement of "process" to "outcomes," with the five domains of the NHS Outcomes Framework (Department of Health 2012) derived from the Darzi (Department of Health 2008) definition of quality: effectiveness, patient experience, and safety, which is now enshrined into the Health and Social Care Act 2012.

The repercussions of "Mid Staffs" continued for "the quality industry" (Klein 2013, pp. 295–298). The final Francis Report (2013) consisted of three volumes of about 1,600 pages and an "executive summary" of 115 pages, which charted the "appalling and unnecessary suffering of hundreds of people," reflecting the failure "of a system which ignored the warning signs and put corporate self interest and cost control ahead of patients and their safety." The 290 recommendations aimed to achieve a "cultural revolution" (Davies & Mannion 2013).

The Quality and Safety Landscape

Raleigh and Foot (2010) state that there is some uncertainty about the respective roles of various agencies (such as the National Quality Board, the NHS Information Centre, the National Institute for Health and Clinical Excellence, strategic health authorities, commissioners, the Care Quality Commission, Monitor, the Audit Commission, and professional regulators) in monitoring and reporting on quality (compare QualityWatch 2013). Gregory, Dixon, and Ham (2012) write that there is much to be clarified under the new NHS structures with regard to patient safety. It could be argued that quality and safety is everybody's business but nobody's responsibility.

The Impact of Reform Efforts on Quality and Safety of Care

There have been a number of studies which have charted changes in quality, and explored the relationship between reforms and quality. First, there are "official" documents by the Department of Health (DH) and other agencies such as the National Audit Office (NAO). DH (2006) contained a Foreword by Chief Medical Officer Sir Liam Donaldson, which stated that since OWAM (Department of Health 2000b) in 2000, "important and necessary steps have been taken on the journey to improve patient safety across the NHS. There is much greater awareness among clinicians, managers and policymakers that patients are not as safe as they should be ...," but "the pace of change has been too slow." NAO (2005) revisited the issue of the scale and nature of the problem and showed that there were around 974,000 reported incidents and near misses in England in 2004 and 2005 (excluding hospital-acquired infections), with around 2,180 of these incidents resulting in death. Although Darzi was on the whole positive about what had been achieved, nevertheless, he reported that "local clinical visions found unacceptable and unexplained variations in the clinical quality of care in every NHS region" (Department of Health 2008, p. 48).

DH (2009) claims that the NHS has made "huge progress over the last decade," with the care the NHS provides to patients having demonstrably improved, moving in the broadest sense from sometimes poor and occasionally good, to largely good and occasionally great. The document continued that challenge is to accelerate this quality improvement, creating services that are not just good, but universally great. It concluded that the NHS is "building on firm foundations" in terms of: lower mortality rates, HCAIs, waiting times, and patient satisfaction.

Berwick (2013) notes that the NHS in England can become the safest healthcare system in the world. Even while asserting unblinkingly what is amiss, it is important to notice and celebrate the strengths of the NHS: "Big changes are needed, but we do not believe that the NHS is unsound in its core. On the contrary, its achievements are enormous and its performance in many dimensions has improved steadily over the past two decades" (Berwick 2013, p. 9).

Second, there are a number of independent commentaries on quality and safety. There are several reports from Leatherman and Sutherland (2003, 2008). Leatherman and Sutherland (2003) broadly defined "quality of care" to include issues of access, effectiveness, equity, responsiveness, safety, and capacity. Within each dimension they examined: a snapshot (a look at a particular quality measure at one point in time), trend data (measured at two or more time points, presented longitudinally to indicate the presence or absence of progress), and international benchmarks making comparisons between countries. They aimed to provide a mid-term assessment of Labour's quality plan on the basis of some 50 indicators. They argued that qualitative and quantitative data indicate that overall performance was trending in the right direction, particularly in salient areas of appropriateness of care, use of effective interventions, and patient outcomes. Performance improved in many areas such as access to inpatient and outpatient care, as well as appropriateness of process and patient outcomes in cardiovascular and cancer care.

Leatherman and Sutherland (2008) later modified, to some degree, their optimistic 2003 verdict. They concluded that given the ten-year time horizon, the generous increase in resources dedicated to healthcare, and the ongoing goodwill on the part of the public, patients, and health professionals, there are many who question whether progress has been as marked, as rapid, or as predictable, as might have been expected.

In a Kings Fund audit of New Labour health policy, Thorlby and Maybin (2010) note that there has been a great deal of policy activity since 1997, including 26 Green and White Papers, and 14 Acts of Parliament. They set out eight criteria for a high-performing health system, including access; safety; clinical effectiveness; patient experience; and equity. They note "huge progress" in improving speed of access to hospital treatment which represents "a major achievement for the NHS;" "substantial progress" and "considerable" achievements in tackling HCAIs; mortality decline within the key areas of cancer and cardiovascular disease; and little change in overall measures of patient experience, but since 1993 overall satisfaction with the NHS has improved. They point to "a mix of achievements and disappointments," concluding that there is no doubt that the NHS is closer to being a high-performing health system now than it was in 1997. It is capable of delivering high-quality care to some patients, in some areas, some of the time (see also Propper and Venables 2013).

Gregory, Dixon, and Ham (2012) update this template to conduct a mid-term assessment of the Coalition Government. They conclude that the performance of the NHS is holding up despite financial pressures and the disruption of reforms. However, cracks are emerging—for example, with a deterioration in waiting times in accident and emergency (A&E)—and significant variations remain by geography and socioeconomic status in access to care, health outcomes, and the quality of care received. While mortality from two of the biggest killers, cancer and cardiovascular disease, continues to fall, England still has higher levels of avoidable mortality than many other countries. Finally, while patient experience of NHS adult inpatient services showed no change overall between 2009/10 and 2011/12, levels of public satisfaction with the NHS have declined.

QualityWatch (2013) draws on work by Leatherman and Sutherland (2008) to group indicators into six domains. Their main findings are that waits for elective outpatient and inpatient care, urgent care in A&E, diagnostic tests, ambulances, and cancer treatment remain consistently low compared to a decade earlier, and that while several safety and effectiveness indicators improved in the past few years, and national patient surveys show that patients generally report a positive experience of NHS care, there is no evidence to suggest that health inequalities have narrowed over the past decade. They conclude that over the past decade the overall picture is of improvements in many important aspects of quality of health and social care in England, but there are some causes for concern.

While most commentators conclude that quality and safety has improved, it is more difficult to causally link specific reforms with particular improvements. Evaluation is complicated by the confluence of multiple reforms, all being pursued in parallel, thereby making attribution to individual elements impossible. In few cases was good baseline data collected prior to the implementation of change. It is almost impossible to attribute causality where performance has changed, either positively or negatively, for these two principal reasons (Leatherman & Sutherland 2008, pp. 18, 21; compare Dixon, Mays & Jones 2011, pp. 140–141).

Dixon, Mays, and Jones (2011) explored the different components of Labour's market-based reforms. They found relatively few studies, with limited evidence, and few studies focused on "quality" per se. In broad terms, the limited studies on provider diversity found no significant differences in clinical quality between Independent Sector Treatment Centres (ISTC) and NHS providers, with patient experience similar or better. Studies on PbR found little impact on quality. The regulation system changed significantly, but failed to pick up some appalling cases of lethally unsafe care. Studies on competition constituted "probably the most discussed and controversial finding" (p. 136), with some studies reporting that hospital death rates after admission for acute myocardial infarction (heart attacks) and all-cause mortality were lower in markets where more competition was possible, but these findings have been heavily disputed (see also Propper & Venables 2013).

Propper and Venables (2013) suggest that the QOF did not lead to large changes in performance. Quality was improving rapidly before payment for performance was introduced. The scheme may have led to a further small, but possibly transient, increase in quality; and the targets may shift the focus of the practice away from harder-to-reach patients.

Moreover, while it is not fully clear if particular mechanisms work to improve quality, it is even less clear *how* they improve quality (for example "selection," "change," and "reputation" pathways (Raleigh & Foot 2010)).

The Current Situation

The current situation reflects a possible paradox of largely positive studies pointing to improvements in quality (above) with reports highlighting widespread problems, with the Francis Report (2013) perhaps reflecting a tipping point. According to the House of Commons Health Select Committee (2013), the failings at Stafford General Hospital have cast a shadow over the reputation of the NHS for safe, high-quality patient care. Similarly, Clwyd and Hart (2013) note that public confidence has been eroded by evidence of poor care and treatment and subsequent failures of the complaints system to acknowledge or rectify shortcomings.

A series of reviews on aspects of NHS care and treatment followed the Francis report (Berwick 2013, Cavendish 2013, Clwyd & Hart 2013, Keogh 2013), with a total of about 500 recommendations (including Francis). Cavendish (2013) suggested appointing on healthcare assistants and support workers. Berwick (2013) stated that in some instances, including Mid Staffordshire, clear warning signals abounded and were not heeded, especially the voices of patients and carers. This report made ten recommendations, but the most important recommendations for the way forward envision the NHS as a learning organization. Keogh (2013) examined 14 NHS Trusts (of which 11 were in "special measures") with high mortality, and showed a positive correlation between safety incident reporting data and a high hospital standardized mortality ration (HSMR) score. Clwyd and Hart (2013) focused on complaints. In January 2014, NHS England (2014) launched "the biggest patient safety initiative in the history of the NHS" creating a countrywide network of "collaboratives" to improve patient safety across England.

Conclusions

Most studies point to improvements in quality and safety over time. Moreover, there has been a shift over time from quality being a predominantly clinical, to a largely managerial, issue; to the use of explicit financial incentives to reward quality; from confidential data on provider quality to the public disclosure of quality data in the form of league tables; and from a focus on process indicators to outcome metrics indicators. Nevertheless, given the "seminal document" of OWAM (Department of Health 2000b), the "Ten-year Quality Agenda" of 1997–1998 (Leatherman & Sutherland 2003), and that the NHS seems to be the only healthcare system in the world with a definition of quality enshrined in legislation (Keogh 2013), scandals such as Mid Staffordshire and other recent reports are difficult to explain. This has possibly been associated with greater transparency and scrutiny. According to QualityWatch (2013), the quality of NHS care in England has been scrutinized more in the past year than in any other since 1948, due to a number of high-profile failings in care and concern about other potential lapses. However, there are a number of barriers and obstacles to reform, not least professional cultures and working practices which have been affirmed over decades and woven into the fabric of healthcare delivery and have remained stubbornly resistant to change.

Since its inception, the NHS has been characterized by continual reform and change and this means that it has been methodologically difficult to disentangle the effects of health policy reform on quality of care. During the last 15–20 years or so there has been a massive shift in focus and resources directed at healthcare quality and patient safety and the issue is now clearly in the public domain. However, there are resonances "deja vu all over again" as history repeats itself as tragedy rather than farce. Quality is periodically rediscovered such as by Darzi, and after Mid Staffordshire (see for example Klein 2013, pp. 259, 296), and solutions sometimes reinvent the wheel. For example, the NAO (2005) conclusion that "organisational learning is key to improving patient safety" is similar to that of Berwick (2013). Likewise, some of the recommendations of Bristol and Mid Staffordshire are similar. At times the NHS appears to be an organization without a memory. "Sorry" may be the hardest word, but learning and implementation appear to be the hardest activities.

Chapter 22
Germany

Holger Pfaff, Tristan D Gloede, and Antje Hammer

Abstract

The German healthcare system is characterized by a principle of subsidiaries, which implies a decentralization of power, as well as by a strong separation of different sectors of care such as inpatient and rehabilitation care. These conditions may impede the successful implementation of healthcare reforms that address quality of care and patient safety. However, since the 2000s, several reforms have been introduced. Among these are: obligatory quality management (QM) in the outpatient and inpatient setting, hospital quality assurance with publicly available quality reports, disease management programs (DMPs) for chronic diseases, and integrated care contracts to overcome sectoral separation. These reforms have transformed the quality and safety landscape where new institutions have emerged. However, whether these reforms have made an impact on patient outcomes remains controversial. The most important barriers for future development of the quality and safety landscape lies in the fragmentation of the healthcare system, limited transparency, access to data, and, on a more general level, the lack of a patient safety culture and a lack of system thinking in German healthcare.

Background

Germany currently has a population of about 80.6 million inhabitants. In 2012, more than 18.5 million inpatients and 18 million outpatients were treated in approximately 2,000 German hospitals and about 2,200 ambulant care settings. Approximately 2.8 million employees including 342,000 physicians and 826,000 nurses provide care to patients in inpatient and outpatient healthcare settings (Statistisches Bundesamt 2013).

After a sharp decline from a ranking of six in 2009 to a ranking of 14 in 2012, Germany reached a reasonable seventh ranking in the Euro Health Consumer Index 2013. With 796 out of 1,000 points, Germany is only 74 points behind the leading country, the Netherlands (Björnberg 2013). In addition, with regard to the selected Organisation for Economic Cooperation and Development (OECD) quality indicators, Germany reached a ranking of eighth (Organisation for Economic Cooperation and Development 2013a, Penter 2014). However, compared to other European countries, Germany takes the third ranking with regard to expenses in healthcare. In Germany, almost 11.3 percent of the GDP is invested in healthcare (Penter 2014).

Table 22.1   Demographic, economic, and health information for Germany

Population (thousands)	82,800
Area (sq. km)*	348.570
Proportion of population living in urban areas (2011)	74
Gross Domestic Product (GDP US$, billions)^	3,425.9
Total expenditure on health as % of GDP	11.3
Gross national income per capita (PPP intl $)	42,230
Per capita total expenditure on health (intl $)	4,617
Proportion of health expenditure which is private	23.7
General Government expenditure on health as a percentage of total expenditure on health	76.3
Out-of-pocket expenditure as a percentage of private expenditure on health	50.8
Life expectancy at birth m/f (yrs)	78/83
Probability of dying under five (per 1,000 live births)	4
Maternal Mortality Ratio (per 100,000 live births) (2013)	7
Proportion of population using improved water and sanitation	100/100

Source: Unless otherwise stated data are for the year 2012 and taken from the World Health Organization 2014. * Area from the World Bank 2014a. ^GDP from the World Bank 2014b.

Notes: PPP is purchasing power parity, intl $ is international dollar which has the same purchasing power as US$ in the US.

Introduction

Health insurance is mandatory in Germany and around 90 percent of the population is publicly insured. A very important rule in the German healthcare system is the principle of subsidiarity: The Federal Joint Committee (G-BA), which represents insurers and healthcare providers, defines the catalogue of benefits. According to this catalogue healthcare has to be delivered by all providers and reimbursed by all insurers. The healthcare providers from a certain sector (for example outpatient physicians) then jointly negotiate with all public insurers for a budget for their sector. The subsidiarity principle assures that the lowest level of the healthcare system, which is able to solve an existing healthcare problem, is in charge of the problem. This decentralization of power is an important strength of the German system, since it reduces the influence of the Government and allows providers and insurers to tailor solutions around their requirements. This structure represents a middle ground between market and hierarchical or state coordination (in particular the Bismarck model compared to the market or Beveridge model). However, the structure also incorporates elements of competition. Patients are free to choose between different insurers and among providers of healthcare. This decentralized structure enables the system to be innovative and counterbalances the different forces within the system. The public health insurers have evolved from the self-help workers movement of the nineteenth century, which shows that the idea of community is built into the system. Hence, social capital and solidarity are essential long-standing pillars of the German healthcare system.

On the other hand, an important weakness of the German healthcare system is partly related to its strength: there are multiple actors in the system. Decentralization combined with a multi-payer system and a multi-sector provider system involves many actors with conflicting interests, which may result in difficult and time and energy consuming decision making. As a result, it sometimes takes too long to react to environmental changes. Often the decision has to be a compromise between the different interest groups and lacks the power to solve healthcare problems in a concerted manner. Another weakness of the German system is its fragmentation, as it is configured into different sectors (specifically outpatient, inpatient, rehabilitation, and long-term care) and it lacks coordination between these sectors (Ommen et al. 2007, Gloede et al. 2013). This leads to several problems with regard to process coordination and information flow between the sectors. Data from the Commonwealth Fund supports this assumption and shows that when compared to patients from other countries, German patients more often face problems with the coordination of their care (Schoen & Osborn 2011).

Particular Quality and Safety Challenges Facing the German Healthcare System

The German healthcare system is currently facing particularly important challenges with regard to quality and safety. Most important are: (1) the fragmentation of the system, (2) a poor implementation of evidence-based guidelines, (3) a poor safety culture, and (4) a lack of system thinking.

With regard to the fragmentation of the healthcare system into different sectors—mentioned above—quality and safety problems occur when information on transitioning patients is not appropriately transferred across sectors (Ommen et al. 2007). In such a system, patients can fall through the cracks.

A second factor to be considered is a deficit in guideline implementation in the German healthcare system. For example, only a small proportion of general practitioners have the necessary knowledge to treat hypertension in accordance with guideline recommendations (Hagemeister et al. 2001, Flesch et al. 2008). Often the mere knowledge of the guidelines does not lead to a better therapy (Karbach et al. 2011). One result from a recent workshop on guideline implementation was that more information is needed about the reasons for physicians deviating from guidelines. (For more information see http://www.netzwerk-versorgungsforschung.de).

The third issue in the German healthcare system is the lack of a patient safety culture and the lack of development of error reporting systems. Healthcare professionals still have problems with reporting and discussing near misses or errors. One problem is that the effectiveness of error reporting systems is based on voluntary error reporting by frontline staff. However, a culture of mistrust and fear of penalties persists, which reduces the effectiveness of critical incident reporting systems with regard to error reporting, analysis, and feedback. Therefore, establishment of the key aspects of safety culture—such as communication openness, non-punitive responses to error, and supervisor and leadership commitment to patient safety procedures—is needed to encourage healthcare professionals to discuss near misses, errors, and systematic problems (Pfaff et al. 2005, Hammer 2012).

One last—but none the less important—issue in the German healthcare system is a lack of system thinking throughout the hospitals and among general practitioners and specialists. Too often care providers blame individual actors for causing quality and safety problems. The possibility that the hospital, as a system, may carry blame for failures is often beyond people's current conceptual framework. As a result, a lot of measures in quality and safety management are individual measures. Actors in the German healthcare system lack appropriate system-based measures to improve quality and safety in Germany.

Key Participants in the Health System

The G-BA is the highest decision-making body in the German healthcare system and oversees and promotes the implementation of quality assurance systems in the German healthcare system. It is supervised by the Federal Ministry of Health and oversees several self-governing organizations that are responsible for initiating and monitoring healthcare reform efforts. Table 22.2 provides an overview and a brief description of the key participants and main actors in Germany, as well as their duties.

Successful drivers for improving quality and safety in German healthcare have been the implementation of guidelines and the institutionalization of state-based, and state-wide, quality institutes like IQWiG, BQS, and AQUA. We are distinguishing two quality realms: one is the realm of diagnosis and therapy; the other is in the context of care, like the hospitals and the patient reported outcomes (PRO). In the realm of diagnosis and therapy, the combination of the implementation of guidelines and the institutionalization of the IQWiG have been the most important steps with regard to quality assurance. The vision of IQWiG is to deliver evidence-based information to the G-BA with regard to the clinical efficacy of therapies and diagnosis. The aim is to make sure that the decision of the G-BA is not only policy-driven but also evidence-driven, thus fostering the quality of the health insurance-paid therapies and diagnostics in the long run. To foster the quality of the healthcare institutions, the German Government has established additional quality institutes. In the first phase, the BQS was founded. Initially, the task of the BQS was to look at the quality of German hospitals,

Table 22.2   Key participants and main actors in German healthcare

Institution	Description and tasks
Federal Ministry of Health (*Bundesgesund-heitsministerium*) (BMG)	*Tasks:* responsible for the drafting of bills, ordinances, and administrative regulations; oversees several Government agencies such as the Robert Koch Institute, responsible for disease control and prevention (http://www.bmg.bund.de).
Federal Joint Committee (*Gemeinsamer Bundesausschuß*) (G-BA)	Committee of the joint self-Government of physicians, dentists, hospitals, and health insurance funds in Germany. *Tasks:* issues directives for the benefit catalogue of the statutory health insurance funds (GKV); specifies which services in medical care are reimbursed by the GKV; is in charge of specifying quality measures in inpatient and outpatient areas of the German healthcare system; decides on the contents, extent, and data format of the hospitals' regularly structured quality reports (*Qualitätsberichte*) (http://www.english.g-ba.de).
National Association of Statutory Health Insurance Funds (*GKV-Spitzenverband*) (GKV-SV)	*Tasks:* representation of interests of the health insurance funds at the federal level; advises parliaments and ministries with regard to law-making procedures (http://www.gkv-spitzenverband.de).
German Medical Association (*Bundesärztekammer*) (BÄK)	Joint association of the 17 State Chambers of Physicians. *Tasks:* represents the interests of physicians related to professional policy, opinion-forming processes with regard to health and social policy and in legislative procedures; promotes continuing medical education and quality assurance in healthcare (http://www.bundesaerztekammer.de).
Institute for Quality and Efficiency in Health Care (*Institut für Qualität und Wirtschaftlichkeit im Gesundheitswesen*) (IQWiG)	Independent organization (similar to the United Kingdom's, National Institute for Health and Care Excellence (NICE)). *Tasks:* prepare evidence-based reports on the benefit of new health technologies that are to be included in the catalogue of benefits; accountable for the provision of, for example, "easily understandable" information on quality and efficiency for patients and the general community (https://www.iqwig.de).
Institute for Applied Quality Improvement and Research in Health Care GmbH (*Institut für angewandte Qualitätsförderung und Forschung im Gesundheitswesen*) (AQUA)	Independent and impartial corporation that provides services for quality assurance. *Tasks:* in 2009 AQUA took on the responsibilities of the Federal Office for Quality Assurance (*Bundesgeschäftsstelle Qualitätssicherung*) (BQS) for the nationwide cross—sectoral healthcare quality assurance mandated by the G-BA (http://www.aqua-institut.de).

Institution	Description and tasks
German Hospital Ferderation (*Deutsche Krankenhausgesellschaft*)	Federation of national and state representing interests of about 2,000 German hospitals. *Tasks:* support and encouragement of members in fulfilling their tasks in the hospital sector; works to sustain and improve hospital performance; promotes the exchange of knowledge; supports scientific research in healthcare; votes as a member of the G-BA (see below); represents German hospitals at the European and international level as a member of the International Hospital Federation and the European Hospital and Health Care Federation (http://www.dkgev.de).
National Association of Statutory Health Insurance Physicians (*Kassenärztliche Bundesvereinigung*) (KBV)	Consists of the 17 Associations of Statutory Health Insurance Physicians (ASHIP). *Tasks:* represents the political interests of doctors and psychotherapists; ensures access to outpatient care (*Sicherstellungsauftrag*); (http://www.kbv.de).
Institute for the Hospital Remuneration System (*Institut für das Entgeltsystem im Krankenhaus*)	*Tasks*: supports contractual partners and their formed committees with regard to introduction and development of the diagnosis related groups system (DRG) in accordance to the law (http://www.g-drg.de).
Evaluation Committee (*Bewertungsausschuss*)	Joint self-administration of doctors and health insurance companies. *Tasks*: specifies the uniform value standard, which is the basis for billing of medical services under the statutory health insurance; decides on provisions for contractual medical compensation (reference price) (https://www.institut-des-bewertungsausschusses.de).
Association of the German Health Insurance Medical Service (*Medizinische Dienst der Krankenversicherung*)	Community of the health insurance companies and care funds, which is organized in each state as an independent community. *Tasks*: advises the healthcare funds on matters of general medical and nursing care; examines individual cases; is involved in the quality developments in healthcare, the justification of the performance decisions of the health insurance, and the prevention of immature, unnecessary, dangerous, or uneconomical performances in healthcare (http://www.mdk.de).
German Agency for Quality in Medicine (Ärztliches Zentrum für Qualität in der Medizin)	Owned by the German Medical Association and the National Association of Statutory Health Insurance Physicians. *Tasks*: initiates quality programs in the German healthcare system with specific focus on evidence-based medicine, medical guidelines, patient empowerment, patient safety, and QM (http://www.aezq.de).

Table 22.2   Key participants and main actors in German healthcare *concluded*

Institution	Description and tasks
German Coalition for Patient Safety (GCPS) (*Aktionsbündnis Patientensicherheit*)	*Tasks*: it is dedicated to research, development and dissemination of appropriate methods to improve patient safety in healthcare. The GCPS work program comprises specific projects acquired within different multidisciplinary working groups, which meet regularly and publish their results in the form of recommendations for action (http://www.aps-ev.de).

primarily with regard to certain procedures and operations. In the second phase, the AQUA Institute followed the BQS Institute. The aim of AQUA was to study the quality of care process between hospitals and the ambulant sector for certain typical illnesses and indications. One of the most powerful instruments of AQUA is that they visit those hospitals that had inferior or suspicious results. There are now plans underway to build up a large German quality institute with the objective of delivering quality and transparency for all players; this institute would probably replace AQUA.

Another successful driver of improvement in the safety of care in Germany has been the institutionalization of the GCPS. The GCPS is an association of private and public institutions that aspires to improve patient safety in Germany. This initiative was important to promote the idea of patient safety within Germany, within the hospitals and within the mind of the physicians. One target was to build up a safety culture (error-admitting culture) by showing the physicians that even very famous physicians admit that they had caused some medical errors in their careers.

Reform Initiatives and Procedures in Healthcare

While previous healthcare reforms, prior to the 2000s, were focusing on cost containment, current reform initiatives have aimed at increasing efficiency, quality, and safety.

Since 2000, hospitals and outpatient physician practices have been obliged to implement an internal QM system. In 2001, DMPs were introduced for certain chronic diseases. Between 2003 and 2004, policymakers endeavored to target hospital efficiency and introduced a DRGs-based reimbursement system for hospitals. In addition, starting in 2004, hospitals were required to participate in a national quality assurance program. The so-called quality reports of this program have been made publicly available, first on a biennial basis and now (since 2013) on an annual basis. Another major healthcare reform of 2004 addressed the contractual relationship between healthcare providers and the conditions for providing integrated health services. This reform established the legal basis for selective contracts between individual insurers and providers. In 2007, allowing long-term care providers to participate in integrated care activities further strengthened integrated care. Enacted in 2012, a new reform targeted access to outpatient care, for instance by setting financial incentives for physicians who settle in undersupplied, mostly non-urban areas. In 2013, a new law was enacted which was intended to improve patients' rights. A significant change under this law is that the process of requiring informed consent from the patient is now codified within the civil law code.

Impact of Specific Healthcare Reform Efforts on the Quality and Safety of Care

Amongst these healthcare reform initiatives, several have sought to improve the quality of care. The following are most relevant: (1) the introduction of DMPs, (2) the facilitation of integrated care, (3) the introduction of DRGs for hospital reimbursement, and (4) the implementation of QM systems for hospitals in 2000 as well as the accompanying obligation of hospitals to participate in national quality assurance. These reforms have clearly made an impact on the quality and safety landscape in Germany. However, whether they have made an impact on actual patient outcomes remains controversial.

DMPs for patients with type 2 diabetes were introduced in 2001. In an effort to facilitate evidence-based care according to clinical guidelines and patient education with close monitoring and quality assurance, all public health insurers may issue DMPs. DMPs were expanded to other chronic diseases such as breast cancer, coronary heart disease, and chronic obstructive pulmonary disease.

The integrated care reform of 2004 established the legal basis for selective, integrated care contracts between individual health insurers and healthcare providers (whereas before they were only able to negotiate collectively and contract as collectives). Under this law, health insurers may contract with hospitals and outpatient physicians to provide integrated care, whereby healthcare providers share accountability for quality and reimbursement. Thereby, actors in the healthcare system may act more dynamically and may respond faster to the needs of patients. To facilitate integrated care contracts, 1 percent of the budget for hospitals and outpatient physicians between 2004 and 2006 was used to provide seed funding.

The use of case-based flat payments, based on DRGs, to reimburse hospitals has incentivized hospitals to use resources more efficiently. Even though this reform has been successful in improving hospital efficiency, the authors of several studies have argued that there are also adverse effects for some patients (Reinhold et al. 2009). Under the DRG regime, the marginal revenue of a day spent in the hospital is zero, hence, it is economically rational to reduce the average length of stay. In this regard, the reform has been successful, but there is consistent evidence that many patients are being discharged too early (Reinhold et al. 2009).

Further adjustment to the reimbursement system is needed to overcome these adverse effects.

With regard to safety assurance in the stationary healthcare sector, several initiatives have been initiated since the 1970s (Böcken, Butzlaff, & Esche 2003). However, it took another two decades for quality assurance procedures in hospitals to be established by law (in 1989, §§135–137 of the Fifth Social Code). These laws mandated that German hospitals implement successful QM arrangements. To facilitate this in ambulant and stationary healthcare settings, the Federal Ministry of Health funded and supported several pilot projects on QM. In 1993, the National Association of Statutory Health Insurance Physicians, the German Medical Association, the German Hospital Federation, and the Central Federal Association of Health Insurance Funds founded the Association for the Promotion of Quality Assurance in Medicine (*Arbeitsgemeinschaft zur Förderung der Qualitätssicherung in der Medizin*). The Association was responsible for reporting on the development of quality assurance in healthcare settings. With the healthcare reform in 2000, healthcare providers became obliged to establish organizational QM (Böcken, Butzlaff, & Esche 2003). In 2004, the G-BA took on the responsibilities of the Association for the Promotion of Quality Assurance in Medicine. Since 2005, German hospitals must, by law, regularly publish (biennial) structured quality reports (§137 of the Fifth Social Code). These reports are considered a tool to measure and describe hospital quality and were published for the first time in 2004. In order to ensure more transparency for patients regarding quality of care, the reports have been envisaged to serve patients and healthcare professionals with sufficient information on hospital quality performance in order to give guidance for hospital selection. In turn, hospitals are required to make their achievements and quality performance transparent.

In January 2014 the G-BA announced a resolution regarding amendments to §137 of the Fifth Social Code. Amendments included: a stronger focus on patient safety as well as a new paragraph on the implementation and development of clinical risk management and error reporting systems, the number of indicators to be published increased from 182 to 286, and hospitals with more than one site have to provide separate reports for each site (Gemeinsamer Bundesausschuss 2014).

Implementation: Barriers and Solutions

The most important barriers to the implementation of QM measures in Germany are the lack of transparency, unequal access to quality-related information, lack of "know-how" in evidence-based medicine, lack of time for training in quality issues, quality documentation overload, financial burden due to QM, strong doubts as to the efficacy of QM, lack of feedback, communication and competence problems between quality-relevant actors, and resistance to change, especially with regard to the autonomy of the profession (Helou 2003). Further barriers for QM implementation arise from the segmentation of the German health system, the large number of players who have to be coordinated to improve QM, the decentralized political system in Germany (central Government with 16 states responsible for healthcare in their region), the professional attitude of "we are doing high quality work and therefore we don't need quality management," a high amount of saturation of demand with regard to QM, economic pressure which replaces quality orientation and a restrictive protection of data privacy (Nothacker et al. 2013).

As solutions to the problem of implementation, the German quality community is considering several measures: participation and involvement of all actors and stakeholders in the process of planning the QM project, personal involvement of the decision maker, clear communication and communication channels, goal-oriented incentives, and adequate methods for monitoring the QM process—the Plan–Do–Check–Act (PDCA)-cycle—and the QM results (Nothacker et al. 2013, Helou 2003). Other measures are targeted at reducing segmentation, diminishing the number of stakeholders (for example health insurance companies), centralizing core activities, working on the professional culture, and reducing economic pressure where possible to gain more money and time for quality. One example of trying to realize some of these solutions in practice is the National Cancer Plan (NCP). The aim of the NCP is to establish a PDCA-cycle, involving important stakeholders and, in the near future, to use the German-wide clinical cancer registry to get data into this cycle (Beckmann 2009).

Prospects for Success and Next Steps

What more needs to be done to achieve a safe, high-quality health service in Germany? The next steps could be to establish a nation-wide quality institute with the aim to gather all subjective and objective data necessary to improve quality within and between the different health sectors. These data should be pseudonomized and open for scientific inquiry. In Germany we need more professorial posts and university chairs in the realm of QM and health services research in order to develop the capacity to do sound research in this field and to educate specialists on QM and quality-oriented health services research. We also need more nation-wide clinical registries for important diseases, such as the German clinical cancer registry. What is also needed is increased public reporting. What might the reform levers be for the future? Future reform levers could be establishing pay for performance programs in Germany. In that case quality would become an economic necessity. What are the timeframes involved? The new quality institute will be installed within the next two years. The German clinical cancer registry will likely be fully operational in three to five years. It will take five to ten years to establish enough professorships in QM and HSR. Probably it will take five years to establish pay for performance in pilot projects and to evaluate them.

Conclusion

The measures for improving quality and patient safety in German healthcare are numerous. However, despite the big efforts and positive results so far to improve quality, there are still a considerable number of problems to solve. The most important conclusion is that in a healthcare system like Germany where there is a mix of market, self-government, and state regulation, state regulation is essential to achieve a concerted effort to enhance quality assurance and QM. This is necessary because it is difficult to coordinate numerous actors with regard to QM. It will take the central Government to initiate this and to set the frame for the different stakeholders to act on quality and patient safety.

Chapter 23
Italy

Americo Cicchetti, Silvia Coretti, and Valentina Iacopino

Abstract

Italy's healthcare system is a regionally-based National Health Service (INHS) that provides universal coverage. Services are free of charge at delivery and this gives rise to several forms of non-price rationing. Quality and safety are considered major policy concerns even in a period, as is currently the case, in which the public healthcare system is suffering from a striking economic and financial crisis. Many healthcare reforms have been launched since the establishment of the INHS in 1978, with the aim of setting structural, professional, and technological standards, managing quality, and assessing performances. Along with healthcare reforms both at the national and regional level within the public system, several emergent initiatives have been promoted at a local level. These are currently in place and promote quality and safety in the whole healthcare sector. Nevertheless, in this scenario, quality and safety assurance in the healthcare system could be improved in the near future by implementing policies that fill some of the existing gaps. A greater involvement of patients and citizens in assessing the performance of the system, a clearer link between publicly available evidence and policymaking, the establishment of a national framework for health technology assessment, and the definition of organizational standards for hospitals and other healthcare services are major priorities for the INHS.

Introduction and Methodology

Italy's healthcare system is a regionally-based NHS that provides universal coverage free of charge at the point of service. The INHS is organized into three layers:

- National, which is responsible for ensuring the general objectives and fundamental principles of the national healthcare system;
- Regional and Local which, through the regional health departments, are responsible for ensuring the delivery of a benefits package through a network of population-based Local Health Organizations (ASL) and through a network of accredited public and private hospitals (Lo Scalzo et al. 2009).

Table 23.1   Demographic, economic, and health information for Italy

Population (thousands)	60,885
Area (sq. km)*	294,140
Proportion of population living in urban areas (2011)	68
Gross Domestic Product (GDP US$, billions)^	2,013.4
Total expenditure on health as % of GDP	9.2
Gross national income per capita (PPP intl $)	32,920
Per capita total expenditure on health (intl $)	3,040
Proportion of health expenditure which is private	21.8
General Government expenditure on health as a percentage of total expenditure on health	78.2
Out-of-pocket expenditure as a percentage of private expenditure on health	92.7
Life expectancy at birth m/f (yrs)	80/85
Probability of dying under five (per 1,000 live births)	4
Maternal Mortality Ratio (per 100,000 live births) (2013)	4
Proportion of population using improved water and sanitation	100/

Source: Unless otherwise stated data are for the year 2012 and taken from the World Health Organization 2014. * Area from the World Bank 2014a. ^GDP from the World Bank 2014.

Notes: PPP is purchasing power parity, intl $ is international dollar which has the same purchasing power as US$ in the US.

The progressive devolution of powers and responsibilities concerning healthcare to regional authorities has strongly characterized the history of the INHS in the last 20 years. This process was initiated by Legislative Decree 299/1999 and Constitutional Law 3/2001, and culminated in Law 42/2009, which formally established fiscal federalism in the healthcare sector (Cicchetti 2011). Devolution made even more urgent the systematic monitoring of care delivered at local levels to safeguard all citizens' right to receive an adequate response to their healthcare needs (Vasselli, Filippetti, & Spizzichino 2005).

In order to reach a clear understanding regarding major past, current, and future initiatives in the INHS to enhance quality of care and patient safety, we have adopted an approach based on the traditional Donabedian model (Donabedian 1980), whereby efforts undertaken to attain enhanced "quality" are aimed at setting structural, technological, and professional standards (structure), managing quality (process), and assessing results (outcomes).

In order to better understand the implementation of Italian reforms for quality and patient safety, the institutional–legislative, economical, technological, and cultural background of the INHS will be presented. In particular, we are convinced that the success of any reform is closely related to cultural factors: resistance to change often impedes the implementation of reforms, whereas the presence of a managerial view, the propensity to work in teams, and a multidisciplinary approach often facilitate the realization of these initiatives. Moreover, from the political and economic point of view, the current pressures to contain costs, together with the necessity of safeguarding universalism, and equity in access to healthcare facilities, call for measures aimed at rationalizing healthcare expenditure rather than putting in place cost-cutting measures. In addition, technological innovation plays a central role in supporting reforms aimed at monitoring and assessing quality, and providing adequate information systems. Finally, in a regionally-based healthcare system, cooperation and collaboration between national, regional, and local institutional levels are essential for the successful implementation of reforms.

Background

Law 833/1978, which established the INHS, attempted to standardize the provision of care across the country, introducing technical standards for hospital construction. However, major reforms in the 1990s were enacted to improve the efficiency of the system through decentralization and competition. The process of regional devolution was formalized by the Constitutional Law 3/2001, whereby the national level sets the general objectives and defines the basic package of healthcare services be available to all citizens (LEAs) and regional Governments are responsible for their provision through accredited public and private hospitals (Lo Scalzo et al. 2009). The devolution process culminated in Law 42/2009, which formally established a form of fiscal federalism (Cicchetti 2011).

A clear policy for addressing the quality of health services emerged only during the 1990s, starting from a "structural" approach. A range of efforts to set structural, technological, and professional standards were made. In particular, starting with Legislative Decree n. 502/1992 (known as the "second reform"),[1] institutional accreditation was established to guarantee structural, technical, and organizational quality standards for hospitals. This enables public and private hospitals to be funded by the INHS and is granted by regional authorities following a prior assessment of specific quality requirements set by a National Commission (Vasselli, Filippetti, & Spizzichino 2005). Moreover, "voluntary accreditation" and "accreditation for excellence," granted by private providers, such as Joint Commission International, can be obtained. The second reform introduced "managerialism" into the Italian NHS (Anessi-Pessina & Cantù 2006), while competition among public and private providers was facilitated via the Diagnosis Related Group (DRG)-based payment scheme. At the end of the 1990s, with Legislative Decree n. 229/1999 (known as the "third reform"), the focus in the INHS shifted from "efficiency" to "quality,"

---

1   The establishment of the INHS, with Law n. 833/1978, is considered the "first reform."

and from "competition" to "cooperation." Diverse initiatives were launched to implement a "clinical governance" framework within INHS following the example of the British NHS (Spandonaro, Mennini, & Atella 2004). This new approach to ensure quality in healthcare was sustained by envisioning a new organizational model based on "clinical directorates" (CDs) to be introduced in Italian public healthcare organizations (Mascia, Morandi, & Cicchetti 2014). Through CDs, higher involvement of physicians in administrative and quality management was pursued. At the beginning of the millennium, attention shifted to the diffusion of the health technology assessment (HTA) approach as a tool to manage the introduction of new health technologies in the INHS resulting in quality of care improvement, higher level of appropriateness, and better outcomes. But only in 2007 was the National Agency for Regional Health Services (Age.Na.S.) made for national coordination of regional and local HTA bodies that had flourished in the meantime. The setting of professional standards and continuous education in medicine was accomplished by Decree 229/1999 and reformed in the 2000s (Vettore 2008).

Several attempts to manage quality (process) were also introduced in the same period. Legislative Decree 502/1992 created conditions for the diffusion of clinical practice guidelines within a National Plan for Clinical Practice Guidelines (PNLG) established within the National Institute of Health. The quality of clinical processes were also ensured through the establishment of a national drug vigilance framework. In the process area, a clear policy for patient safety emerged in 2003 when a National Technical Committee on Clinical Risk was established. The National Observatory for Monitoring Sentinel Events started in 2005 and only in 2007, a National System for Patients Safety was implemented. More recent reforms aimed at assessing quality are discussed in the next sessions. An overview of the major healthcare reforms affecting quality and dating from the institution of the NHS to the present is presented in Table 23.2.

The Current Situation

Nowadays the INHS is a Beveridge–model health system based on universalistic principles and ensuring free access to healthcare facilities. It was established within a welfare state system in which funding is ensured by general taxation. Three main principles govern the system: (1) universal coverage of citizens and guarantees, (2) solidarity in contribution and funding, (3) equality in accessing healthcare services (Damiani & Ricciardi 2005). The affirmation of these principles during the first 35 years of activity (1978–2013) should be considered a strength of the system compared to other systems, which are based on different principles. Moreover, INHS guarantees large pharmaceutical coverage, a well-performing national network for organ transplantations, free pediatric care, high-tech diagnostics, and high levels of vaccination coverage (Italian National Health Plan 2011–2013, Ministero della Salute 2010a) which all contribute to Italy reaching adequate levels

Table 23.2   Major reforms affecting quality in Italy

Major reforms	Quality and patient safety
1978: A national health service was established by Law 833/1978.	Introduction of **homogeneous technical standard** for hospital construction (nationwide).
1992–1994: The Government approved the first reform of the INHS, which started a devolving healthcare powers to the regions and simultaneously delegated managerial autonomy to hospitals and local health units (public trusts).	**Accreditation** mechanisms introduced for both public and private providers; Establishment of national **drug vigilance framework;** First national program for the development of **clinical practice guidelines.**
1999: Legislative Decree 229/1999 launched a new reform package, which deepened the regional devolution process, envisaged the reorientation of the internal market reforms introducing the concept of **Core Benefit Package** (CBP).	**Continuous medical education** (ECM) national framework introduced.
2000–2001: Constitutional Law n. 3, 18 October 2001, modified the second part of the Italian Constitution (Title V), providing regions with more powers.	**Hospital accreditation framework** devolved to Regions.
2003: Establishment of a **National Technical Committee on Clinical Risk.** **2007**: the Ministry of Health (MoH) initiated the National System for Patients Safety.	Regions were pushed to establish a **Regional System for Patient Safety.**
2007: First attempt to introduce a national framework for HTA.	Age.Na.S. created **a national coordination for regional HTA** bodies.
2009: National Law n. 42/2009 modified the financing systems creating a real federal system in healthcare sector.	Tuscany Region launched a **regional performance management program (PMP)** for healthcare trusts including quality indicators.
2011: MoH started the Clinical Outcomes National Plan and PMP goes nationwide.	Age.Na.S. designed and tested the new system; Tuscany PMP extended nationwide to monitor CBP.
2012: Decree on **organizational standards** proposed by the MoH.	The application of new organizational standards is delayed to 2014.

in key health status indicators such as life expectancy at birth (second highest in the world) and low infant mortality rates. Conversely, several criticisms can be made, including the inappropriateness of certain services provided in hospital settings and within emergency care because of an inadequate organization of territorial settings. For instance, often patients prefer to turn to an emergency department, even if their clinical condition is not urgent, because they cannot find adequate response to their needs in primary care setting. Second, concerns over waiting times must be recognized. Third, the cross-regional differences in terms of prompt access to innovative drugs and the quality of healthcare facilities, which result in inter-regional mobility, deserve mention (Italian National Health Plan 2011–2013, Ministero della Salute 2010a).

The INHS has reached, on average at national level, good performance on indicators (compared with major Organisation for Economic Cooperation and Development (OECD) countries) with public health expenditures that are lower than the average of 25 major OECD countries (see OECD Health Data 2013b). The latest available comparative data (2012) show that total healthcare expenditures equal US$3,071.1 per capita (OECD average US$3,322), accounting for 9.3 percent on GDP (that is, at the OECD average). Nevertheless, all major initiatives dedicated to the assessment of the performance of the INHS such as Osservasalute,[2] show significant heterogeneity in accessibility, quality, and economical performance of regional health services.

Challenges facing the Italian system are listed in the National Health Plan, which is realized by the National Government under the proposals of the Minister of Health, the Ministry of Economy and Finance, having consulted the regions. It provides a general framework for national planning and includes the declaration of future actions. The National Health Plan 2011–2013 identified several challenges directly related to quality and safety improvement, namely the update of LEAs, the promotion of appropriateness in service delivery through guidelines, the definition of diagnostic, and therapeutic patterns and standards, with the final goal of achieving a uniform provision of the basic package across the country. Another relevant challenge relates to long waiting times for treatment, which are a major policy concern in countries with public health insurance, zero, or low-cost sharing, and constraints on supply (Siciliani and Hurst 2004, Siciliani and Hurst 2005). Finally, further worries relate to cost containment measures, which led to an increase of copayments on diagnostics and specialist care, which currently accounts for 16.3 percent of the overall cost. In 2013, nine million Italians declared to give up necessary health services because they could not afford copayments. Not surprisingly, the demand for publicly funded services decreased on average by 8.5 percent (Cittadinanzattiva 2013).

At a national level, several actors are responsible for quality and safety improvement. Primarily, the MoH encompasses a technical body explicitly devoted to monitoring and managing quality. The Italian Agency of Medicines (AIFA), in charge of pharmaceutical approval and policies, monitors the safety of drugs, whereas Age.Na.S. manages quality by monitoring waiting times and continuous education in medicine. Regional authorities are autonomous in setting

---

2   Osservasalute is a joint effort of more than 200 independent researchers in the area of public health and health economics. Since 2002, it has been publishing an annual national report containing demographic, epidemiological, health status, organizational, and economic indicators from the 21 regional health systems which constitute the INHS (http://www.osservasalute.it/).

specific projects to improve quality and safety within the framework provided by the National Health Plan. Finally, citizens are increasingly interested in quality issues, thus some citizens' associations such as Cittadinanzattiva are currently contributing to quality monitoring reports (http://www.cittadinanzattiva.it/).

Detail of Current Reform Initiatives

In the INHS different initiatives have been undertaken recently to improve patient safety and quality of care from structural, process, and outcomes perspectives.

Recent reforms have attempted to improve professional and technological standards. In 2012 the Standing Conference on the Relations between the State, the Regions, and the Autonomous Provinces attempted to improve the quality of ECM. The agreement set guidelines for the accreditation of ECM providers and two surveillance bodies. ECM providers need to earn two-year accreditation and be listed in the national register. Health professionals must reach 150 training credits every three years. Quality of clinical pathways and healthcare systems are indicated as the most relevant contents of ECM programs. The Decree 95/2012 established a control room for HTA at the MoH, with the aim of providing a national framework for several regional HTA initiatives. Such a measure acknowledges the political relevance of HTA in rationalizing investment and disinvestment decisions. This is particularly important in regard to medical devices, which are still lacking a strict regulation for their market access.

Some efforts have been undertaken from a "process" point of view, in particular to tackle the challenge of waiting times. The National Plan to manage waiting lists 2010–2012 designed a new information system for monitoring waiting lists, setting central booking points, and compelling regions to define their maximum waiting times. A well-structured monitoring system (NSIS) was established involving information flows about outpatient care, inpatient care, patients' pathway in oncology, private service delivery, and suspension of delivery. Furthermore, accredited public and private hospitals are supposed to publish information about their waiting times on their own website (Fattore and Ferrè 2012).

Recently, a major emphasis has been placed on performance measurement and health system outcomes. The National Plan for Outcome Assessment (PNE), managed by Age.Na.S., started in 2010 to identify aspects of the healthcare pathways affecting outcomes and to promote internal and external auditing. PNE assesses outcomes of inpatient care. Its aim is to favor clinical audit rather than to produce judgments or rankings, while a possible pitfall is the heterogeneous quality of data deriving from hospital discharge forms. Moreover, some initiatives to assess quality are currently running at regional level.

In addition to these reforms, promoted by the public side of the system, some emergent initiatives deserve mention. For instance, some hospitals have implemented the lean model (Kim et al. 2006) to make pathways fluid and cut costs. However, no published evidence is available on the effects of this approach on quality. Interestingly, in recent years the Italian Federation of Health Clinics and Hospitals (FIASO) established an observatory to systematically collect and share best practices to encourage the uptake of measures to improve performance and contain costs (Italian Federation of Health Clinics and Hospitals 2012).

Table 23.3 summarizes the main reforms concerning quality and safety which occurred within the INHS and provides a classification based on an adaptation of the Donabedian model.

Table 23.3   Majors programs for quality and patient safety in Italy

Setting standards	Healthcare organizations (Accreditation, Clinical directorates model)
	People (Continuous medical education)
	Technology (Clinical guidelines national program and HTA network)
Managing quality	Patient safety framework (National and regional bodies)
	Clinical governance framework (Regional and local level)
	National drug vigilance framework (AIFA)
Assessing outcomes	National patient safety framework (MoH)
	National and regional performance management programs (MoH, regional Department of Health)
	National clinical outcomes program (MoH)

The Quality and Safety Landscape

Responsibilities for quality and safety improvement are shared among the national, regional, and local level. At national level, several actors are responsible for quality and safety improvement. The MoH provides the regulation framework, ensures national planning, and monitors quality by means of its own Quality Department (Lo Scalzo et al. 2009). This technical body is crucial in the definition of LEAs. Quality and safety of pharmaceuticals are guaranteed by AIFA, which ensures the standardized access to drugs and their safe and appropriate utilization. AIFA is also in charge of ensuring innovation and governing drug expenditure. It cooperates with the European Medicines Agency, and other national authorities, and favors investments and research activities. Age.Na.S. plays a central role in monitoring quality and safety, assessing the efficacy of LEAs. It formulates proposals for the organization of healthcare services, analyzes quality, costs, and safety of innovations, and monitors waiting times and ECM. It also carries out national programs connected to quality and safety, such as the programs on HTA, on clinical risks and patients' safety, and on organizational and clinical guidelines.

Regions progressively acquired political power in planning local activities and monitoring quality in the delivery of healthcare services. The same occurred at local level, where the Management Team of the Local Health Enterprises and

Hospital Enterprises became responsible for resource allocation and the quality of services (Lo Scalzo et al. 2009).

Citizens are scarcely involved in national initiatives to improve quality. Some examples of civic audit can be sporadically observed at the local level (Vasselli, Filippetti, & Spizzichino 2005). Often citizens are not adequately informed of the measures to improve quality that are currently in place. In fact, reforms recently introduced, and primarily aimed at containing public expenditure, seem to erode the quality and quantity of services that the INHS is supposed to guarantee. Thus, while out-of-pocket expenditures paid by citizens increase, they perceive no extension in the range of services delivered (Censis 2013).

Impact of Reform Efforts on Quality and Safety of Care

Even though the assessment of the impact of health reforms on quality of care and patients safety poses both methodological and technical problems, it should be considered as crucial for any public healthcare system. In Italy, until now, no systematic assessment of the impact of major healthcare reforms implemented in INHS is available. Nevertheless, in some areas, it is possible to draw some conclusions thanks to both public and private initiatives focused on assessing the impact of specific policies.

Among these initiatives, a recent study by the MoH reported the results achieved by the National Observatory for Monitoring Sentinel Events in its first five years of activity, highlighting a strong reduction in non-specified sentinel events (from 41 to 17 percent). Cases in which some action plans have been developed have doubled during the observation period. Moreover, the Observatory produced a manual on root cause analysis and eight guidelines addressed to different stakeholders. The success of this initiative was due to the constant cooperation between the state and the regions, as well as the existence of a continuous and reliable information flow, and the involvement of several key stakeholders (Ghirardini et al. 2010). Another initiative explicitly addressed to improve quality was represented by the National Plan to manage waiting lists. Age.Na.S. is now monitoring the impact of this new policy. A recent report shows how 63.3 percent of citizens can currently access information about waiting times in their regions (National Agency for Regional Healthcare Services 2011). Monitoring of policies introduced to reduce waiting times has also been performed by Cittadinanzattiva, a citizens' advocacy organization (2013). According to their study, recent policies have reduced waiting times by 0.6 percent between 2011 and 2012. These results are promising, but specific investigation is needed to understand the extent to which they are a consequence of reforms.

The National Monitoring System of Healthcare Service Effectiveness initiative of the MoH, supporting the diffusion of the National Plan for Performance Management and National Plan of Outcome Measurement (PNE), is also assessing the impact of specific policies on quality of care. As an example, the initiative, with the collaboration of the Graduate School of Health Economics and Management of Università Cattolica del Sacro Cuore, Rome, is assessing the impact of the implementation of the organizational model based on CDs in Italian public hospital trusts. Results reported in a recent study show how the adoption of the model is able to produce better results, in terms of appropriateness and safety, only under specific organizational conditions. The new model, introduced in the 1990s, was aimed at achieving strategic, organizational, clinical, and economic objectives within hospitals. CDs were meant to enhance quality by encouraging the application of diagnostic–therapeutic patterns and reducing the variability in clinical outcomes through implementing a clinical governance approach in Italian hospitals. The introduction of directorates induces better results in terms of clinical appropriateness only if the adoption of the model fosters the use of clinical governance tools such as clinical practice guidelines and patient-based Information Technology solutions (Cicchetti 2012).

Little evidence is available on the unintended impact of fiscal federalism on quality and safety. A recent analysis exploring the degree of satisfaction in the Italian population concerning hospital admissions between 1997 and 2009, provided a positive appraisal for medical and nursing assistance and an increasingly negative appraisal of non-core aspects, such as food, since the beginning of the devolution process (Gargiulo et al. 2011). Moreover, as a consequence of fiscal federalism, regions are entitled to modify DRG tariffs, adapting them to the providers' characteristics. A recent study investigated the impact of this arrangement on the quality of hospital assistance based on data from the PNE. It demonstrated that hospitals located in regions utilizing perspective payment more extensively are characterized by better performance (Cavalieri, Gitto, & Guccio 2013).

Implementation of Reforms: Barriers and Solutions

Resistance to change often threatens the successful implementation of reforms and policies aimed at improving safety and quality. However, even when stakeholders' commitment exists, technical difficulties can occur. For example, in Italy, a large variety of indicators to monitor quality and patients' safety have been developed both at the national and the local level, yet one of the major obstacles to the development of an effective monitoring system is the lack of consistency between the features of such measurement frameworks and their actual aim, that is satisfying the informational needs of the stakeholders. Another complicating factor is that information flows have been designed without a systemic view; this occasionally impedes the comparison of data across regional jurisdictions and leaves some areas uncovered (Vasselli, Filippetti, & Spizzichino 2005).

On the other hand, several factors can encourage or accelerate the uptake of measures for quality improvement. Unfortunately, often the main driver of such initiatives is the occurrence of malpractice cases, which is frequently considered as the warning that some measure to manage quality and safety needs to be undertaken. Moreover, the current economic crisis forces policymakers to put in place policies aimed at improving efficiency. The effect of such policies on quality and safety depend on the means used to achieve the objectives: if the improvement of efficiency is sought through cutting costs indiscriminately, then the policy will yield unintended negative effects on quality. Conversely, policies aimed at improving efficiency through the rationalization of healthcare expenditure are likely to improve quality and safety as well.

Technological innovation is another driver of quality improvement since it makes safer technologies available both for patients and for healthcare professionals. In addition, the improvement of information technology makes well-structured information systems increasingly available. This facilitates the exchange of information and the creation of networks allowing the systematic monitoring of quality. Finally, as documented from experiences reported in the White Paper of FIASO, the presence of receptive organizational culture is what makes initiatives possible. More specifically, all the local initiatives considered as successful in improving quality were characterized by willingness to change. Nonetheless, other attributes such as a multidisciplinary approach to care reportedly contributed to the successful implementation of these initiatives (Italian Federation of Health Clinics and Hospitals 2012).

Prospects for Success and Next Steps

Policymakers in Italy consider quality and patient safety priority issues. Nonetheless, a round of fresh initiatives should be promoted to improve the current regulatory framework. So far, institutional accreditation has been playing a central role in the definition of INHS structural standards. However, little work has been done to set organizational standards for providers. Law 135/2012 delegated to a further regulation to be approved by the MoH, the Ministry of Economy and Finance and the Standing Conference on the Relations between the State, the regions, and the autonomous provinces jointly, which would define the minimum and maximum standards for facilities (for example, number of beds in an hospital) in each clinical area (for example, number of cardio-surgery units per 1,000,000 of the population), minimum volumes of surgical procedures, and risk and outcomes targets. The regulation is still debated between regional authorities and the MoH and a set of organizational standards is still lacking in the INHS. Still, from the perspective of improving the quality standards for healthcare facilities, a wider dissemination of HTA practices would be desirable. As a matter of fact, in Italy HTA initiatives are very heterogeneous and their degree of formalization is variable. In this regard, the forthcoming institution of a control room for HTA at the MoH could represent a means of input for more widespread dissemination of HTA as well as a chance of coordinating research efforts.

Referring to the monitoring of quality, a deeper involvement of patients and citizens would be beneficial (Ministero della Salute 2010b). So far, only sporadic initiatives have been undertaken to collect the patients' judgments on the INHS and this form of assessment has traditionally been considered as an optional rather than an effective tool to monitor quality. Some measures in this sense would be desirable, but to this point no reforms have systematically addressed this issue despite the increasing relevance of patients' associations.

Finally, it would be desirable for the data from the outcomes of the PNE to be extended, as those currently available focus on a limited number of procedures. Policies to improve the quality of care should be informed by these results, so that the monitoring system will not remain an ineffectual activity. Moreover, clearer patient information from this data would certainly orient citizens' choice of provider. These improvements could be achieved quickly once the practice of data collection and processing has been established within the PNE framework.

Conclusion

The current economic crisis calls for a more rational allocation of scarce healthcare resources. Quality and safety are currently perceived as major policy concerns in Italy. Many healthcare reforms have been launched in recent years to improve quality and patient safety. The most successful initiatives are characterized by cooperation and agreement among institutional levels and supported by effective information systems. Nevertheless, all major indicators measuring the quality of healthcare system and patient safety show variation across regions, driving concerns regarding the equity of the INHS. At the local level, a managerial view and a multidisciplinary approach proved to be key factors facilitating the effective implementation of quality improving initiatives. The forthcoming measures focus on the design of organizational standards to be fulfilled, in order to support equal levels of safety and quality to all the citizens across the country, and on the establishment of a control room for HTA to coordinate local efforts.

Chapter 24

Norway

Ellen Catharina Tveter Deilkås, Tor Ingebrigtsen, and Ånen Ringard

Abstract

Healthcare in Norway has been seen as a public responsibility since the end of the Second World War. The overarching aim has been to ensure "equal access to healthcare of good quality." Taxation and public sources account for almost all health expenditure. Healthcare delivery is semi-decentralized. Responsibility for specialist care lies with the state. The municipalities are responsible for primary care. Since the beginning of the millennium emphasis has been given to structural changes in delivery and organization, and to policies intended to empower patients and users. Quality and patient safety have, over the past few years, emerged on the health policy agenda, as well as efforts to improve coordination between healthcare providers. The chapter aims to describe how the Norwegian healthcare system has developed in relation to quality and patient safety issues.

Background

Norway is a small country with a population of just above five million. The public healthcare system can trace its roots back to the ending of the Second World War. Healthcare is currently delivered via two distinct administrative tiers: specialist care by the state and primary care by municipalities. The problem of coordination has loomed large on the health policy agenda for some time (Ministry of Health and Care Services 2005). The coordination reform, which came into effect in 2012, consisted of new legislation and financial incentives (for example municipal co-financing of secondary care) designed to engage municipalities more fully in the care of chronic and elderly patients (Ministry of Health and Care Services 2009).

Health policy focused in the first decades of the post-war period on improving equal access (Ringard et al. 2013). Access is still regarded as a crucial component of quality care in Norway. More recently the concept has been developed also to include effectiveness, safety, patient centeredness, coordination, efficiency, equity, and accessibility (Norwegian Directorate of Health 2005). There have also been several initiatives, mainly carried out by the Norwegian Board of Health, underpinning quality of care. One example of an early initiative was the national system for reporting hospital adverse events, which began in 1994.

Table 24.1   Demographic, economic, and health information for Norway

Population (thousands)	4,994
Area (sq. km)*	304,250
Proportion of population living in urban areas (2011)	79
Gross Domestic Product (GDP US$, billions)^	500.0
Total expenditure on health as % of GDP	9.1
Gross national income per capita (PPP intl $)	66,960
Per capita total expenditure on health (intl $)	5,970
Proportion of health expenditure which is private	14.9
General Government expenditure on health as a percentage of total expenditure on health	85.1
Out-of-pocket expenditure as a percentage of private expenditure on health	90.1
Life expectancy at birth m/f (yrs)	80/84
Probability of dying under five (per 1,000 live births)	3
Maternal Mortality Ratio (per 100,000 live births) (2013)	4
Proportion of population using improved water and sanitation	100/100

Source: Unless otherwise stated data are for the year 2012 and taken from the World Health Organization 2014. * Area from the World Bank 2014a. ^GDP from the World Bank 2014b.
Note: PPP is purchasing power parity, intl $ is international dollar which has the same purchasing power as US$ in the US.

Various initiatives to support improvement of patient safety and quality have been introduced by the Government since 2005. They will be described further, later in the chapter.

Due to oil production and aquaculture, Norwegian GDP has, despite the financial crisis in much of the western world, continued to grow. The same holds true for total healthcare expenditures. Continuing increase in health expenditure has made cost containment a natural focus of Government policy over the past few decades. As in other countries, the increasing cost has been attributed to factors such as: an aging population, technological development, introduction of new treatment opportunities, and rising expectations on behalf of the citizenry towards the healthcare system. Rising awareness of waiting times and the occasional reporting on adverse events in healthcare have fuelled public and political interest in quality and safety. The recently regained financial control, especially in hospitals, has made it possible to further pursue this interest.

Introduction

The Norwegian healthcare system was, as mentioned above, established in the period from 1945 to the mid 1970s (Johnsen 2006). In the 1970s the focus was primarily on organizing services so that they were effectively distributed geographically. "To treat patients at the lowest effective level of care," became a guiding principle to increase resource effectiveness. Specialist care could only be accessed by referral from a general practitioner. The 1980s reforms aimed at cost containment. Hospitals were no longer financed per diem. Instead, funding depended on hospital population characteristics and estimated needs (Nerland 2001). Queues for elective care and deficits in the hospitals financial balances emerged on the political agenda. This resulted in additional Government funding and hospital expenses continued to increase. Activity-based payment was introduced in the late 1990s to reduce queues and increase efficiency. The system was based on Diagnosis Related Groups (DRGs). Hospitals were simultaneously required to report on process measures, like waiting times. As an incentive to improve both quality and efficiency, patients were, in 2001, given the right to choose which hospital to go to for elective care.

Hospital ownership was transferred from the counties to the state in 2002. The aims of this reform were, amongst others, to rationalize management and enhance the quality of care (Ministry of Health and Care Services 2001). The reform has consequently been labeled as both "an ownership" and "a leadership reform." A follow-up report pointed out that the reform succeeded in increasing political governance, but at the expense of leadership autonomy at lower hierarchical levels (Hippe & Trygstad 2012). The hospital reform gave the regional health authorities and hospital trusts independent financial responsibility. After several decades of budget deficits, in 2009, the regional health authorities finally managed to balance the financial situation in specialist healthcare (Ringard et al. 2013).

The Current Situation

The Parliament serves as the main political decision-making body, and has the responsibility for approving new legislation and the State budget (also including the overall public spending in healthcare). The Ministry of Health and Care Services sets the national health policy agenda, and provides day-to-day decision making. It prepares major reforms, proposals for legislation, and the budget for specialist healthcare. It also provides a limited amount of funding to support specific initiatives in primary healthcare. The Ministry[1] owns four regional health authorities (RHAs), which in turn own 19 hospital trusts. RHAs and hospital trusts are currently financed by a combination of activity-based (50 percent), and block

---

1   The official name is the Ministry of Health and Care Services. We will, however, in the text also use the shorter form the Ministry of Health or the Ministry interchangeably.

funding (50 percent). The activity-based component is, so far, only implemented for somatic hospital care.

Four hundred and twenty-eight municipality councils have independent responsibilities for the healthcare budgets for primary healthcare. Municipalities are responsible for the provision of primary care (mainly provided by self-employed general practitioners (GPs)), nursing homes, rehabilitation, physiotherapy, nursing, and after-hours emergency services.

Several agencies assist the Ministry in both the planning and the implementation of national policies and quality and patient safety initiatives. Knowledge about patient safety and quality is provided to a large degree by these agencies, which are listed in Table 24.2.

Table 24.2   National institutions and agencies with a particular responsibility for quality and patient safety

Name	Task related to quality and safety
Ministry of Health and Care Services	Sets national health policy, prepares major reforms and proposals for legislation and the national budget for the Parliament. Monitors implementation and assists the Government in day-to-day decision making.
Directorate of Health	Monitors and publishes national quality indicators. Implements national policies through ordinances, national guidelines, and campaigns.
National Board of Health Supervision	Provides general supervision of healthcare services both at the national and local level (the latter is done through health departments of the Offices of the County Governors).
Norwegian Medicines Agency	Supervises and monitors new and existing medicines and the supply chain (for example, entry to market, reimbursement). Runs the national registry for pharmacovigilance.
Knowledge Centre for the Health Services	Promotes and monitors patient safety through the Patient Safety Programme and the National Reporting and Learning System for adverse events in hospitals. Monitors quality of services through developing quality indicators and measuring patient's experiences with the health services.
Norwegian System of Patient Injury Compensation	Provides compensation for patient injury.
Centre of Clinical Documentation and Evaluation	Provides organizational, technical, and methodological support for development and operation of clinical quality registries.

RHAs are governed by legislation and an annual letter of instruction from the Ministry of Health. The annual letter of instruction stipulates the hospital budgets and sets activity goals for each RHA. The number of parameters and special reports was reduced by the Ministry, from 40 in 2012 to 16 in 2014. The Ministry holds regular meetings with the RHA to monitor if targets are met. The hospital trusts are governed by annual letters of instruction from the regional health authorities. The trusts have to report to, and meet with, the regional health authorities to report on their activities and results.

By setting goals for different aspects of quality and safety of care, and demanding regular reports, the Ministry of Health motivates and governs improvement efforts. Analysis of the annual letters of instruction since 2007 demonstrates a shift in the focus on quality and patient safety. The 2007 document is the first to mention the concept of patient safety, and the new definition of healthcare quality, in particular that healthcare should be effective, safe, patient centered, coordinated, resource effective, and accessible (Norwegian Directorate of Health 2005). More recently, the letters of instruction have emphasized the role of leaders in promoting a good patient safety culture, and the significance of learning from adverse events. Participation in preparation and implementation of the national campaign, and the later program for patient safety, was made mandatory from 2010.

Examples of dimensions of quality emphasized by the Ministry in the letter of instruction for 2014 are: access to healthcare, patient centeredness, healthcare effectiveness, and safety. Examples of data reported to monitor these aspects are: average waiting time for planned treatment (goal <65 days), ratio of colon cancer patients to get treatment within 20 working days after first referral to hospital, patients' experiences with hospital care, and 30–days hospital mortality rate. The letter of instruction for 2014 also sets a long-term goal for the health trusts: to reduce preventable adverse events by 50 percent within five years (from 2010 estimates).

Financial incentives to promote quality and patient safety in hospital care were introduced from 2014. The pilot program will run for three years. About 1 percent of the hospital budgets will be redistributed based on hospital scores on process, outcome, and patient experience indicators. Examples of process indicators are the proportion of stroke patients receiving thrombolytic treatment and mean times from referral to treatment for some cancers. The outcome-indicators are based on results from the clinical quality registries, such as five-year survival rates for common cancers and 30-day survival rates for cardiovascular disease. Patient experience indicators are, for example, patients' perceptions of coordination of care and information received. An evaluation is planned after three years, and distribution of an increasing proportion of the budget based on quality indicators will be considered (Directorate of Health 2013).

In primary aged healthcare, the Directorate of Health provides quality indicators for nursing homes. Examples of quality indicators monitored in the municipalities are: physician hours per resident in nursing homes per week, rate of readmissions of elderly patients, and rate of residents that involuntarily share rooms with other residents and/or do not have their own bath and toilet.

With the intention to improve healthcare access, policies over the last 25 years have aimed to limit physician employment in urban areas. The intention has been to make it easier to recruit physicians to urban areas. According to the 2013 Organisation for Economic Cooperation and Development (OECD) report, "Health at a glance," the density of Norwegian physicians is 7.2 per 1,000 citizens in urban areas versus 3.8 in rural areas (Organisation for Economic Cooperation and Development 2013a).

The Quality and Safety Landscape

In 1984 a new law was enacted which instructed all healthcare facilities to tighten systematic controls to ensure that their practices are in accordance with rules and regulations (Ministry of Health Norway 1984). The same year, hospitals were required to report adverse events to the Norwegian Board of Health. The Board also initiated a project entitled "National strategy for quality development in healthcare." The project ran from 1995 to 2000, and focused on the introduction of internal control systems and quality routines in all healthcare facilities. Moreover, improvement projects initiated by both organizations and institutions were supported by project funding. National networks of quality advisors were established in both specialist and primary healthcare. Evaluation showed that although the hospitals and municipalities had established internal control systems, they had problems in making the systems function in order to learn from adverse events (National Board of Health 2002).

A few years later, in 1998, the Norwegian Medical Association started its Breakthrough Series Program. The program was based on the Collaboration model, developed by the Institute for Healthcare Improvement in the United States of America (US) (Norwegian Medical Association 2009). The projects introduced methodologies of continuous system improvement, such as Deming's circle and statistical process control, to different healthcare settings.

In 2005 the Directorate of Health, which was established in 2002, launched a second national strategy for quality improvement for the period 2005–2015 (Norwegian Directorate of Health 2005). The current strategy chose, in line with the international trends at the time (Institute of Medicine 2001), to define healthcare of good quality as effective, safe, patient centered, coordinated, resource effective, and accessible. The strategy emphasizes the continuous process of quality improvement above control, based on Deming's theory (Kenney 2008).

In the aftermath of the new strategy, several initiatives have been undertaken with respect to enhancing quality and patient safety. In 2007 the National Unit for Patient Safety was established by the Government, as part of the Norwegian Knowledge Centre for Health Services. The first national conference on patient safety was initiated and organized in 2008 by the Norwegian System of Patient Injury Compensation. The following year, a program for the development of clinical quality registries was established by the Ministry of Health. It has coordinated 45 national clinical quality registries in a network, with both technical and methodological support. The registries have steering committees comprising members from all the health regions, and information about treatment rates, complications, and outcomes are provided to all hospitals through annual feedback reports. Clinical leaders are expected to utilize the results for service improvements (Nasjonalt folkehelseinstitutt 2009).

Necessary legislation was provided in June 2011 to move the system for reporting adverse events from the Norwegian Board of Health to the Norwegian Knowledge Center. The move was motivated by the increasing international evidence on the advantages of having a non-sanctioning, rather than a punitive system for reporting adverse events. The new learning center opened in July 2012 (Ringard et al. 2012). It receives confidential reports from healthcare staff. Clinicians and safety experts analyze the reports to identify common risks to patients. In addition, advice is offered in some individual cases. During the first nine months the center received approximately 6,400 reports.

In 2011, a three-year national patient safety campaign was launched by the Government. The aims of the campaign are: to reduce patient harm, to implement administrative and clinical routines for patient safety, and to improve the patient safety culture. The conceptual framework of the patient safety campaign is based on Donabedian's quality assurance model and organizational psychology research (Zohar et al. 2007, Zohar & Luria 2005). Initially, stakeholders were invited to identify clinical target areas, such as safe surgery, and medication reconciliation. Tools for the target areas, and for leadership of patient safety, were piloted and spread by the collaborative approach (Institute for Healthcare Improvement 2003), organized by the regional health authorities.

In 2012 the Government at the time put forward the first White Paper explicitly addressing quality and patient safety (Ministry of Health and Care Services 2012). This mandated, amongst others, a five-year national program for quality and patient safety in healthcare, which started in 2014. One of its main goals is to strengthen healthcare leaders' roles in improving the culture for patient safety. Another initiative currently being developed is a more systematic approach to ensure a safer and more efficient introduction of new technologies (for example pharmaceuticals and medical devices) in hospitals.

Impact of These Reform Efforts on Quality and Safety of Care

There remains paucity of data available to evaluate the impact of previous reforms on quality and safety. There are, however, some pieces of information available to illuminate some of the aspects of quality identified by the national strategy for quality improvement (Norwegian Directorate of Health 2005). Regarding efficiency, Norway's health expenditure as a proportion of GDP, matched the OECD average of 9.3 percent in 2011 (Organisation for Economic Cooperation and Development 2013a). Norway's numbers of hospital beds per 1,000 citizens were 3.3 percent, while the European average was 5.3 percent. Hospital discharges per 1,000 citizens were the same in Norway as in the European Union (EU). Annual growth in healthcare expenditure was 2.9 percent, compared to the EU average of 4.1 percent, from 2000–2009. These data indicate that the efficiency in Norwegian hospital care has improved over time.

With respect to equal access, hospital care is free of charge for inpatients, independent of income. For outpatient and physician consultations, patients have to pay a part of the cost out-of-pocket. Shorter waiting times for access to planned hospital care, has been an issue for many years. Data from Statistics Norway show that the average waiting times for planned somatic hospital treatment increased from 74 days in 2008 to 95 in 2012 (Statistics Norway 2014). This indicates that accessibility to elective hospital care in Norwegian hospitals has somewhat decreased over the past few years.

Five-year relative cancer survival may be an indicator of treatment "effectiveness" in Norwegian healthcare. These survival rates have reduced since 2001. Compared to other OECD countries these rates are above average for cervical, breast, and colorectal cancer (Organisation for Economic Cooperation and Development 2013a).

Regarding patient safety, rates of adverse events are estimated at the national level, based on reviews of randomly selected samples of medical records in all hospital trusts (started by the patient safety campaign in 2011). The procedure is standardized, since the data were planned to be aggregated at the national level, as well as to be available at the hospital trust level (Deilkås 2013).

National estimates rated urinary tract infections, adverse drug reactions, and surgical complications as the most frequent adverse events (Deilkås 2013). That corresponded well with the campaigns clinical target areas. The estimated reduction, in 2012, of adverse events that require intervention, lead to prolonged hospital stay, permanent harm, or that contribute to patient death, was statistically significant (13.9 percent in 2012 versus 16.1 percent in 2011, <0.05). The estimated reduction of iatrogenic urinary tract infections (1.7 percent in 2012, compared to 2.8 percent in 2011), and reoperations, related to adverse events (0.7 percent in 2012, compared to 1.2 percent in 2010 and 1.3 percent in 2011) were also statistically significant (Deilkås 2013). The estimates indicate that a possible decline in adverse events in Norwegian hospitals has coincided with the national patient safety campaign.

The campaign coordinated patient safety culture surveys in all hospital trusts in 2012, these will be repeated in 2014 (Nasjonalt Kunnskapssenter for Helsetjenesten 2014). Data from the 2012 survey have been used in local improvement efforts, but have not yet been made available at the national level. Comparison of the results may show if frontline personnel perceive that the patient safety culture has improved simultaneously with the campaign. The information gives leaders a chance to intervene in unsafe pockets in their organizations. It also contributes to understanding the validity of data on quality and adverse events from other sources.

Table 24.3   Estimated rates of admissions with adverse events 2010, 2011, and 2012

	Percent of all admissions (95% CI)		
Indicators/year	2010*	2011	2012
Admissions with at least one adverse event that required intervention, prolonged hospital stay, or had more serious consequences.	15.8% (13.9–18%)	16.1% (14.6–17.6%)	13.9% (12.5–15.3%)
Admissions with at least one adverse event that led to prolonged hospitalization or more serious consequences.	8.9% (7.3%–10.5%)	8.8 % (7.8–9.8 %)	7.6% (6.6–8.5%)
Numbers of admissions reviewed.	7,819	10,288	11,728

Source: Deilkås 2013.
Notes: *The period March to December 2010.

Implementation: Barriers and Solutions

Through the annual letters of instruction, the Ministry of Health is able to enhance the attention paid to how quality and safety issues should be prioritized in hospital care. The same opportunity still does not exist to the same extent for primary healthcare. The 428 municipalities are politically and financially independent in their day-to-day decisions, within the framework of legislation. This may explain why hospital care has been subject to more monitoring and goal setting than we have seen in primary healthcare. A result of this is that more data regarding quality and safety are currently provided by hospitals and hospital trusts than by municipalities.

There are, however, reasons to be optimistic about the future as many municipalities did decide, on a voluntary basis, to participate in the patient safety campaign. The project targeting medication routines in nursing homes involved municipalities in all 17 counties. Involving the municipalities has demanded more effort, but has also provided opportunities for individual municipalities to act as opinion leaders and offer guidance to other municipalities. One municipality, for instance, initiated a survey of patient safety culture in its nursing homes. The survey was combined with what they called "the patient safety talk," as a way to follow up results.

Lack of good access to quality and patient safety data at the ward and department level is an immediate barrier to patient safety and quality improvement in Norwegian hospitals. Electronic systems for continuous and automatic production of routine quality and safety data are hampered by lack of legislation, financial will, and in some instances even leadership and knowledge. Initiatives to provide data more easily, by structuring electronic records, are emerging, but still in an uncoordinated fashion. Such processes rely heavily on clinicians' time to ensure that the records comply with clinical logic. To limit the use of clinicians, as well as administrative personnel's, time, this area would probably benefit from more national coordination.

Lack of leadership support is, to some extent, a second barrier to improving patient safety and quality. Leaders' priorities have been found to have a significant impact on patient safety and quality outcomes (Jiang et al. 2008). A recent report on behalf of the Ministry of Health stated that the most important leadership challenge is to deliver care of high quality within given limits of resources. The report also presented data from a survey of Norwegian leaders, stating that they are motivated to support patient safety and quality improvement, but lack knowledge about how to do it (Schumacher 2012). The Government-funded program for patient safety addresses this by focusing on the topic of patient safety leadership. Examples of leadership tools are patient safety walk rounds, multidisciplinary patient safety meetings, and initiatives aimed at getting the boards "on board." What the leadership tools have in common is that they facilitate dialogue regarding quality and patient safety.

Lack of consensus between professional groups, patients, and leaders may undermine safe clinical processes. One example may be if a nurse thinks that a guideline should be followed, while the physician considers it to be contradicted by a specific patient condition. Another example could be when members of a transfusion department find members in intensive care to be reckless when they do not follow the strict transfusion rules, while those in intensive care may indicate that the safety procedures are not adapted to their needs to be able to deliver blood on short notice.

Bringing clinicians and leaders together to address misunderstandings, disagreements, and priorities is a solution for progress. Such meetings need to be informed by both patient stories and data that reflect critical situations, how often they occur, and the human factors and risk factors that contributed to the event. Models to facilitate dialogue amongst leaders and different professional groups have been published (Schilling et al. 2011, Pronovost et al. 2005). The aim is to develop consensus on patient safety issues amongst clinicians, both within and across units at the lowest organizational level. A similar model was included in the patient safety campaign, but has not been fully implemented. It is therefore continued as a part of the patient safety program (Nasjonalt Kunnskapssenter for Helsetjenesten n.d.).

How leaders react to and handle adverse events defines the patient safety culture in their facility (Deilkås 2010). In order to contribute with relevant information in the analysis, the people involved in adverse events need to be present when the events are analyzed. If the leader manages to address the conditions in the organization that contributed to the adverse event, rather than the human contribution, the leader will build trust and subordinates will feel safe to report new adverse events.

Prospects for Success

Traditionally, patient safety and quality has been regarded as the responsibility of clinical professionals. Increased Government attention in recent years gives reason for future optimism regarding how quality and safety issues will be prioritized at all levels in Norwegian healthcare. The annual letters of instruction have given hospital managers larger responsibility for quality and patient safety. This may facilitate more open dialogue between managers and clinicians regarding priorities and practices, which in turn hopefully will provide opportunities for increased mutual understanding and trust. Addressing clinical quality and patient safety in the annual letters of instruction may help in developing a shared logic throughout the healthcare system. We are, however, not there yet.

Bringing clinicians, managers, health and financial administrators, and politicians together on a more regular basis may also be a way of addressing misunderstandings, disagreements, and priorities. Through dialogue regarding patient safety routines, risks, priorities, decisions, and results, healthcare workers and managers together can develop a learning community across professional and hierarchic boundaries. Mutual understanding of risks and the necessity of safety precautions and routines, amongst clinicians who depend on each other's input to provide safe patient care, is the foundation of a productive patient safety culture.

Recent health reforms have intended to strengthen leadership responsibility and involvement in setting goals for quality and patient safety. This has been achieved without changing legislation, which still holds clinicians responsible for adverse patient outcomes. A possible consequence of the new policy where leaders set priorities in patient care is to also make leaders legally responsible for patient results.

Concluding Remarks

To solve the challenges of quality and safety, politicians, clinicians, and patients need to share in the understanding of what the problems are. Clinicians need to be supported by well-functioning clinical routines, priorities, and infrastructure to do their jobs effectively. Good interpersonal skills are necessary to function well in teams. Problems related to practical conditions and teamwork need to be sorted out together with leaders and fellow employees. To analyze and improve quality and patient safety, clinicians and leaders need relevant data and time to tell and discuss stories that demonstrate how conditions, priorities, and practices affect their patient care. They also need to make decisions on what routines to change, or who to involve in solving problems. To do this they must meet regularly, in multidisciplinary settings. Responsiveness from leaders in the hierarchy is required to help address problems that cannot be resolved at the frontline. Leaders at all levels require the same responsiveness. Progress and success will depend upon the fora that can be facilitated to share it.

Chapter 25
Scotland

Andrew Thompson and David R Steel

Scotland is a small nation within the United Kingdom (UK) that has recently had a high degree of autonomy over health policy, such that it has adopted a very different direction, not only from England, but also many other health systems around the world. Under a narrative of mutuality, Scottish health policy is based on partnership; working across Government, health and social care services, professions, and civil society to deliver nationally agreed health outcomes, increasingly through prevention and anticipatory care, aiming for social solidarity and equity. It faces similar drivers for change as other countries, but adopts a distinct vision of its goals and direction. Its Quality Ambitions focus on person-centeredness, safety, and effectiveness. Stability of the quality infrastructure, clinical leadership, and strong networks facilitate clarity of purpose and communication. There have been many substantive improvements in life expectancy, morbidity, and mortality, as well as in healthcare associated infections and waiting times—although it is difficult to be sure about attribution of causes. The major current challenge is in reducing health inequalities, for which policy is focused on sustainable economic growth and improved effectiveness and efficiency.

Introduction

In this chapter we aim to show how the major national reforms of healthcare in Scotland have impacted on the quality and safety of services for patients, carers, and staff. In many ways, when considering the underlying ideas and logic of the way these reforms have been fashioned, Scotland can be seen as a deviant case, in the sense of choosing not to adopt the current orthodoxy of neo-classical economic thinking that has permeated most other developed health systems around the world. It is not as though Scotland is lacking a clear vision of where it wants to get to, nor of how it should get there, but rather it has set its face against neo-liberal ideology and towards a partnership approach that attempts to offer social solidarity and equity of outcomes to its population.

In order to understand the reform agenda in Scotland, it is important to take account of the general drivers for change that affect all healthcare systems, as well as the specifics of how these manifest themselves within the nation itself.

Table 25.1   Demographic, economic, and health information for United Kingdom (*Scotland alone data not available*)

Population (thousands)	62,783
Area (sq. km)*	241,930
Proportion of population living in urban areas (2011)	80
Gross Domestic Product (GDP US$, billions)^	2,475.7
Total expenditure on health as % of GDP	9.4
Gross national income per capita (PPP intl $)	37,340
Per capita total expenditure on health (intl $)	3,495
Proportion of health expenditure which is private	17.5
General Government expenditure on health as a percentage of total expenditure on health	82.5
Out-of-pocket expenditure as a percentage of private expenditure on health	56.8
Life expectancy at birth m/f (yrs)	79/83
Probability of dying under five (per 1,000 live births)	5
Maternal Mortality Ratio (per 100,000 live births) (2013)	8
Proportion of population using improved water and sanitation	100/100

Source: Unless otherwise stated data are for the year 2012 and taken from the World Health Organization 2014. * Area from the World Bank 2014a. ^GDP from the World Bank 2014b.

Notes: PPP is purchasing power parity, intl $ is international dollar which has the same purchasing power as US$ in the US.

Moreover, there are additional factors relating to the geography, politics, culture, history, and leadership style of Scotland which, it is argued, have important determining effects on what is deemed to be appropriate and effective within any reform initiative.

While evidence is much vaunted as being the engine of policy development, it is clear that ideas provide the narrative through which we develop a vision of the nature of welfare in society and what shape it should take. Crises, such as the recent global economic one, can provide an opportunity to make changes that are otherwise unthinkable, or they may inhibit innovation and change due to path dependency (Peters 2011). As Kuisma (2013) states, strategic choices need to be made about which aspects to tackle and on the timescale for achieving the benefits. In a withering attack on the arational and sometimes irrational developments in the English National Health Service (NHS), Paton (2013) points to the garbage-can theory (Cohen, March & Olsen 1972) of applying policy-based solutions to ill-defined problems in an ideological context of anti-statism and pro-market competition. By contrast, Scotland's narrative reflects a wide consensus across political parties, professionals, and civil society about how to achieve public service improvements, based on support for public sector organizations, in collaboration with local communities and voluntary groups, who can offer innovation based on trust and obligation (Housden 2014). This "progressive localism" is in stark contrast to neo-liberal ideas about "personalization" as individualized, commodified care (Hall & McGarrol 2013). Scottish policy ideas have in part been drawn from international models, such as the Nordic countries, with divergence from England since the market reforms of the 1990s and a rejection of the linear and centrist thinking of New Public Management, which gave rise to organizational fragmentation and a "disembodied view of human and organisational behaviour" (Housden 2014, p. 71).

It is generally agreed that Scotland, despite being in political union with the rest of the UK since 1707, has maintained a distinct identity and culture, which were being harnessed to promote the referendum for independence in September 2014 by the Scottish Government. Greer (2009) has argued that health policy in Scotland is more important than at the UK level due to the relative lack of competing policy areas under its control and, furthermore, that professionals are respected and central to policymaking (Greer 2008), such that clinicians head, or feature prominently in, most health service institutions. The geography of Scotland comprises large rural and remote areas (including 99 inhabited islands), and is home to a relatively small population of around 5.2 million people, the majority of whom live in the narrow central belt between the principal cities of Glasgow and Edinburgh. This factor, together with the small number of senior civil servants across the Scottish Government as a whole—around 250—enables collegiality (Fox 2013, p. 505), even at the risk of "groupthink," through frequent and inclusive meetings with politicians and civil society to agree on policy developments.

The Current Situation

Ostensibly, healthcare reform is focused on tackling the major health challenges that face a nation. In this regard, Scotland has some of the most startling and urgent problems facing any developed country. It has the lowest life expectancy of all of Western European countries (Scottish Public Health Observatory 2013). It suffers from the highest mortality in Western Europe among working-age adults since the late 1970s. It also exhibits amongst the highest mortality in Western Europe from circulatory diseases. There is clear evidence of increasing mortality from chronic liver disease, associated with high levels of consumption of alcohol. It has one of the highest levels of obesity in the world, which increasingly affects the younger generations (Scottish Government 2011a). Scotland also has a population characterized by a history of a relatively poor diet, lack of exercise, and, until recent legislation to ban it in public buildings, high rates of smoking. Of further concern is the high and increasing level of inequality across the country, with healthy life expectancy 22.3 years lower in the most deprived decile of the population compared to the least deprived decile in 2009–2010 (Steel & Cylus 2012).

Based on Wendt's (2014) taxonomy of Organisation for Economic Cooperation and Development (OECD) healthcare systems, Scotland, which is subsumed under the political union of the UK, continues to exhibit many of the same characteristics of financing, healthcare provision and regulation since devolution of the competence for health policy in 1999. It has had an NHS system since 1948, offering universal coverage mostly free at the point of use, financed largely by taxation and with minimal out-of-pocket payments (mainly for dentistry and optician services), but with free pharmaceutical prescriptions, eye tests, and personal care for older people. Its total per capita health expenditure (US$2990 PPP in 2007) is close to the mean of all OECD countries, with public expenditure as a proportion of the total in the UK (mirrored in Scotland) rising from 80.4 percent in 1998 to 87.3 percent by 2010 (Thompson 2009). The indices of health service provision in the UK for primary and secondary care are slightly below the average for the OECD in 2007 (Wendt 2014). Regarding regulation, hospital personnel are salaried, while most general practitioners (GPs), dentists, opticians, and pharmacists are self-employed, providing services to the NHS under contract. Patients are free to choose their GP, but are required to register with a general practice. GPs receive capitation fees for patients on their lists and act as gatekeepers for specialist referrals.

Brief History

Until devolution in 1999, healthcare policies in Scotland were determined by the Scottish Office, a department of the UK Government, and reforms in structure and management tended to reflect those in the rest of the UK (Hunter 1982, Keating & Midwinter 1983). This included two major developments of the 1980s: the introduction of general management following the Griffiths Report in 1983 (Department of Health and Social Security 1983) and competitive tendering of ancillary services. Similarly, the replacement of the hierarchical model of organization of the NHS since its inception by the so-called "internal market," with separation of purchaser and provider functions, was announced in 1989 at the same time as in the rest of the UK (Scottish Office 1989). However, its implementation was significantly slower, reflecting a general reluctance—in a country which returned a majority of Labour ministers throughout the Thatcher years of Conservative Government—to adopt policies "imposed" from London. However, by 1996 NHS Trusts were in place across all of mainland Scotland and 43 percent of the Scottish population were registered with GP fundholders (who could purchase certain services from NHS Trusts on behalf of their patients) (Steel & Cylus 2012).

In 1997, following the election of a Labour Government, broadly similar steps were taken across the UK to dismantle this internal market. GP fundholding was abolished, but initially the organizational distinction between purchaser (Health Board) and provider (NHS Trust) roles was retained, albeit with an increased emphasis on collaboration and integration (Scottish Office 1997).

In 1999 health was one of the functions devolved to the Scottish Parliament and Scottish Executive (now called the Scottish Government), which decided to unify all boards and trusts, thus removing the purchaser–provider separation (Scottish Executive 2000). Since 2004, 15 geographically-based boards (reduced to 14 in 2006) have had responsibility for both planning and delivering services to meet the healthcare needs of their catchment populations. Within each, Board operational functions are delegated to operating divisions for acute services and community health partnerships (CHPs) for community and primary care services, including linking with local authorities responsible for social care (Steel & Cylus 2012).

In 2005, a route map committed the NHS to continuing development as an integrated service to shift the balance of care away from acute care in hospital, increasingly as a result of emergency admissions, to an emphasis on preventative medicine, self-care, and targeting of resources on those at greatest risk through anticipatory medicine (Scottish Executive 2005). In contrast to the fragmentation caused by internal markets, there have been progressive moves towards greater integration, both vertically within the NHS and horizontally with local authorities (Ham et al. 2013). Scotland has also banned new private contracts for hospital catering and cleaning, to reintegrate them with clinical services and reduce healthcare associated infections, as well as private firms operating GP practices and hospital car parking charges, except where there is an existing obligation under the Private Finance Initiative.

Since 2007 the organizing motif for health policy in Scotland is "mutuality," by which is meant the partnership between the different stakeholders—Government, professions, and the public—to improve the health of the population, and the quality and experience of healthcare through a person-centered (users and staff) approach. The strengths of the system are in guaranteeing access to all services for everyone, irrespective of the ability to pay, with guaranteed maximum waiting times. While patients and carers are the focus of services, the emphasis is on establishing publicly agreed provision, rather than individual choice, in order to avoid distortions in resource allocation. The design of the system is aimed to remove any barriers to care, but the wide disparities between sub-population groups suggest that equity remains the major challenge to be tackled, albeit probably largely through action outside healthcare.

Current Reform Initiatives

The key strategy document of the Scottish National Party (SNP) Government (in office as a minority administration from 2007 to 2011, and with an overall majority since 2011), *Better Health, Better Care: Action Plan,* published in December 2007, was built around what it described as "the existing strengths of NHS Scotland—a collaborative, integrated approach built upon our traditional values" (Scottish Government 2007, p. 3). It committed the Government to a publicly provided service with a focus on mutuality and on quality as a key organizing principle for healthcare.

Whilst the use of the term "mutuality" was novel, in other respects the Action Plan confirmed and extended the direction of travel since devolution. It also reinforced the diverging paths of the NHS in Scotland and England in its rejection of solutions based on market forces or internal competition.

The Action Plan contained proposals, subsequently implemented, to:

- strengthen patient and public involvement in the NHS, including a pilot of direct election of a proportion of non-executive directors on two boards;
- strengthen partnership working with NHS staff and with voluntary and community organizations;
- strengthen clinical leadership of service planning and delivery;
- improve quality across all six dimensions of quality identified by the US Institute of Medicine (Institute of Medicine 2001); viz. patient centered, safe, effective, efficient, equitable, timely.

The commitment to enhance quality and to place it at the heart of NHS activity was further developed in *The Healthcare Quality Strategy for NHS Scotland*, published in 2010 (Scottish Government 2010). It set out three Quality Ambitions relating to: (1) partnerships with patients, carers, and those delivering services which respect individual needs and values and demonstrate compassion, (2) the avoidance of injury and harm in a clean and safe environment, and (3) the provision of clinically appropriate treatments, interventions, and support.

Implementation of the strategy has been seen as the means by which longer-term transformational challenges are addressed and in the shorter term greater efficiency and productivity achieved. As well as building upon existing initiatives, the strategy recognized the need "to do some new things (and) to do some things differently" (Scottish Government 2010, p. 8), but within the context of "NHS Scotland's integrated delivery arrangements, encouraging whole system improvement through mutually beneficial partnerships between clinical teams and the people in their care" (Scottish Government 2010, p. 8) and in partnership with other bodies.

This approach was consistent with the Government's policy for the public sector generally. To articulate a distinctive Scottish approach, in a context of rising demand for public services in an environment of constrained public spending, the Government established in 2010 a Commission on the Future Delivery of Public Services, chaired by Campbell Christie. Its report called for substantial reform of how public services are delivered to make them "outcome-focused, integrated, and collaborative. They must become transparent, community-driven, and designed around users' needs. They should focus on prevention and early intervention" (Scottish Government 2011b, p. 22).

These themes were highlighted the same year in the Government's strategic vision for achieving sustainable quality in healthcare which reiterated the focus on prevention, anticipation, and supported self-management, and stressed the need to extend integration to encompass social care as well as healthcare (Scottish Government 2011c). This led in 2013 to the introduction of legislation requiring NHS boards and local authorities to integrate health and social care arrangements, initially for adults, by creating new corporate bodies with integrated budgets and a single point of oversight and accountability to replace CHPs (Scottish Government 2013a).

The Quality and Safety Landscape

Since devolution there has, therefore, been a high degree of continuity in health policy and structures, facilitated by relative consensus across political parties regarding means and ends in healthcare. This is particularly apparent in relation to quality. Whilst there has been a steady growth in the range and focus of action to improve quality across all the dimensions identified by the Institute of Medicine, policy has generally developed in an evolutionary manner.

The current landscape, as set out in the *Healthcare Quality Strategy*, has three priority areas for intervention, linked to the Quality Ambitions:

Person centered: Since 2008 the *Better Together Programme* has been designed to embed patient experience in NHS practice, initially based on patient feedback through surveys and various qualitative techniques, but since 2011 including more interventionist approaches (Better Together 2013). This is underpinned by the Patient Rights (Scotland) Act 2011, which led in 2012 to production of a charter of patient rights and responsibilities (Scottish Government 2012) and put the 12-week guarantee for planned inpatient and day-case treatment on a statutory footing.

Safe: Also in 2008, the *Scottish Patient Safety Programme* (SPSP) was launched, in partnership with the Institute for Healthcare Improvement, in all acute hospitals—the first national initiative of this kind—with the aims of reducing adverse events and avoidable mortality (Haraden & Leitch 2011). Encouraging results led to extension of the original five-year program to 2015 and to the development of four complementary programs for primary care, mental health, maternity and children's services, and sepsis and venous thromboembolism. SPSP reinforced earlier work on healthcare associated infection; continuing public concern led the Government to establish a Healthcare Environment Inspectorate in 2009 to undertake a program of announced and unannounced inspections of hospitals.

Effective: The Scottish Intercollegiate Guidelines Network (SIGN)—a network of doctors and other healthcare professionals, funded by Government—has produced over 130 evidence-based guidelines since its inception in 1993 (Harbour,

Lowe & Twaddle, 2011). Its work forms the basis of the strategies and clinical standards developed for all major conditions, supported currently by around 130 managed clinical networks. SIGN has been an enduring feature of the landscape for the last 15 years (Ham et al. 2013).

Even more striking, particularly in comparison with England, has been the stability of the quality infrastructure. Developments have generally added to what was already in place rather than sweeping away institutions that had a track record with the service and the public. At the national level, although initially a number of separate bodies had been established, five were merged in 2003 to form NHS Quality Improvement Scotland (QIS), charged with responsibility for developing and implementing a coordinated quality strategy. Two years later two further bodies (SIGN and a statutory Scottish Health Council to promote *Patient Focus and Public Involvement* (Scottish Executive 2001), and to support and monitor Health Boards' efforts in this area) were added to QIS, which in 2011 became Healthcare Improvement Scotland (HIS), when it took on responsibility also for regulation and inspection of independent (private and non-profit) healthcare. The remit of QIS/HIS combines: advice, guidance, and standards; implementation and improvement support; and—in a break with normal practice—assurance, scrutiny, measurement, and reporting.

HIS provides support to the territorial boards in fulfilling their responsibility for maintaining and improving the quality of healthcare. Boards' duty in this regard was set out in the Health Act 1999, which underpins the development of *clinical governance* ("corporate accountability for clinical performance"), which remains a key part of their governance framework (Scottish Office 1998).

Implementation of the interventions in the *Healthcare Quality Strategy* is monitored though a Quality Management Framework with 12 national quality outcome indicators. This provides a structure for relating the wide range of measurement that goes on across the NHS to the Quality Ambitions and is part of the system of performance management for the NHS, which is directly linked with the Government's overall Purpose and National Outcomes (Steel & Cylus 2012).

Impact of These Efforts on the Quality and Safety of Care

Scotland has, in many respects, been a pioneer in the development of interventions such as clinical audit, clinical guidelines, and clinical standards, and in their use as the basis for improving and reviewing clinical performance. None of these developments is unique to Scotland but they have been taken forward in a distinctive manner, which reflects the prevailing culture of the NHS, with an emphasis on clinical leadership and ownership, working in close partnership with Government and NHS management.

These initiatives are, however, only worthwhile if they result in improved standards of care and better outcomes for patients. During the period under review most of the key quality indicators have been moving in the right direction. This is particularly so in relation to access and safety, and there have also been significant improvements in mortality and morbidity. Despite recent efforts, inequalities in health have proved more intractable.

However, measuring quality over time, comparing performance across different healthcare systems, and attributing causality are complex processes. On measurement, a composite proxy that is now widely used, although not universally accepted, is the hospital standardized mortality ratio. Against a baseline of 2007 this had decreased in acute hospitals by around 12.5 percent by mid 2013 (Information and Statistics Division Scotland 2014).

Two areas of particular public concern have been waiting times and healthcare associated infections. Waiting times have fallen progressively over the last decade and in March 2013 90.6 percent of patients were treated within 18 weeks of referral (Scottish Government 2013b). On healthcare associated infections, in comparison with 2007–2008 there was a reduction in methicillin-resistant *Staphylococcus aureus* and methicillin-sensitive *Staphylococcus aureus* bacteraemia cases among all patients of 37 percent by mid-2013. Equivalent figures for Clostridium difficile infections in patients aged 65+ showed a reduction of 77 percent (Scottish Government 2013b).

Other specific measures of health service outcomes (or their proxies) that are commonly used include:

- an increase in life expectancy between 1981 and 2013 of males from 69.1 years to 76.9 and of females from 75.3 to 80.9 (Scottish Public Health Observatory 2013);
- 25 percent reduction in levels of premature mortality (deaths of those aged under 75) since 2001 (Scottish Government 2013b);
- 48 percent reduction in deaths of those aged under 75 from stroke and coronary heart disease since 2001 (Scottish Government 2013b);
- 15 percent reduction in emergency bed days per 100,000 people over 75 since 2002 (Scottish Government 2013b).

However it is much more difficult either to attribute these improvements to specific interventions or to gauge the effect of the context in which they have been implemented, including the overall approach to healthcare reform. The challenges of evaluating large-scale interventions have been well-documented and definitive claims for particular interventions such as SPSP need to be based upon rigorous and independent evaluation (Health Foundation 2011).

Prospects for Success

The major challenges for Scottish health policy are in improving population health while reducing health inequalities. Research shows that poor health is strongly associated with poverty (Dorling 2013). The Chief Medical Officer (Burns 2011) believes health inequalities are the biological consequences of socioeconomic factors relating to deindustrialization, community and family breakdown, and other adverse events that create chronic stress and remove a sense of coherence (Antonovsky 1979). The solution for both challenges is seen in linking the two, through making public services more effective and efficient, while boosting economic growth, employment, and income (Fox 2013). Changes in lifestyles, such as smoking, alcohol consumption, diet, and exercise, will also be necessary, but evidence suggests that harmful decisions on these stem from poor environments, rather than being a simple matter of choice.

For the current SNP Government, the prospect of independence by 2016 offered the chance to change the tax framework to grow the economy, provide more jobs, and ensure a decent standard of living for those in and out of work (Scottish Government 2013c). However, given the relatively narrow margin by which the Scottish people voted to stay in the UK, there are current uncertainties about whether and how the current devolved settlement will be changed and with what impact on the level of resources available to meet the challenges outlined above.

The emphasis within the health services is on person-centeredness, acknowledging the importance, not only of ensuring that patients are at the center of service delivery and involved as much as they wish to be, but also that this should extend to "lay" carers and staff. Research has long shown the positive correlation between the treatment of those who care and those who are cared for (Revans 1972).

The current refocusing of services on improved outcomes through prevention and anticipatory care, recommended by the Christie Commission (Scottish Government 2011b), has established a line of travel, but needs to extend the salutogenetic, asset-based approach to individuals and communities to enable them to build resilience and manage the stressors they face if they are to overcome the negative effects. This requires a major reorientation from traditional disease and deficiency models of healthcare. Working in partnership across all the stakeholders within a consensual model of the goals of public policy provides a sound basis on which to make progress. This is not something that can be achieved overnight and it will require consistent and sustainable effort if it is to be realized by future generations in Scotland. However, it will take place in a stable policy context in which, whichever party is in power, the broad tenets of social democracy and belief in the communitarian ideas of collectivism, fairness, and social justice are likely to prevail.

Conclusion

This chapter has shown that in an independent minded country, with a distinct identity, culture, history, and politics, alternative ideas can promote politically rational and innovative public policy that challenges some of the current dominant beliefs found elsewhere. This is not simply a matter of "what works," but also of what the citizens and those involved in governance want for their society. Scotland's relatively small size has allowed strong networks to emerge that foster partnerships and collaboration across the public, voluntary, and community sectors. The private sector has little take-up beyond supplying acute care through voluntary health insurance for the small minority who desire it, medical products and nursing home care. The Government has attempted to give more focus through setting fewer priorities than before and bringing all parts of the public sector and its third sector partners together in a common aim to meet (currently) 16 National Outcomes, without being micromanaged to achieve them. There is a remarkable degree of consensus, across the political spectrum and different stakeholders, for the collective model of public provision, avoiding the service and social fragmentation, and transaction costs associated with markets and competition.

This context, and the stability of health policies and structures associated with it, have provided fertile territory for quality and safety initiatives. Moreover, the emphasis on collaboration and integration has facilitated progress, for example, through clinical leadership of initiatives, the provision of mutual support and sharing of ideas, and good practice. There is plenty of evidence that quality and safety in the NHS in Scotland are improving. The challenge, however, is to demonstrate whether progress is as fast, equitable, and sustainable as it would have been had Scotland not chosen to eschew the levers and incentives that have been widely adopted in other, more market-driven health systems to promote quality and efficiency. Recent attempts to explore this have been inconclusive and their findings challenged, not least due to problems of data comparability even within the UK (see Nuffield Trust 2010, Centre for Public Policy in the Regions 2010). However, such comparative analysis is essential, both to assess the effectiveness of the approach adopted in Scotland and to increase our understanding of what drives quality improvement in healthcare.

Chapter 26

Sweden

John Øvretveit, Magna Andreen Sachs, and Marion Lindh

Abstract

National and local reforms in Sweden have focused on reducing waiting times, increasing efficiency, containing costs, choice, and competition, and introducing more private providers. Quality and safety is comparable to many western countries, possibly slightly higher for clinical quality, and lower for aspects of patient-centered care. Evidence of the effects of reforms locally and nationally is limited, and especially of their effects on quality and safety. The future is likely to see more emphasis on patient empowerment, performance measurement, and national and international comparisons, performance-related financial incentives, new payment systems, and care coordination for older people.

Introduction

The proponents of healthcare reform commonly present one of the aims as being to improve the quality or safety of healthcare, as a part or sole aim of the reform. In a reform where quality or safety is not an aim, its impact on quality and safety is of interest to patients and others. Assessing this impact can increase the accountability of policymakers and implementers and can provide useful lessons to others. But is such an assessment possible? Can changes in safety and quality be attributed with any certainty to a healthcare reform and could lessons be generalized to other health systems? These two questions are only partially addressed by this chapter, which rather seeks to assess the evidence of how recent health reforms have affected quality and safety in Swedish healthcare.

Background

Swedish healthcare is mostly tax-based, publicly funded, and publicly provided by 21 local county councils, within a national regulatory framework with national grants to the counties to reduce inequities. The independence of counties is similar in some respects to that of the 16 German Länder, and to the United States of America (US) and Australian states: significant health reforms are made at both a county and national level. In addition, as Sweden has 21 geographic integrated service delivery and financing systems, and a history of emphasizing public health

Table 26.1   Demographic, economic, and health information for Sweden

Population (thousands)	9,511
Area (sq. km)*	410,340
Proportion of population living in urban areas (2011)	85
Gross Domestic Product (GDP US$, billions)^	523.9
Total expenditure on health as % of GDP	9.6
Gross national income per capita (PPP intl $)	43,980
Per capita total expenditure on health (intl $)	4,158
Proportion of health expenditure which is private	18.3
General Government expenditure on health as a percentage of total expenditure on health	81.7
Out-of-pocket expenditure as a percentage of private expenditure on health	88.1
Life expectancy at birth m/f (yrs)	80/84
Probability of dying under five (per 1,000 live births)	3
Maternal Mortality Ratio (per 100,000 live births) (2013)	4
Proportion of population using improved water and sanitation	100/100

Source: Unless otherwise stated data are for the year 2012 and taken from the World Health Organization 2014. * Area from the World Bank 2014a. ^GDP from the World Bank 2014b.

Notes: PPP is purchasing power parity, intl $ is international dollar which has the same purchasing power as US$ in the US.

measures, a conception of quality and safety beyond that of individual providers is used in this chapter. "Health system quality" is defined here as: The ability of a set of services which a patient needs to cooperate to assess and meet the requirements of the patient, at the lowest costs, without duplication or errors and in a way in which the patient experiences care as one continuous episode.

"Health system quality" also includes the extent to which services reach out and are accessible to people who do not ask for services, but who have health problems, or are at risk, but who may be in greater need of caring, curative, or preventative services than those who do use services. These definitions include equity as a property of "health system quality," a feature not so prominent in provider definitions, but which are a key aspect of Sweden's social welfare history.

The 18 county councils, plus two regional bodies and one island municipality, referred to here as the 21 counties, are responsible for providing health services (primary, secondary, and public health) and for "a good standard of health" in their population. In 1992, the responsibility for long-term inpatient healthcare and care for older people was transferred to local municipalities. This was later expanded to include care for the physically disabled and people with long-term mental illnesses, in 1996. The municipalities either directly run or contract public nursing homes, or home care services. In addition the 290 municipalities provide social services financial assistance, childcare, school health services, and environmental health, as well as non-health services for roads, water, sewerage, and energy. Both the county councils and municipalities raise tax from residents. Healthcare is financed 59 percent from county taxes, 23 percent from national insurance and state grants, 11 percent from patient charges, and 7 percent by payment from communes to county councils for some functions they have taken over.

Relevant also to the context for the reforms, and for quality and safety, is the high use of information technology (IT): Sweden is a country which invested early in broadband and the population is "computer and mobile literate." However, healthcare lags behind, as in other countries, in its effective use of digital technologies and the internet, and especially in connections between providers; an IT-related reform will be mentioned later in this chapter. Also relevant is a lack of consumerism in patient attitudes, passivity, at least compared to many US patients, and a relative weakness in organized patient advocacy groups, as well as in understanding patient-centered care.

Reforms

In the early 1990s, nine county councils introduced a form of purchaser–provider reform with Diagnostic Related Group-based contracts, and allowed some hospitals to become more independent as public companies—a few were fully privatized (Jonsson 1994, 1995, Gerdtham et al. 1999, Øvretveit 2001). Special purchasing units were formed, usually with a political board. Two-thirds of the county councils have contracted out some of their activities. Social care is provided by smaller municipalities, which, as a consequence of reforms in the 1990s, took over from the counties in providing, or funding, care for older people, non-medical mental health services, and services for people with disabilities. To finance these changes, about 20 percent of county council healthcare expenditure was transferred to municipalities.

In the 2000s, national initiatives were taken to improve primary, psychiatric, and aged care, and especially to enhance cooperation with municipalities. Pharmacy sector reforms were also introduced including privatization and competition, and devolved drugs budgets, as well as changes in patient copayments. Counties have tested different models in primary care including cooperatives, not-for-profit, and private providers.

A waiting time guarantee for elective services was introduced in 2005 with targets for same day "contact" for primary healthcare centers (PHCCs), doctor visits within seven days, within 90-day specialist appointment after PHCC referral, and within a 90-day window from specialist decision to treatment. The penalties for not meeting these were that the county had to offer care at an alternative

provider (expected times are given on the publically accessible website: www.
vantetider.se). To this "guarantee" was added, in 2008, a Government grant to
those counties that met the targets.

Reforms between 2009 and 2013 included:

2009: Half of the pharmacies owned by the public national provider were
   privatized and certain painkillers and other pharmaceuticals could be sold
   in ordinary shops. Also patients had to pay the full cost for a non-generic
   medication, or for one not prescribed by the physician.

2010: A law gave patient choice of PHCC, not of individual primary care
   provider (PCP) (specifically general practitioner), from an approved list
   of public and private centers. This was a change from patients previously
   being allocated a PHCC depending on their geographic area of residence,
   although some counties had previously introduced this reform. Public
   finance is paid to the doctor or center depending on patients choosing that
   center. (In 2013, Government grants totaling €7 million were given to
   counties to develop systems of choice of care).

2011: A new law defined healthcare providers' responsibility for patient safety.
   There was also a series of restructurings:

   • Nationally, in 2011, six regional cancer centers were further developed
     to support cancer prevention, treatment, and care.
   • Most counties are consolidating clinical and other services in fewer
     hospitals and specialist centers, and closing, or "repurposing,"
     small hospitals.
   • In Stockholm, a major restructuring of healthcare was carried out to
     provide, "The right care when and where you need it." The aims are:
     – "for patients to get the right care including a clearer role for
        family doctors;
     – investment in hospitals with specialist care so that more care is
        available closer to patients;
     – more e-health services to facilitate dialogue and greater participation
        and make it easier for caregivers to provide effective care and have
        more time for the patient;
     – for healthcare to function as a network around the patient, which
        is accessible and close. The patient's ability to choose healthcare
        providers will increase" (Stockholms läns landsting 2013a).

And performance reforms were made to improve measurement and monitoring:

   • This refers to a set of changes nationally, locally, and many pilots,
     some about measurement and providing comparative performance
     information, and some with financial incentives related to performance
     (Pay for Performance (P4P) schemes). Initiatives to increase efficiency

and performance included public comparisons of performance measures, which started in 2006 with "Öppna jämförelser" (transparent regional comparison) and strengthening and extending the national clinical quality registers for different diseases and patient groups (Sveriges Kommuner och Landsting 2010). The Balanced Score Card is a popular tool (Funck 2009).

- Different counties have linked payment to performance figures for services—Anell et al. (2012) reports that P4P in primary care is two to four percent of total payments based on 20 process indicators. There are few clinical outcome indicators.

Influences and Stakeholders

One influence on these reforms was a political move to the right in national and county elections, with parties which put a greater emphasis on choice, internal competition between public services, and encouragement for more private services. Politicians and managers were also influenced by the United Kingdom (UK) healthcare market reforms of the 1990s, as well as concerns about rising costs causing rising taxes and public dissatisfaction with waiting times. To address the latter, reforms have included contracting private providers, privatization, new payment systems, targets, and waiting time guarantees, as well as Government grants.

Institutions other than the counties and municipalities which have a significant interest, influence, or role in reforms, and in quality or safety initiatives, include:

- Ministry of Health and Social Affairs (*Socialdepartementet*).
- The National Board of Health and Welfare (*Socialstyrelsen*) (NBHW): general responsibilities for quality and safety.
- The Swedish Association of Municipalities and Counties (*Sveriges Kommuner och Landsting*) (SALAR).
- Swedish Medical Association and specialty groups and other professional associations such as Swedish Society of Nursing.
- Private healthcare service providers association (*Vardforetagena*).
- Swedish Insurance Federation (public no-fault insurance scheme—pays for injury to patients caused by healthcare).
- Swedish Council on Technology Assessment in Health Care (SBU)—similar, in some respects, to the UK National Institute for Health and Care Excellence).

Other stakeholders with an interest in quality and safety include patients' organizations, which are mostly defined by disease group. Those most prominent include the Swedish diabetes patients association, the Swedish heart disease association, and the Swedish cancer patients association.

Quality and Safety Challenges and Initiatives

Indicators and Information about Safety and Quality

Evidence of some of the challenges comes from routinely collected and reported indicators of poor quality and safety. Since 2006 SALAR has collected and published 169 performance indicators, which include some quality and safety indicators reported by hospitals: any hospital acquired infections, hygiene and dress code compliance, patient falls, pressure ulcers, any overcrowding, as well as other indicators, for example adverse events detected using the Institute for Healthcare Improvement global trigger tool (publically available and nearly all hospitals report every six months, see Sveriges Kommuner och Landsting 2013, 2011).

There is also evidence of patient's and citizen's perceptions of healthcare from a set of questions posed to samples in each county every six months (111,000 people total) and published by county in the "Vårdbarometern" health survey. The health center survey covers experience of recent visit: overall impression, attitude, participation, information, trust, accessibility, perceived usefulness, and if the patient could recommend the clinic to others. Other non-public data can be found in around 100 Swedish, disease-based, quality registers (clinical databases holding individual patient details including treatment and outcomes (Sveriges Kommuner och Landsting 2010)).

The Challenges

The particular quality and safety challenges facing Sweden are mostly similar to those in other countries. The national patient record medical error study which many countries have undertaken found similar rates of about 8.6 percent of hospital patients experiencing an adverse event (Soop et al. 2009).

Some challenges however, are slightly different and there are different priorities and programs for addressing these. One is the higher proportion of older people in the Swedish population, often with multiple chronic conditions, combined with under-developed coordination of providers and of self-management support to patients and carers. Waiting times also are longer than for many other Organisation for Economic Cooperation and Development (OECD) countries. Closure of maternity units has resulted in longer distances to travel. Many emergency rooms are over-crowded and "trolley-waits" by patients in corridors, while a bed is found in a ward, are not uncommon. There are also access problems for some patients: as for most countries, those in urban areas have shorter distances to travel than those in remote rural areas, but there are access (and response) problems for some immigrant groups in the cities due to linguistic, cultural, and financial hindrances (copays discourage use in low-income groups).

Impact of Reforms on Quality and Safety of Care

Because of the decentralized nature of Swedish healthcare in 21 different health systems, and because most of the population live in a few large counties, the following considers both the impact of national reforms and of reforms carried out by some of the larger counties, such as Stockholm (with 20 percent of the Swedish population). It also considers access and equity issues to be part of "health system quality."

The following considers possible evidence of impact on quality and safety outcomes, processes, and structure of those changes made by the reforms listed earlier, and then notes challenges in assessing how much these "impacts" may have been due to reforms and how much may be due to other changes, such as those pursued by professional associations or other non-reform influences.

Purchaser Provider Split and Service Agreements

Studies on the mid and late 1990s suggest that these reforms had little impact on the indicators studied and assessed by care providers (Alban & Christiansen 1995, Bergman 1998).

More Private Providers and Competition

This has increased the choice aspect of quality, and in part influenced more quality indicator reporting. However, information about quality for the public has limited publicity and is incomplete, difficult to access, spread over many different databases, and there are few comparisons over time or between providers. An innovative private initiative created a website which brought together the disparate indicators to present them in a meaningful way for members of the public (http://www.omvard.se/).

Waiting Time Targets

After three years, the number of patients waiting longer than 90 days for elective treatments had been reduced by 50 percent. Often it was extra finance and contracting private providers for elective care which explained the changes, as well as "list management." Physicians argued that many initiatives to reduce waiting times are insensitive to patient need and that patients with greater needs may have to wait even longer if waiting time targets are to be fulfilled (Winblad & Andersson 2010). Waiting times continue to be an issue, and are carefully monitored; but it is often unclear how much long waiting is caused by efficiency and process problems, limited capacity in already efficient systems, or by times being used to negotiate extra finance. The National Patient Survey in 2013 reports that 17 percent of emergency department patients had waited four to six hours and 15 percent had waited for six hours or more (Nationella Patientenkäten 2013).

Pharmacy Deregulation and Privatization

These reforms aimed to increase access to pharmacies and medicines by encouraging additional pharmacies to open with longer opening hours, as well as lower prices for over the counter drugs and other medicines. There is some evidence that access was increased (Swedish Competition Authority 2010), but less evidence of significantly lower prices. Copayments have been found to discourage purchase by low-income groups but there is no evidence of a significant worsening of this element of inequity in Swedish healthcare since these and other reforms.

Patient Choice of Primary Care

Insofar as patient choice might be considered an aspect of quality—at least the quality of a health system, if not an aspect of the quality of a service—in this respect reforms have raised quality (Sveriges Riksdag 2012, Stockholms läns landsting 2013b). This reform made PCPs and other health center staffs' incomes dependent on patients choosing them, and there is some evidence that centers provided more information about services and may have made their services more attractive to patients in different ways. There was a 23 percent increase in the number of PHCCs, and most of these were established in the three large urban county–regions. In these, a third of the private providers are owned by three private corporations.

It is possible that this reform made clinical coordination more difficult between PCPs and other geographically-organized providers such as some nurses and municipalities. Before the choice reform, PCPs, nurses, and other care providers served patients in one geographical area. After the reform some patients chose doctors outside of the area which continued to be served by some nurses and social service personnel who remained organized on a geographic basis. These geographically-organized personnel found themselves having to liaise with many more doctors, often with information systems which were not easily accessible, and it is possible that clinical coordination was poorer as a result.

An evaluation of this reform in Stockholm found a 10 percent increase in productivity, mostly due to an increase in patient consultations, but which reduced in subsequent years (Rehnberg et al. 2010). However, results may be different in other counties which made more use of capitation-based payments and required more responsibilities for PHCCs (Anell, Glenngård, & Merkur 2012). Also, the content and quality of the visits is unknown. Utilization increased in all age groups, and more in patient groups with multiple chronic illnesses and in low-income areas. This may suggest the reforms increased equity by encouraging more services in low-income areas and for patient groups more in need.

Performance Reforms

These initiatives aim to collect, report, and use data on different aspects of performance of services and county systems to enable performance improvement. Janlöv (2010) found that counties which were high in traditional cost-based productivity measures also were high on measures of health outcomes. As regards effects of P4P initiatives, there is little evidence; one study found improvements in care process quality for P4P for heart failure patients (Olsson, Kullberg, & Landgren 2010).

Improvement: Barriers, Solutions, and Prospects

This overview has shown some evidence of improved quality and safety as detected in changes in process quality and outcome indicators, and which can be attributed to both generic reforms and specific quality initiatives at a national and county level. Current barriers and possible solutions for the future are noted below (Table 26.2), based on our understanding of the research and our experience working and advising on quality and safety programs and projects in Sweden since 1990:

Overall Assessment

Have the generic or quality-specific reforms in Sweden improved the quality of care for patients? The limited evidence and varied evidence for different reforms makes this a difficult question to answer. Any response needs to be qualified and will be partial, and to some extent, subjective. There were differences between the authors in their overall assessments of whether generic or quality reforms had improved quality and safety for patients, or had reduced quality. One view was that if the time, money, and effort spent on some of the changes had been allocated directly to quality improvement projects and developing health provider capability for improvement, then patients would have benefitted more.

Another view was that some of the reforms created the conditions, with more competition, choice, and incentives, for those who could use quality methods to gain an advantage, which would benefit patients. Yet another view was that some of the quality-related reforms did have a greater impact on quality, but there were differences between the authors about whether the efforts could have been better spent on other types of quality reform, such as improving data, measurement and competence in use of project teams, and quality methods.

Overall, perhaps the biggest positive impact of the reforms in the last ten years has been to give patients more choice (of hospitals, and local health centers), and waiting time guarantees for visits and treatments. There is mixed evidence of impact on costs, which are considered here an aspect of "management quality" (Øvretveit 1992).

Table 26.2　Key barriers and solutions

Current barriers to improving quality and safety	Possible future solutions
Measurement: lack of credible valid and cost-effective indicators at each level of the health system.	**Investment** in practical research and information systems to define and gather indicator data automatically from medical records, databases, and quality registers.
Use of data for quality improvement: despite quality methods and ideas now being widespread, methods and discipline to use data to assess changes is under-developed.	**Training** to demonstrate the benefit and methods to use available data cost-effectively to assess the effect of improvement changes. Publication and emphasis on large **variations** in quality of care within and between counties, and on methods for improvement.
Attitudes: Under-developed understanding of patient centered care and of working with patients in co-service.	Evidence and examples of benefits of a more patient centered care approach, increase capability to design PCC services which enable providers to give PCC.
Patient acquiescence and under-developed responsibility for own health: especially older patients, who are not "demanding consumers."	Publicity and media information to raise patient awareness of self-care, of rights, and of what they should expect from providers. Patient advocates and navigators to advice and strengthen patient influence. Development of patient associations and of direct to patient information, and personal health records or portals.
Inter-connectivity: no or poor connections between electronic medical records in PHCC and hospitals, or with social care.	Healthcare Information Exchanges and faster progress on national strategy (Sveriges Kommuner och Landsting 2009), reforms to privacy and access laws.
Under-Coordination: communication does not always bring collaboration and coordination, especially for frail older patients, cancer patients and those with multiple morbidity. Most quality and safety problems are in the "in-betweens," but many providers do not have the time, support systems, or understand the need to communicate and coordinate their work with that of others.	Measures showing the improvement opportunities for between-provider coordination, financial penalties, and incentives, and better designed systems for communication and coordination between providers helping one patient and informal carers.
Insufficient incentives to overcome barriers: time, personal benefit, and demonstrated benefit to patient.	**Feedback** from patients to providers about their experience of quality and safety, professional associations giving quality and safety higher priority, more comparative performance data, which is credible, and P4P incentives.
Opposition to restructuring: local services provide access and are preferred by many patients, but may be of lower quality and higher cost. In the past concentration has reduced access and been of uncertain quality and safety benefit.	When services are restructured in fewer concentrated centers, local services, and arrangements to provide fast access are needed including telemedicine to PHCCs.

Conclusion

The aim of this chapter was twofold: first, to assess possible impact of reforms on quality and safety, and second, to consider how future assessments could be made to increase the accountability of politicians and implementers to the public for the effect on their reforms on the quality and safety of care which the public receives.

Sweden has 21 county integrated health systems, mostly public, within a national framework. National and county reforms in recent years have focused on reducing waiting times, increasing efficiency, and containing costs, choice, and competition, and introducing more private providers. There have been initiatives to improve care for older people and for people with mental health problems. Quality and safety is comparable to many western countries, possibly slightly higher for clinical quality, and lower for aspects of patient-centered care.

Evidence of the effects of reforms locally and nationally is limited, and especially of their effects on quality and safety. However, no or limited evidence does not mean no impact. Future reforms in the last ten years have given patients more choice (of hospitals, and local health center) and probably reduced waiting times compared to what they would otherwise be without the reform. It is likely other clinical improvements have taken place and been driven by professionals. It is possible direct investment in quality improvement capability would make better use of resources to improve quality and safe guarantees, for visits and treatments.

Reform planning, implementation, and research could pay more attention to theorizing how possible pathways of influences may flow from the reform change, through different mediators, to affect different aspects of provider behavior and organization, which are themselves likely to impact quality and safety indicators.

The future is likely to see more emphasis on patient empowerment, performance measurement and comparisons, performance-related financial incentives, and new payment systems and care coordination for older people.

Chapter 27

Discussion: Integrating and Synthesizing the Evidence Across Countries

Jeffrey Braithwaite, Yukihiro Matsuyama, Russell Mannion, and
Julie Johnson

In this book we aimed to offer a global perspective on healthcare reform and its relationship with efforts to improve quality and safety. We examined the way reforms developed in multiple countries and the prospects for reforms, and specifically looked at the impact that national reform initiatives have—and have had—on the quality and safety of care. Our interest was in how reforms drive quality and safety improvement, and as a corollary, how they might inadvertently serve to undermine or negate such goals.

We recognize that healthcare systems can be more complex and dynamic than simple, linear, cause-and-effect rationalities sometimes suggest (Braithwaite et al. 2013, Plsek & Greenhalgh 2001, Tan, Wen & Awad 2005). On-the-ground improvement can occur purposefully, or as a byproduct of meeting other objectives, and poor quality services might be an unintended outcome of other health systems activities, outside of attempts to enact reform. But in the main, reforms and improvement activities are well intentioned and designed and funded by those aiming for, and striving to enact, positive change.

When we started out we knew that there was no book of this type available, and there was a unique opportunity for cross-fertilization of ideas to the mutual benefit of countries involved in the project, and other international colleagues. As such, the book fills a gap in our knowledge, and serves a wide range of groups (patients and the public with an interest in health systems, and more particularly Governments, policymakers, managers and leaders, interested clinicians, teaching academics, researchers, and students). Even though we did not include 100 percent of health systems internationally, the book nevertheless forms a compendium of the current "state of the art" of global healthcare reform and its putative effects. It includes chapters as different as Niuyun's China (population 1.4 billion) and Al-Mandhari's Oman (population 3.3 million), and those as large in square kilometers as Johnson and Bierman's United States of America (US) (9.1 million) and as small as Yeoh and Fung's Hong Kong (1,104).

What is it That People do When Reforming Systems and Improving Quality of Care and Patient Safety?

There are some common patterns across the countries enrolled in the book which readers will have discerned as they take in the breadth of scholarship over the chapters. Armed with the chapters' detailed, nation-level analyses, we can now see much more clearly than previously that every country has invested, virtually continually, in reform and improvement processes. Each takes place in the particular historical, social, cultural, economic, and developmental context of that country, leading to distinctive emphases and reports of varied progress. Furthermore, they are path-dependent (Wilsford 1994, Bloom, Standing & Lloyd 2008): where they start, and how the journey progresses, determines where each health system is now, at the time of this assessment in 2014.

There are striking similarities across the countries. Most importantly is the universal aim—underlying the efforts in all represented countries—towards enhancing the ability to deliver quality healthcare and thereby improve the health of society. Methods for tackling common objectives include modifying financial allocations, enacting legislation, strengthening regulatory regimes, promulgating policy measures, reorganizing ministries or sectors, introducing, modifying, or removing policy institutions in the form of ministerial committees, commissions, and authorities, making infrastructure available to providers, freeing up or stimulating market forces, developing and using performance indicators, recruiting and training workforces, exploiting new IT capabilities, and providing incentives, education, and training. Indeed, while there is a unique mix of reform approaches adopted by each country in our cohort, they are drawn from what can now be seen as a core list of measures recurring throughout the book. Collectively, these are what people mean by, and what constitutes, "reform."

To view the range of reform measures in use across the sample of countries, we created a word cloud—a picture giving prominence to the most frequently occurring words across the texts in the reform sections of the chapters—using Wordle (www. wordle.net; the clouds were made with the exclusion of "healthcare," "health," "care," "system," "quality," "safety," and "reform(s)" as these words were overwhelmingly recurrent throughout the text). This shows a concentration on hospitals, patients, and public issues, with national matters and Government at the heart of reform, and a focus on specified reform issues such as accreditation and insurance (Figure 27.1).

In regard to quality and safety, there is too, an identifiable set of commonly-articulated mechanisms. These include (after the obvious listings of patients, hospitals, medical, and improvement), striving for more evidence-based practice, designing accreditation programs, applying standards, conducting incident reporting, developing and using clinical guidelines, and instituting programs and projects such as root cause analysis, hand hygiene, and handover initiatives, through to industrial approaches to quality improvement such as lean methodologies. As a whole, these are what people mean by, and what constitute, "quality and safety improvement." The word cloud for this illuminates the key concepts (Figure 27.2).

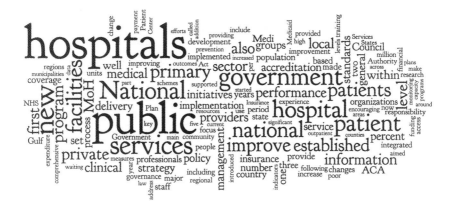

Figure 27.1   Key words in health reform

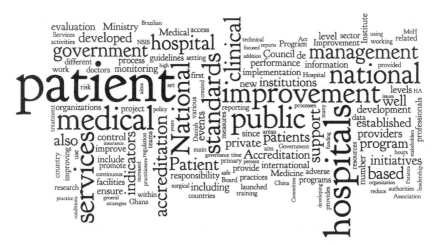

Figure 27.2   Key words in quality and safety

The Relationship between Reform and Quality and Safety

Turning to the content of the chapters centered on the relationships between the core reform and quality and safety constructs at the heart of the book, we present a word cloud synthesizing what chapter authors said about this question (Figure 27.3). It shows similar themes to those in Figure 27.1 and 27.2, but distinctively highlights not only words such as improvement, but also impact, providers, performance, delivery, indicators, information, measures, deaths and mortality, community, and evidence.

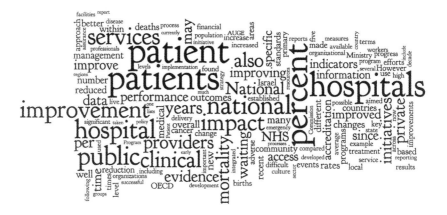

Figure 27.3   Key words at the nexus of reform and quality and safety

However, the most immediate answer to the question we asked chapter authors about the extent of the relationship between reform measures and quality and safety is that, in general, it is *weak at best* and *situation-dependent*. By that is meant that there is no guarantee that any particular reform measure, or packages of measures, whether it involves revamping the organizational chart of the health ministry such as reported in Powell and Mannion's chapter on England, reorganizing specified sectors or sub-sectors, for example in de Noronha, Grabois, and Gomes' chapter on Brazil, promulgating improved legislation, for example in Arce and Elorrio's chapter on Argentina, or issuing new policy (all chapters), will have the desired effect in improving quality of care or making things safer for patients. The chapter authors as a whole are saying that reformers ubiquitously seek to enhance the health system by their actions. Virtually every reform comes with an optimistic stance arguing that the initiative or program proposed will lead to some kind of progress, improvement, or streamlining of the provision of healthcare to its citizenry. Yet the barriers and obstacles to progress and the enhancement of health systems are considerable.

Indeed, there is a view held by researchers such as Coiera (2011), Braithwaite et al. (2006), and Scott et al. (2003) indicating that health systems are characterized by deep forces (for example, frozen or hard-to-change cultures, sectional interests, politics, and rigid extant resource allocations) which act concertedly to impede change. As a result, a common property of health systems is inertia (or even entropy, where things degrade, become less organized and less effective, and health systems go backwards). Where there are strong inertial forces or resistant practices anchoring behaviors to the status quo, there is no real prospect of above-down transformation initiatives, regardless of how well designed or implemented, having an effect. These chapters act in part to reject such a proposition. No health system has, to any extent, surrendered to this view, and all continue to hold to a tenet that says change is not only possible, but that the initiatives that those in authority are sponsoring or enabling, described so extensively in these chapters, will have a positive effect. This stance is universal. *No chapter author wrote about any country which held that change was not feasible, that they had given up, or that trying to improve the public's health through reform wasn't worthwhile.*

Thus, reformers and improvement agents have a great deal of faith that their activities will bear fruit. They specify programs, projects and activities, fund and authorize them to proceed, and intend for them to "roll out" flowing from decisions made in the upper echelons of the system. According to this perspective, legislating, policymaking, or initiating change will result in a considerable shift in localized behaviors and practices—that, is, they will streamline, improve, or increase the quality of care across services and micro-systems, nation-wide.

However, all is not smooth sailing. Chapter authors specify in detail numerous obstacles to implementation, showing significant barriers have been faced by every country. Sometimes changes end up being overturned as in the case of Cumming's report of New Zealand's efforts in the 1990s. Many of the barriers are common, such as healthcare finances and costs, medical professional politics and intransigence, infrastructure support, deeply embedded and entrenched ways of doing things that have been woven into the fabric of healthcare delivery, and poor leadership, governance, and management.

Moreover, although authors discussed the need for better leadership or more patient-centered care, they recognized that many clinician and patient groups remain disenfranchised from reform and improvement measures (Audet et al. 2005, Crawford et al. 2002, Grol et al. 2013). A central theme throughout the book (and specifically in the chapters by Yeoh and Fung (Hong Kong), and Zimlichman (Israel)) is the importance of engaging staff and patients in reform and improvement processes, as they are the agents with whom successful reform at the coalface ultimately rests.

Evaluation as a Tool for Feedback and Improvement

A striking feature of the book, riven throughout the chapters is that, across the world, there is little by way of prospective, planned evaluation reported at the time of the instigation of reform or quality and safety initiatives. Thus, when nations design and then sanction a new regulatory regime, or agency to manage accreditation, or authority to report on systems-level performance, or they institute a hand hygiene, root cause analysis, or incident monitoring system, they rarely establish a parallel, prospective evaluation framework at the time of starting the initiative or project. Consequently, they are obliged to rely on retrospective evaluation, if evaluation is to occur at all. Anyone with even a cursory knowledge of how *hindsight bias* operates will know that this is highly problematic.

Going further, it seems to us that our chapter authors struggled to see good examples of reforms at the origination stage being accompanied by baseline measurement, or with plans to measure progress against a basket of indicators at intervals, as the reform program unfolded. Both formative and summative evaluation frameworks seemed missing. (And at least in some systems, evaluation often takes the form of politically-initiated, big-stage investigations—as the experience with the English National Health Service exemplifies, with multiple inquiries over many years, such as the Bristol (Teasdale 2002, Coulter 2002) and Francis (Francis 2013) inquiries). (For a discussion of a wide range of inquiries in six countries, see Hindle et al. (2006)).

Our own experience supports this interpretation of the evidence from the chapters: we have observed many reforms over the decades, and researched or worked with multiple health systems, and it is rare that policymakers take baseline measures at the time of instigating their reforms, or ensure that their reform initiatives are evaluated over time to measure progress (see Clay-Williams et al. 2014). Instead, policymakers will often call for an evaluation after they see a reform initiative or project come close to its endpoint and exhibit signs of success. They will often then fund a retrospective evaluation, typically engaging one of the well-known management consulting practices. No politician or bureaucrat who does this can escape from the criticism that they are guilty of *positive hindsight bias*: they select from the reform initiatives they have sponsored one which has produced what they judge to be a good outcome after the event, ask an evaluator to confirm their views and then include an argument in the minister's next speech or distribute a media release indicating how effective the project was, and by extension how good the health system is, on their watch. They may even argue that they knew all along that the selected initiative would do well.

With such assumptive approaches to policy analysis there is less learning from those initiatives that were simply less successful. In one sense this can be attributed to politics (after all, which politician or party official, whether under a democratic model such as those of Europe, or centrally governed arrangements such as that of China, wants the electorate or citizens to think they did not design and deliver effective outcomes, and which bureaucrats or regulators want their minister, colleagues or the public to know they have presided over reform or implementation failure?). But in a very real sense this is inexcusable: we spend billions of dollars, pounds, euros, yen, rupees, yuan, francs, pesos, and related currencies on health reform and quality and safety, most of it funded from the public purse, and we know very little about what the *range* of successes and failures look like. That is why this book is critical: authors endeavored to give an honest, clear-eyed appraisal of change mechanisms, past and current, and how they have performed.

All in all, several authors, including Cicchetti, Coretti, and Iacopino (Italy), Whittaker, Marshall, and Labadarios (South Africa), Deilkås, Ingebrigtsen, and Ringard (Norway), Øvretveit, Sachs, and Lind (Sweden), and Duckett (Australia), directly or indirectly call for better studies measuring progress. Pfaff, Gloede, and Hammer (Germany) go further than most, suggesting a nation-wide quality measurement institute.

Overall, we would argue that if care is actually improved, and this can be attributed to the reformers' or improvement agents' actions, these successes will be best understood with reference to what things were like at the starting point, that is, from the baseline. It would lead to much more tangible and transferable knowledge if carefully, arm's length, dispassionate evaluators were undertaking more regular assessments based on a basket of qualitative and quantitative indicators of the reforms and improvement initiatives in every country. It might create a virtuous feedback loop of considerable utility to the individual systems, and valuable international comparative information.

Drilling Deeper into the Heart of Change

To build on the chapter authors' aggregated wisdom further, we might draw a distinction here between wealthier countries (for example, those in Northern Europe) and less wealthy countries (for example, Gyani's India, or Adu-Krow and Sikosana's Papua New Guinea). It is true to say that in the main, in higher income, Organisation for Economic Cooperation and Development (OECD)-type health systems, many of the most basic problems have already been solved. Care is provided by comparatively well-trained and appropriately resourced professionals, and services are typically provided across-the-board with satisfactory levels of equity, via delivery mechanisms that are organized and funded, and are more likely than not to work. There is relatively good access to clinical and communications capacity and technology, expensive medications, and serviceable infrastructure.

In less well-endowed countries the systems' capacities and delivery mechanisms are profoundly different. Modern healthcare is expensive to provide. There is often a dearth of trained, skilled health professionals and a mal-distribution of them in rural or remote parts of the country, contrasted with urban areas. Indeed, across the book, developing country chapters such as those provided by Al-Mandhari (Oman), Gyani (India), and Adu-Krow and Sikosana (Papua New Guinea) talked more about reform in terms of enhancing the availability of health services, increasing and training the workforce, and improving the overall health of their populations. Several authors were able, in this respect, to demonstrate progress, such as the examples provided in Sodzi-Tettey's Ghana chapter regarding eradication of guinea worm disease and improvements in child and maternal health indicators.

Yet it seems that once a country passes a development and income threshold, and occupies a GNI per capita bracket at, or approaching, OECD-levels, there is more likely to be a focus on things like efficiency, safety, and quality, particularly in acute settings, and an increasing ability to embrace initiatives which involve taking the needs of patients into account or measuring patient experience. They are also more likely to be able to afford expensive technology such as IT and diagnostic technology.

Relatively poorly resourced systems—though lacking expensive infrastructure and informatics support, and information support richer health systems take for granted—do have a notable advantage over their higher-income counterparts. The margin of possible improvement is much wider amongst the poorer compared with the richer countries: an additional dollar of resources will go much further in a less wealthy health system, all other things being equal, and assuming it is used wisely.

Let's provide an example of this, drawing from ideas strewn throughout the book. Say there is a move to conduct some financial restructuring of a health system, starting with decisions taken at the peak level, to fund one set of services at the expense of another. In a lower-income country this may mean that newly allocated resources, even if relatively slight, to provide community-wide vaccinations for children under five, for example, or to build a hospital in a peripheral but growing township area removed from the central business district, may result in significant benefits at both the individual and population levels.

Financial restructuring in higher-income countries, within a health system in which every sub-sector is already quite well supported—say by moving funding allocations from acute to chronic diseases, or moving resources from general practice to a specific purpose such as more services for HIV/AIDS patients—is markedly different. All sub-sectors (aged, acute, community-based, primary, tertiary, and quaternary care) start from a relatively well-resourced base. Redistribution decisions may typically confer few additional benefits beyond marginal gains. There is no real net effect on the quality of people's lives, the quality of care, or the safety of patients across-the-board.

So, a notable paradox emerges from reading chapters where the authors across less wealthier health systems were asked to look for a relationship between reform and quality and safety. Typically, with a little effort, these kinds of outcomes can be measured fairly readily—and they frequently are, especially as the World Health Organization (WHO) and the donors who fund such programs prefer to see indicators of progress or, better still, formalized, measurable success. A wealthier country could operationalize the same kind of reforms and even pump many more resources into reducing infant mortality or improving maternal health but would likely achieve no substantive improvement in either of these because the levels of achievement are already so high.

There are echoes here with the economic concept of marginal utility. In healthcare, we usually try to measure health gains of this type through quality adjusted life years (QUALYs) (La Puma & Lawlor 1990, Mortimer & Segal 2008), but quite simply if you have a measurable problem like this example, and come from a low base, you are much more likely to achieve more QUALY benefits than if you already have demonstrably high levels of success.

Building on this distinction, a related issue is well known to public health specialists, and also differentiates wealthier and less wealthy countries. If your goal as a health reformer is to enhance the health status of a poorly resourced population you may be much better off allocating resources to activities outside the health system, not spending money directly on the quality and safety of patients in acute settings. So providing sanitation to a great number of people in the community, making money available to fund law and order services, or enhancing farming practices, could improve the economic quality of lives and the well-being, and safety and security, of citizens (Marmot et al. 2008, Prüss-Üstün & Corvalán 2006, Tilman et al. 2002), adding substantial QUALYs to the population. There is much more to be gained this way than attempting to provide diminishingly small increases in hand hygiene rates, or training yet more people how to do root cause analyses after adverse events occur in inpatient settings in the hospitals of rich countries with little benefit to the systems of care, which is where much new expenditure is committed.

Another recurring theme running through the chapters, and distinguishing lower- and higher-income countries, is that of equity. This manifests quite differently in the various systems. Clearly, equity—whether we are talking about vertical or horizontal equity, equity of access, utilization, or outcome (Mooney 2000, Mooney & Jan 1997)—is a reform and quality and safety issue. For example, if resources are not distributed relatively fairly and widely across a population then those who do not receive a share, such as members of marginalized groups, will receive sub-standard care. This is the spirit level idea, which says that the more equity in society, the better the nation's health. Yet, in under-resourced health systems, there is the problem of spreading the available resources too thinly. If there are insufficient healthcare resources across-the-board the risk is that everyone gets sub-standard care, although equally. Similarly, as Solimano and Valdivia (Chile) point out, setting priority targets to focus limited resources runs the associated risk of de-prioritizing other conditions, potentially creating new marginalized populations. Healthcare economic and quality-of-care problems, as always, are replete with potential tensions and paradoxes.

We might note in passing on the equity question, that the US has historically been an exception to the general rule. Every other country seems to embrace equity as a key feature of providing quality care to its citizens. The US, however, has a strong tradition of not promoting universal equity, although, as Johnson and Bierman show, under Obamacare this has begun to change. The policy landscape since the Affordable Care Act's (US Congress 2010) promulgation in 2010 has meant that finally, a reasonable standard of care is now being made available to a much bigger proportion of the American population. But for far fewer resource inputs than those provided by the US, other countries produce better results, and greater levels of equity prevail. Indonesia's goal of creating its first universal healthcare system (see Hermawan and Blakely's chapter), Hong Kong's policy that "no one should be denied of adequate healthcare through lack of means" (see Yeoh and Fung's chapter), and Brazil's progress towards more equitable care (see Noronha, Grabois, and Gomes' chapter), drawn from countries with a range of income levels, illustrates the priority most countries place on this principle. Promoting greater amounts of equity, particularly to vulnerable populations, remains a recurring feature of every other health system canvassed in this book.

Continuous Reform and Improvement, or Punctuated Equilibrium?

We said earlier, and it is confirmed in every chapter, that health systems are undergoing multi-faceted and multi-level reform and improvements. With the publication of this book, it no longer appears tenable to think that there are periods when health systems undergo reform and then periods when they are stable and not reforming. Instead, a lesson from the book is that health systems-strengthening is an ongoing, never-ending stream of activities and supporting strategies. Certainly, there may be times of more intense and less intense change; but even in relatively quiet periods, where, for example, the top-level structure is not being drastically reorganized, nevertheless there are various policy refinements, updated legislation, fresh procedures, new safety projects, and fine-tuning of budgetary allocations going on all the time. Reform and improvement should be seen as occurring in continuous evolution rather than following a "punctuated equilibrium" model, whereby there are long periods of no reform followed by short bursts of "big bang" reform. Duckett even suggests that in the Australian context there have been no real "big bang" attempts, but that all reforms could be better characterized as "slow and steady." In addition, almost every country felt there was still "more to do."

The other lesson in terms of the continuous flow of reforms and improvements is how every country's history of health reform and improvement displays what we might call *concordant resonance* across the last 20 years or so. For instance, all reforms were reported by chapter authors as being led from the top, typically through the minister, ministry, or department of health, although some such as Sodzi-Tettey's chapter on Ghana, Powell and Mannion's chapter on England, and Thompson and Steel's chapter on Scotland do speak of the connections between bottom-up and top-down initiatives.

Another striking similarity is that changes are dominated by the *structural* (new bodies to manage things or changes in organizational arrangements), and the *procedural* (new laws, policies, or incentives to influence, enable, or constrain behaviors in the aggregate). There was also mention of the need to change or reinvigorate cultures and values within healthcare organizations and across systems (such as in Khoja and Kamel's chapter on The Gulf, Al-Mandhari's chapter on Oman, Niuyun's chapter on China, Matsuyama's chapter on Japan, Cumming's chapter on New Zealand, Ruelas, Gómez-Dantés, and Morales' chapter on Mexico, and Knudsen, Engel, and Eriksen's chapter on Denmark, amongst others). But most changes were almost always evolutionary rather than revolutionary. They represent the gradual encroachment and pervasion of ideas rather than anything radical being introduced.

There are common constraining factors and obstacles to change. Key barriers to overcome to achieve progress were identified as healthcare finances and costs, medical professional politics and intransigence, infrastructure support, entrenched ways of doing things, and poor leadership. There are also counter cultures which resist and circumvent the dominant discourses of reform. Integration—of teams at the clinical coalface, or beyond that, of services or whole sectors—was identified across many countries as being a key reform and improvement ingredient, but is notably hard to achieve. A word cloud (Figure 27.4) summarizes what the authors of chapters said about implementation barriers and solutions.

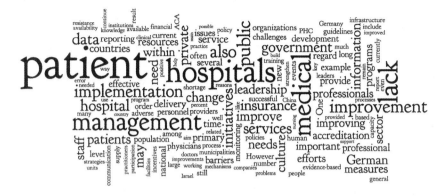

Figure 27.4   Key words concerning implementation barriers and solutions

The Outcomes of Reform and Improvement

In some countries (for example, Australia, Israel, and Ghana) there are hints that the reforms and improvements that authorities design, sponsor or initiate drive tangible outcomes of some form or another. As we have seen, whether or not they do, little robust evidence based on well-designed, objective studies was available to authors across the chapters to substantiate this.

We would also simply underscore the point we made earlier: that when positive outcomes (or negative consequences) do result from reform or improvement strategies, it is possible that they have arisen due to other factors, or to factors outside the health system. Indeed, it is well known, as we indicated above, that improving population health is largely attributable to non-healthcare drivers and there are strong linkages to levels of poverty, provisions of housing, ensuring societal law and order, and providing sanitation and running water (Marmot et al. 2008, Prüss-Üstün & Corvalán 2006, Tilman et al. 2002). These are substantial forces in reducing disease and creating healthy communities beyond the care provided in acute or aged care sectors, especially in vulnerable or less well-endowed societies. Parallel to this is the failure of reforms because of forces outside of the health sector and therefore outside the reach of health system reforms. Arce and Elorrio (Argentina), for instance, show that a succession of economic cycles, based on the differing macroeconomic and ideological policy views of its leaders, led to inequalities in the availability and access to resources between lower- and higher-income populations. Cicchetti, Coretti, and Iacopino (Italy) also noted deleterious effects sustained in the healthcare system as a result of economic turmoil.

Perhaps another key message we can take from this book, then, is that it provides an answer to a question we did not specifically formulate at the start of our journey: how can reformers and improvement agents *optimize the outcomes of their efforts*? An answer appears to be: if agents sponsoring reforms or improvements want to augment their efforts and increase their chances of achieving far-reaching change, they might look beyond the health system for leverage. There is a good case that the best reform and improvement is intersectoral in nature (Adeleye & Ofili 2010, Marmot et al. 2008, Walley et al. 2008), and involves not just the health system, but the education, transport, agriculture, retail, judicial, and telecommunications sectors—to mention only some of the more important sectors which can support improved population health outcomes.

Whether or not intersectoralism is pursued, what is vital, as we touched on earlier, is that reforms and improvement initiatives are evaluated and assessed so that outcomes are thoroughly understood. Optimally, as we allude to above, this is best done at the point of planning the initiatives in the first place, taking baseline measures before intervening, and ensuring independent evaluators are involved in making assessments of emergent change and progress. Nevertheless, we issue a word of caution: even when there is evaluation of reforms and improvements the methods are often not robust nor applied longitudinally—which are key reasons why there is a paucity of sound evidence on the impact of reforms in many countries. Additionally, even when we do see better-quality evaluations, they are often not as well informed by theory as we would like; and simplistic, atheoretical evaluation approaches often fail to generate an explanatory, generalizable framework of broader utility.

Having said that, what are the prospects for success in improving health systems, discernible across the chapters? We created a final word cloud to glimpse this point (Figure 27.5). It shows that success factors are similar to those already discussed by chapter authors in other parts of their chapters.

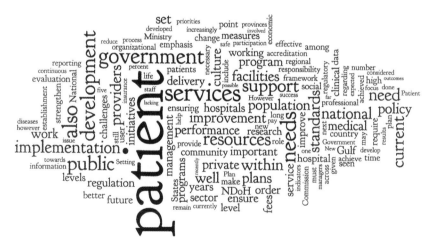

Figure 27.5   Key words regarding prospects for success

The Next Generation of Reform and Improvement

Despite the extensive scholarship displayed by the chapter authors, there are several areas that could do with more attention in the future. Additional work needs to be done to understand the unintended and dysfunctional consequences of reforms and quality and safety improvements. How do health systems anticipate and design ameliorative strategies to mitigate dysfunctional consequences? We have discussed the optimistic bias of the sponsors of change, whether working on reform or improving quality and safety, and that this pervades most thinking. Yet specifying the risks, and analyzing their effects including the potential for progress to be de-railed, would seem to us to be a necessary precondition to any successful change initiative. If there is a generalized neglect of analyzing risks and adverse consequences of change initiatives, then it should be remedied.

There is also work to be done to appreciate more fully the cost savings or efficiencies that accrue from having high quality or safe care (Øvretveit 2009). Several scholars and commentators (for example, Berwick & Hackbarth 2012, Kenagy, Berwick & Shore 1999, Campbell, Roland & Buetow 2000) have articulated an argument which says that getting it right the first time, or more often, and having a well-functioning system in the first place, reduces waste and duplication, and improves outcomes. But this of course is easier said than done.

Another fruitful area for further research is the extent to which health systems learn from other countries or embrace initiatives because they are part of the international "thing to do." Everyone learns from international experience, and there is a great deal of policy transfer. People go to conferences, there are regional political meetings, and bodies such as WHO promulgate various frameworks, projects and approaches believed to be useful. That is the key reason why both the reforms we read about in the chapters, and the quality and safety projects and programs reported on by our authors, begin to exhibit such marked similarities. It's known as *institutional isomorphism*—structures and initiatives start to look the same over time because of pressures including via cross-jurisdictional coercion or international imitation, or the similar constraints under which systems operate (Scott 1987, Scott 2001). Or more simply, reform and quality improvement fads, trends, and fashions are followed (Walshe 2009).

Conclusion

A key message we take from this volume into our future efforts is that a sound goal would be to distil and synthesize the best evidence, taking into account the different contexts of implementation and embracing robust evaluation, perhaps taking a realistic evaluation approach (Pawson & Tilley 1997, Evans & Killoran 2000, Ranmuthugala et al. 2011). We are also advocates for the importance of understanding the contexts of reform and quality and safety improvement, and we believe it is desirable to ensure that the global experiences and the wealth of knowledge represented by the chapters in this book continue to be shared. One option is to do another book of this type every five years or so, and map progress over time.

A final lesson from the book, now that we have a reservoir of the best thinking to tap on this topic, and a contemporary snapshot of reform progress and quality and safety initiatives from a diverse range of countries, is that we can understand much better how international policy and improvement initiatives spread readily across national boundaries. Healthcare is indeed a global undertaking.

References

Aaron, HJ 2014. 'Here to stay—Beyond the rough launch of the ACA.' *New England Journal of Medicine,* vol. 370, no. 24, pp. 2257–9.

Abuelafia, E, Berlinski, S, Chudnovsky, M, Palanza, V, Ronconi, L, San Martín, ME & Tommasi, M 2002. *El funcionamiento del Sistema de Salud argentino en un contexto federal.* Centro de Estudios para el Desarrollo Institucional. Document 77, September 2002.

Adeleye, O & Ofili, A 2010. 'Strengthening intersectoral collaboration for primary health care in developing countries: Can the health sector play broader roles?' *Journal of Environmental and Public Health,* pp. 1–6.

Agência Nacional de Saúde Suplementar 2013. *Caderno de Informação da Saúde Suplementar—Dezembro 2013.* Agência Nacional de Saúde Suplementar: Rio de Janeiro.

Agyepong, IA & Adjei, S 2008. 'Public social policy development and implementation: A case study of the Ghana National Health Insurance scheme.' *Health Policy and Planning,* vol. 23, no. 2, pp. 150–60.

Ahwoi, K 2014. 'Presentation at the Opening Ceremony of the Ministry of Health and its Development Partners.' Health Summit *Working Together Towards Quality Health Care for All in Ghana.* Gimpa, May 12.

Al-Lawati, JA, Al Riyami, AM, Mohammed, AJ & Jousilahti, P 2002. 'Increasing prevalence of diabetes mellitus in Oman.' *Diabetic Medicine,* vol. 19, no. 11, pp. 954–7.

Alban, A & Christiansen, T (eds) 1995. *The Nordic Lights: New initiatives in health care systems.* Odense University Press: Odense.

Alhyas, L, McKay, A & Majeed, A 2012. 'Prevalence of Type 2 diabetes in the states of The Co-Operation Council for the Arab States of the Gulf: A systematic review.' *PloS One,* vol. 7, no. 8, pp. 1–8.

Alpen Capital 2011. *GCC Healthcare Industry Report 2011.* Alpen Capital Group [pdf]. Viewed June 10, 2014: http://www.alpencapital.com/downloads/Alpen Capital's GCC Healthcare report 2011.pdf.

Andrés Bello University 2011. *La Salud del Bicentenario, Chile 2011–2020: Desafíos y Propuestas.* Andrés Bello University: Santiago.

Anell, A, Glenngård, A & Merkur, S 2012. 'Sweden: Health system review.' *Health Systems in Transition,* vol. 14, no. 5, pp. 1–159.

Anessi-Pessina, E & Cantù, E 2006. 'Whither managerialism in the Italian National Health Service?' *International Journal of Health Planning and Management,* vol. 21, no. 4, pp. 327–55.

Antonovsky, A 1979. *Health, Stress, and Coping.* Jossey-Bass: San Francisco.

Aranaz-Andres, JM, Aibar-Remon C, Limon-Ramirez, R, Amarilla, A, Restrepo, FR, Urroz, O, Sarabia, O, García-Corcuera, LV, Terol-García, E, Agra-Varelal, Y, Gonseth-García, JD, Bates, W & Larizgoitia I (on behalf of the IBEAS team) 2011. 'Prevalence of adverse events in the hospitals of five Latin American countries: Results of the "Iberoamerican Study of Adverse Events" (IBEAS).' *BMJ Quality & Safety*, vol. 20, no. 12, pp. 1043–51.

Arce, H 1998. 'Hospital accreditation as a means of achieving international quality standards in health.' *International Journal for Quality in Health Care*, vol. 10, no. 6, pp. 469–72.

Arce, H 1999. 'Accreditation: The Argentine experience in the Latin American region.' *International Journal for Quality in Health Care*, vol. 11, no. 5, pp. 425–8.

Arce, H 2001. *La Calidad en el territorio de la Salud*. ITAES: Buenos Aires.

Arce, H 2010. *El Sistema de Salud; de dónde viene y hacia dónde va.*1st edn. Prometeo: Buenos Aires.

Asante, A & Hall, J 2011. *A Review of Health Leadership and Management Capacity in Papua New Guinea*. Human Resources for Health Knowledge Hub of the School of Public Health and Community Medicine, University of New South Wales [online]. Viewed March 18, 2014: http://www.hrhhub.unsw.edu.au.

Ashton, T 1998. 'Contracting for health services in New Zealand: A transaction cost analysis.' *Social Science & Medicine*, vol. 46, no. 3, pp. 357–67.

Ashton, T, Cumming, J & Mclean, J 2004. 'Contracting for health services in a public health system: The New Zealand experience.' *Health Policy*, vol. 69, no. 1, pp. 21–31.

Aspinall, E 2014. 'Health care and democratization in Indonesia.' *Democratization*, February 26, pp. 1–21.

Assistant Secretary for Planning and Evaluation (ASPE) 2011. *ASPE Issue Brief: Overview of the Uninsured in the United States: A Summary of the 2011 Current Population Survey*. United States Department of Health and Human Services, September 13.

Audet, A, Doty, M, Shamasdin, J & Schoenbaum, S 2005. 'Measure, learn, and improve: Physicians' involvement in quality improvement.' *Health Affairs*, vol. 24, no. 3, pp. 843–53.

Australian Government Department of Health and Ageing 2013. *Medicare Locals Operational Guidelines April 2013*. Commonwealth of Australia [online]. Viewed January 2, 2014: http://www.yourhealth.gov.au/internet/ yourhealth/publishing.nsf/Content/ml-operational-guidelines-toc~strategic-objectives – .UsTtxNIW00I.

Azzam, DG, Neo, CA, Itotoh, FE & Aitken, RJ 2013. 'The Western Australian audit of surgical mortality: Outcomes from the first 10 years.' *The Medical Journal of Australia*, vol. 199, no. 8, pp. 539–42.

Barker, A, Mengersen, K & Morton, A 2012. 'What is the value of hospital mortality indicators, and are there ways to do better?' *Australian Health Review*, vol. 36, no. 4, pp. 374–7.

Barnett, P 2001. *The Formation and Development of Independent Practitioner Associations in New Zealand: 1991–2000*. University of Otago: Christchurch.

Barnett, P, Smith, J & Cumming, J 2009. *The Roles and Functions of PHOs*. Health Services Research Centre: Wellington.

Barraclough, BH & Birch, J 2006. 'Health care safety and quality: Where have we been and where are we going?' *Medical Journal of Australia*, vol. 184, no. 10, pp. 48–50.

Bastias, G & Valdivia, G 2007. 'Reforma de salud en Chile; el Plan AUGE o Regimen de Garantías Explícitas en Salud (GES): Su origen y evolución.' *Boletín Escuela de Medicina UC*, Pontificia Universidad Católica de Chile, vol. 32, no. 2, pp. 51–8.

Bateman, C 2012a. 'Health leadership training academy tackles worst first.' *South African Medical Journal*, vol. 103, no.10, pp. 707–8.

Bateman, C 2012b. 'RWOPS abuse–Government's had enough.' *South African Medical Journal*, vol. 102, no. 12, pp. 899–901.

Beckmann, MW 2009. 'Nationaler Krebsplan des Bundesministeriums für Gesundheit – Strategieplan der Deutschen Krebsgesellschaft.' *Frauenheilkunde up2date,* vol. 3, no. 5, pp. 323–9.

Bergman, S 1998. 'Swedish models of healthcare reform: A review and assessment.' *International Journal of Health Planning and Management*, vol. 13, no. 2, pp. 91–106.

Berwick, D 2013. *The National Advisory Group on the Safety of Patients in England, A Promise to Learn–a Commitment to Act: Improving the Safety of Patients in England*. Department of Health: London.

Berwick, DM & Hackbarth, AD 2012. 'Eliminating waste in US health care.' *Journal of the American Medical Association,* vol. 307, no. 14, pp. 1513–6.

Better Together 2013. *Better Together: Scotland's patient experience programme* [online]. Viewed December 29, 2013: http://www.bettertogetherscotland.com.

Bisang, R & Cetrángolo, O 1997. 'Descentralización de los servicios de salud en Argentina.' *Serie de Reformas de Política Pública*, vol. 47. Comisión Económica para América Latina y el Caribe: Santiago de Chile.

Bismark, MM & Studdert, DM 2013. 'Governance of quality of care: A qualitative study of health service boards in Victoria, Australia.' *BMJ Quality & Safety*, vol. 23, no. 6, pp. 474–82.

Björnberg, A 2013. *Euro Health Consumer Index 2013 Report*, Health Consumer Powerhouse, Täby, Sweden.

Bloom, G, Standing, H & Lloyd, R 2008. 'Markets, information asymmetry and health care: Towards new social contracts.' *Social Science & Medicine,* vol. 66, no. 10, pp. 2076–87.

Bloomberg 2013. *Bloomberg Visal Data.* Bloomberg [online]. Viewed February 27, 2014: http://www.bloomberg.com/visual-data/best-and-worst/most-efficient-health-care-countries.

Blumenthal, D & Tavenner, M 2010. 'The "meaningful use" regulation for electronic health records.' *New England Journal of Medicine*, vol. 363, no. 6, pp. 501–4.

Böcken, J, Butzlaff, M & Esche, A (eds) 2003. *Reformen im Gesundheitswesen. Ergebnisse der internationalen Recherche.* Carl Bertelsmann-Preis 2000. 3rd edn. Bertelsmann Stiftung: Gütersloh.

Bogue, R, Hall, C & La Forgia, G 2007. *Hospital Governance in Latin America; Results from a Four Nation Survey.* World Bank, Human Development Department, Latin America and Caribbean Region: Washington, DC.

Braithwaite, J, Clay-Williams, R, Nugus, P & Plumb, J 2013. 'Health care as a complex adaptive system.' *In:* Hollnagel, E, Braithwaite, J & Wears, R (eds), *Resilient Health Care.* Ashgate Publishing Limited: Surrey.

Braithwaite, J, Shaw, C, Moldovan, M, Greenfield, D, Hinchcliff, R, Mumford, V, Kristensen, M, Westbrook, J, Nicklin, W, Fortune, T & Whittaker, S 2012. 'Comparison of health service accreditation programs in low-and middle-income countries with those in higher income countries: A cross-sectional study.' *International Journal for Quality in Health Care,* vol. 24, no. 6, pp. 568–77.

Braithwaite, J, Westbrook, M, Hindle, D, Iedema, R & Black, D 2006. 'Does restructuring hospitals result in greater efficiency? An empirical test using diachronic data.' *Health Services Management Research,* vol. 19, no. 1, pp. 1–12.

Brammli-Greenberg, S, Gross, R, Yair, Y & Akiva, E 2011. *Public Opinion on the Level of Service and Performance of the Healthcare System in 2009 and in Comparison with Previous Years.* Myers-JDC-Brookdale Institute [online]. Viewed February 28, 2014: http://brookdale.jdc.org.il/?CategoryID=192&Art icleID=251ht.

Brasil 2010. *Constitution of the Federative Republic of Brazil: Constitutional Text of October 5, 1988.* Chamber of Deputies: Brasilia.

Brien, SE, Lorenzetti, DL, Lewis, S, Kennedy, J & Ghali, WA 2010. 'Overview of a formal scoping review on health system report cards.' *Implementation Science,* vol. 5, no. 1, p. 2.

Brown, M & Underwood, B 2013. *Very Low Cost Access Practice Case Studies: Summary Report for the PHO Services Agreement Amendment Protocol Group.* DHB Shared Services: Wellington.

Burns, H 2011. 'Kilbrandon's vision: Healthier lives, better futures.' Lecture to Glasgow University, November 7. Scottish Government: Edinburgh.

Campbell, S, Roland, M & Buetow, S 2000. 'Defining quality of care.' *Social Science & Medicine,* vol. 51, no. 11, pp. 1611–25.

Canitrot, C 1980. *Acreditación de establecimientos asistenciales; aportes para el estudio y puesta en marcha de un programa en la Argentina.* COMRA: Buenos Aires.

Carman, KG & Eibner, C 2014. *Survey Estimates Net Gain of 9.3 Million American Adults with Health Insurance.* The RAND Blog [online]. Viewed June 23, 2014: http://www.rand.org/blog/2014/04/survey-estimates-net-gain-of-9-3-million-american-adults.html.

Carr, S 2008. *A Quotation with a Life of Its Own*. Editors Notebook. Patient Safety & Quality in Healthcare [online]. Viewed May 5, 2014: http://www.psqh.com/julaug08/editor.html.

Cavalieri, M, Gitto, L & Guccio, C 2013. 'Reimbursement systems and quality of hospital care: An empirical analysis for Italy.' *Health Policy*, vol. 111, no. 3, pp. 273–89.

Cavendish, C 2013. *The Cavendish Review: An Independent Review into Healthcare Assistants and Support Workers in the NHS and Social Care Settings*. Department of Health: London.

CENSIS 2013. *47° Rapporto sulla situazione sociale del Paese/2013*. Social Investments Research Center. Franco Angeli: Rome.

Census and Statistics Department HKSAR 2013a. *Hong Kong Annual Digest of Statistics*. Census and Statistics Department HKSAR: Hong Kong.

Census and Statistics Department HKSAR 2013b. *Thematic Household Survey Report No. 50, Doctor consultation*. Census and Statistics Department HKSAR: Hong Kong.

Central Intelligence Agency 2014 [last update]. *World Factbook*. Central Intelligence Agency [online]. Viewed May 15, 2014: https://www.cia.gov/library/publications/the-world-factbook/geos/gh.html.

Centre for Health Protection 2014. *Vital Statistics*. Centre for Health Protection [online]. Viewed February 27, 2014: http://www.chp.gov.hk/en/vital/10/27.html.

Centre for Public Policy in the Regions 2010. *Spending on Health*. Centre for Public Policy in the Regions: Glasgow.

Chernichovsky, D 2009. 'Not "socialized medicine"—an Israeli view of health care reform.' *New England Journal of Medicine*, vol. 361, no. 21, p. e46.

Chigwedere, P, Seage, GR, Gruskin, S, Lee, TH & Essex, M 2008. 'Estimating the lost benefits of antiretroviral drug use in South Africa.' *Journal of Acquired Immune Deficiency Syndromes*, vol. 49, no. 4, pp. 410–15.

Chopra, M, Lawn, JE, Sanders, D, Barron, P, Abdool Karim, SS, Bradshaw, D, Jewkes, R, Abdool Karim, Q, Flisher, AJ, Mayosi, BM, Tollman, SM, Churchyard, GJ & Coovadia, H 2009. 'Achieving the health Millennium Development Goals for South Africa: Challenges and priorities.' *The Lancet*, vol. 374, no. 9694, pp. 1023–31.

Churchyard, GJ, Mametja, LD, Mvusi, L, Ndjeka, N, Hesseling, AC, Reid, A, Babatunde, S & Pillay, Y 2014. 'Tuberculosis control in South Africa: Successes, challenges and recommendations.' *South African Medical Journal*, vol. 104, no. 3, pp. 244–8.

Cicchetti, A (ed) 2011. *Efficacia ed equità nell'assetto federale del Servizio sanitario nazionale*. Vita e Pensiero: Milano.

Cicchetti, A (ed) 2012. *I Dipartimenti ospedalieri nel Servizio Sanitario Nazionale*. Franco Angeli: Rome.

Cittadinanzattiva 2013. *Pit Health Report 2013*. Cittadinanzattiva [online]. Viewed January 25, 2014: http://www.cittadinanzattiva.it.

Classen, D, Resar, R, Griffin, F, Federico, F, Frankel, T, Kimmel, N, Whittington, JC, Frankel, A, Seger, A & James, BC 2011. '"Global trigger tool" shows that adverse events in hospitals may be ten times greater than previously measured.' *Health Affairs,* vol. 30, no. 4, pp. 581–9.

Clay-Williams, R, Nosrati, H, Cunningham, F, Hillman, K & Braithwaite, J, 2014. 'Do large-scale hospital- and system-wide interventions improve patient outcomes? A systematic review.' *BMC Health Services Research*, vol. 14, no. 1, pp. 369.

Clinical Care Division of the Volta Regional Health Directorate 2010. *Volta Regional Health Directorate Clinical Care Division 2010 Annual Report.* Ghana Health Service [pdf]. Viewed June 10, 2014: http://www.ghanahealthservice. org/documents/RHD CLINICAL CARE REPORT.pdf.

Clinical Excellence Commission 2014. *Homepage.* Clinical Excellence Commission [online]. Viewed January 3, 2014: http://www.cec.health.nsw. gov.au/ht.

Clwyd, A & Hart, T 2013. *A Review of the NHS Hospitals Complaints System Putting Patients Back in the Picture.* Department of Health: London.

CMS.gov 2014. *The CMS Innovation Center.* Centers for Medicare & Medicaid Services [online]. Viewed February 6, 2014: http://innovation.cms.gov/.

Cohen, M, March, J & Olsen, J 1972. 'A garbage-can theory of decision-making.' *Administrative Science Quarterly*, vol. 17, no. 1, pp. 1–25.

Coiera, E 2011. 'Why system inertia makes health reform so difficult.' *British Medical Journal,* vol. 343, pp. 27–9.

Committee on Health Insurance Status and Its Consequences, Institute of Medicine 2009. *America's Uninsured Crisis: Consequences for Health and Health Care.* National Academies Press: Washington, DC.

Committee on Quality of Health Care in America, Institute of Medicine 2001. *Crossing the Quality Chasm: A New Health System for the 21st Century.* National Academy Press: Washington, DC.

Commonwealth Department of Health and Family Services 1996. *The Final Report of the Taskforce on Quality in Australian Health Care.* Australian Government Publishing Service: Canberra.

Concha, J 2007. *Sistema Nacional de Acreditación Prestadores Institucionales.* Superintendencia de Salud [pdf]. Viewed May 15, 2014: http://www. supersalud.gob.cl/difusion/572/articles-5355_p_3.pdf.

Congressional Budget Office 2011. *CBO Estimate of the Effects of the Insurance Coverage Provisions Contained in P.L 111–148 and 111–152.* Congressional Budget Office [pdf]. Viewed March 18, 2014: https://www.cbo.gov/sites/ default/files/cbofiles/attachments/HealthInsuranceProvisions.pdf.

Connolly, C 2010. 'How Obama revived his health-care bill.' *The Washington Post*, March 23 [online]. Viewed June 25, 2014: http://www.washingtonpost. com/wp-dyn/content/article/2010/03/22/AR2010032203729.html.

Constitutional and Law Reform Commission of Papua New Guinea 2009. *Review of the implementation of the OLPG and LLG on Service Delivery Arrangements:*

A Six Provinces Survey. Monograph 1. Kalinoe, L (ed). Constitutional and Law Reform Commission of Papua New Guinea: Port Moresby.

Coulter, A 2002. 'After Bristol: Putting patients at the centre.' *British Medical Journal,* vol. 324, no. 7338, pp. 648–51.

Council of Australian Governments 2011. 'National Health Reform Agreement.' Council of Australian Governments [pdf]. Viewed January 2, 2014: http://www.federalfinancialrelations.gov.au/content/npa/health_reform/national-agreement.pdf.

CPC Central Committee & the State Council 2009. *Opinions of the CPC Central Committee and the State Council on Deepening the Reform of the Healthcare System.* China Food and Drug Administration [online]. Viewed March 15, 2014: http://www.sda.gov.cn/WS01/CL0611/41193.html.

CPC Central Committee & the State Council 2013a. *Planning and Implementation Scheme for Deepening Reform of the Healthcare System during the 12th Five-Year Plan.* Central People's Government of the People's Republic of China [online]. Viewed March 15, 2014: http://www.gov.cn/zwgk/2012-03/21/content_2096671.htm.

CPC Central Committee & the State Council 2013b. *Opinions of the State Council on Promoting the Development of the Health Service Industry.* Central People's Government of the People's Republic of China [online]. Viewed March 15, 2014: http://www.gov.cn/zwgk/2013-10/14/content_2506399.htm.

Crawford, MJ, Rutter, D, Manley, C, Weaver, T, Bhui, K, Fulop, N & Tyrer, P 2002. 'Systematic review of involving patients in the planning and development of health care.' *British Medical Journal,* vol. 325, no. 7375, pp. 1263–5.

Crengle, S 1999. 'Māori primary care services.' *In: Discussion Papers on Primary Health Care.* National Advisory Committee on Health and Disability: Wellington.

Crethar, MP, Phillips, JN, Stafford, PJ & Duckett, SJ 2009. 'Leadership transformation in Queensland Health.' *Australian Health Review,* vol. 33, no. 3, pp. 357–64.

Cumming, J 2011. 'Integrated care in New Zealand.' *International Journal of Integrated Care,* vol. 11, p. e138.

Cumming, J 2013. 'New Zealand.' *In:* Siciliani, L, Borowitz, M & Moran, V (eds), *Waiting Time Policies in the Health Sector: What Works?* Organisation for Economic Cooperation and Development: Paris, pp. 201–20.

Cumming, J & Mays, N 2011. 'New Zealand's primary health care strategy: early effects of the new financing and payment system for general practice and future challenges.' *Health Economics, Policy, and Law,* vol. 6, no. 1, pp. 1–21.

Cumming, J, Mays, N & Daubé, J 2010. 'How New Zealand has contained expenditure on drugs.' *British Medical Journal,* vol. 340, no. c2441, pp. 1224–7.

Cumming, J, Mays, N & Gribben, B 2008. 'Reforming primary health care: Is New Zealand's primary health care strategy achieving its early goals?' *Australia and New Zealand Health Policy,* vol. 5, no. 24, pp. 1–11.

Cumming, J, McDonald, J, Barr, C, Martin, G, Gerring, Z & Daubé, J 2013. 'New Zealand health system review' *Health Systems in Transition*, vol. 4, no. 2 Asia Pacific Observatory on Health Systems and Policies & European Observatory on Health Systems and Policies, World Health Organization, Geneva.

Damiani, G & Ricciardi, G 2005. *Manuale di Programmazione e Organizzazione Sanitaria*. Idelson–Gnocchi: Naples.

DATASUS n.d. *Procedimentos hospitalares do sus–por local de internação–Brasil*. DATASUS, Ministério da Saúde [online]. Viewed January 28, 2014: http://www2.datasus.gov.br/DATASUS/index.php?area=0202&VObj=.

Davies, HTO & Mannion, R 2013. 'Will prescriptions for cultural change improve the NHS?' *British Medical Journal*, vol. 346, no. 7900, pp. f1305.

Deilkås, E 2010. 'Patient safety culture—opportunities for healthcare management' [dissertation]. University of Oslo [online]. Viewed March 15, 2014: https://www.duo.uio.no/handle/10852/27907.

Deilkås, E 2013. *Rapport for Nasjonal Journalundersøkelse med Global Trigger Tool i Norge 2012*. Nasjonalt kunnskapssenter for helsetjenesten: Oslo.

Departamento de Estadísticas e Información de Salud 2012. *Indicadores Básicos. Argentina 2012*. Departamento de Estadísticas e Información de Salud, Ministerio de Salud [online]. Viewed February 12, 2014: http://www.deis.gov.ar/indicadores.htm.

Departamento de Estadísticas e Información de Salud n.d., *Homepage*. Departamento de Estadísticas e Información de Salud, Ministerio de Salud [online]. Viewed March 31 2014: http//www.deis.cl.

Department of Health 1997. *The New NHS–Modern, Dependable*. The Stationery Office: London.

Department of Health 1998. *A First Class Service – Quality in the New NHS*. The Stationery Office: London.

Department of Health 2000a. *The NHS Plan – A Plan for Investment, a Plan for Reform*. The Stationery Office: London.

Department of Health 2000b. *An Organisation with a Memory*. The Stationery Office: London.

Department of Health 2001. *Building a Safer NHS for Patients: Implementing an organisation with a memory*. The Stationery Office: London.

Department of Health 2005. *Health Reform in England: Update and Next Steps*. Department of Health: London.

Department of Health 2006. *Safety First – A Report for Patients, Clinicians and Healthcare Managers*. Department of Health: London.

Department of Health 2008, *High Quality Care for All (Final Darzi Report)*. The Stationery Office: London.

Department of Health 2009. *NHS 2010–2015: From Good to Great*. The Stationery Office: London.

Department of Health 2010. *Equity and Excellence: Liberating the NHS*. The Stationery Office: London.

Department of Health 2012. *NHS Outcomes Framework.* The Stationery Office: London, UK.

Department of Health and Social Security 1983. *NHS Management Inquiry Report (the Griffiths Report).* The Stationary Office: London.

Department of Health Republic of South Africa 2011a. *Human Resources for Health South Africa: HRH Strategy for the Health Sector: 2012/13–2016/17.* Department of Health Republic of South Africa: Pretoria.

Department of Health Republic of South Africa 2011b. *National Core Standards for Health Establishments in South Africa.* Department of Health Republic of South Africa: Tshwane.

Department of Health Republic of South Africa 2013. *Annual Report 2012/2013.* Department of Health South Africa: Tshwane.

Department of Provincial and Local Government 2009a. *Determination: Assigning Service Delivery Functions and Responsibilities to Provincial and Local-Level Governments.* Department of Provincial and Local Government, Government of Papua New Guinea: Port Moresby.

Detsky, A 2014. 'Why America is Losing the Health Care Race.' *The New Yorker,* June 13 [online]. Viewed June 14, 2014: http://www.newyorker.com/online/blogs/elements/2014/06/why-america-is-losing-the-health-race.html.

Dewi, WN, Evans, D, Bradley, H & Ullrich, S 2013. 'Person-centered care in the Indonesian health-care system.' *International Journal of Nursing Practice* [online]. November 13, 2013.

DHB Shared Services 2013a. *PHO Services Agreement–31 May 2013 FINAL.* DHB Shared Services: Wellington.

DHB Shared Services 2013b. *Alliance Agreement (Template).* DHB Shared Services: Wellington.

DHB Shared Services 2013c. *Alliance Leadership Team Charter (Template).* DHB Shared Services: Wellington.

DHB Shared Services Agency 2014. *PHO Performance Programme.* DHB Shared Services [online]. Viewed March 5, 2014: http://www.dhbsharedservices.health.nz/Site/SIG/pho/Default.aspx.

Directorate of Health 2013. *Kvalitetsbasert finansiering 2014.* Report No.: IS-2111, Directorate of Health: Oslo.

District Health Boards New Zealand 2009. *PHO Performance Overview Report with Local Targets for the Period Ending 31st December 2009 including Change in Performance since 30th June 2009.* District Health Boards New Zealand: Wellington.

Dixon, A, Mays, N & Jones, L (eds) 2011. *Understanding New Labour's Market Reforms of the English NHS.* King's Fund: London.

Donabedian, A 1980. *Explorations in Quality Assessment and Monitoring Vol. 1. The Definition of Quality and Approaches to its Assessment.* Health Administration Press: Ann Arbor, MI.

Dorling, D 2013. *Unequal Health: The Scandal of Our Times.* Policy Press: Bristol.

Dorrington, RE, Bradshaw, D & Laubscher, R 2012. *Rapid Mortality Surveillance Report 2012*. South African Medical Research Council: Cape Town.

Duckett, SJ 1995. 'Hospital payment arrangements to encourage efficiency: The case of Victoria, Australia.' *Health Policy*, vol. 34, no. 2, pp. 113–4.

Duckett, SJ 2008. 'The continuing contest of values in the Australian health care system.' *In:* den Exter, A. (ed), *Access to Health Care. Solidarity and Justice.* Erasmus University Press: Rotterdam.

Duckett, SJ 2009. 'Accountability, transparency and participation: Process values underpinning the new approach to governance of patient safety in Queensland Health.' *In:* Healy, J & Dugdale, P (eds), *Patient Safety First: Responsive Regulation in Health Care.* Allen & Unwin: Sydney.

Duckett, SJ 2012. 'Designing incentives for good-quality hospital care.' *The Medical Journal of Australia*, vol. 196, no. 11, pp. 678–9.

Duckett, SJ 2014. 'Australia.' *In:* Fierlbeck, K & Palley, HA (eds), *Comparative Health Care Federalism: Competition and Collaboration in Multistate Systems.* Ashgate Publishing Limited: Surrey.

Duckett, SJ, Collins, J, Kamp, M & Walker, K 2008a. 'An improvement focus in public reporting: The Queensland approach.' *The Medical Journal of Australia*, vol. 189, no. 11/12, pp. 616–7.

Duckett, SJ, Daniels, S, Kamp, M, Stockwell, A, Walker, G & Ward, M 2008b. 'Pay for performance in Australia: Queensland's new Clinical Practice Improvement Payment.' *Journal of Health Services Research & Policy*, vol. 13, no. 3, pp. 174–7.

Dwyer, JM 2004. 'Australian health system restructuring—What problem is being solved?' *Australian and New Zealand Health Policy,* vol. 1, no. 6, pp. 1–6.

Econex 2013. *Updated GP and Specialist Numbers: 2011 and 2012.* Health Professions Council of South Africa [pdf]. Viewed June 17, 2014: http://www.hpcsa.co.za/Uploads/editor/UserFiles/downloads/service_fees-tariff/submissions/sappf_f_econex_updated_gp_specialist_numbers_27 03 2013.pdf.

Elbualy, M, Bold, A, De Silva, V & Gibbons, U 1998. 'Congenital hypothyroid screening: The Oman experience.' *Journal of Tropical Pediatrics*, vol. 44, no. 2, pp. 81–3.

Erazo, A 2011. *La protección social en Chile. El Plan AUGE: avances y desafíos.* CEPAL [pdf]. Viewed May 15, 2014: http://www.cepal.org/publicaciones/xml/7/44517/lcl-3348.pdf.

Escobar, LA 2013. 'El Sistema Nacional de Acreditación de Calidad en Salud: Visión de la Superintendencia de Salud.' United Nations Economic Commission for Latin America and the Caribbean. Superintendencia de Salud, Gobierno de Chile [pdf]. Viewed March 31, 2014: http://www.supersalud.gob.cl/portal/articles-8307_p1.pdf.

Evans, D & Killoran, A 2000. 'Tackling health inequalities through partnership working: Learning from a realistic evaluation.' *Critical Public Health,* vol. 10, no. 2, pp. 139–140.

Fair Wages and Salaries Commission 2010. *Fact Sheet on Single Spine Pay Policy*. Fair Wages and Salaries Commission, Ghana [online]. Viewed May 15, 2014: http://fairwages.gov.gh/component/option,com_jefaq/Itemid,30/view,faq/.

Fattore, G & Ferrè, F 2012. 'I tempi d'attesa per le prestazioni del SSN: stato dell'arte e alcune riflessioni.' *In:* Pessina, EA, Cantu, E, Ferre, F & Ricci, A (eds), *L'aziendalizzazione della sanità in Italia. Rapporto Oasi 2012.* Università Bocconi: Milano.

Flesch, M, Hagemeister, J, Berger, HJ, Schiefer, A, Schynkowski, S, Klein, M, Sahebdjami, S, vom Dahl, S, Fehske, W, Mies, R, von Eiff, M, Pfaff, H, Frommolt, P & Hoepp, HW 2008. 'Implementation of guidelines for the treatment of acute ST-Elevation myocardial infarction: The Cologne infarction model registry.' *Circulation: Cardiovascular Interventions,* vol. 1, no. 2, pp. 95–102.

Food and Health Bureau HKSAR 2013. *Hong Kong's Domestic Health Accounts (HKDHA)– Estimate of Domestic Health Expenditure, 1989/90–2010/11.* Government, Hong Kong Special Administrative Region: Hong Kong.

Forgia, GL & Nagpal, S 2012. *Government-sponsored Health Insurance in India: Are You Covered?* Directions in Development, World Bank eLibrary [pdf]. Viewed May 15, 2014: http://www-wds.worldbank.org/external/default/WDSContentServer/WDSP/IB/2012/08/30/000356161_20120830020253/Rendered/PDF/722380PUB0EPI008029020120Box367926B.pdf.

Fox, DM 2013. 'Health inequality and governance in Scotland since 2007.' *Public Health,* vol. 127, no. 6, pp. 503–13.

Francis, R 2013. *Report of the Mid Staffordshire NHS Foundation Trust Public Inquiry.* The Stationery Office: London.

Francis, R 2013. *Report of the Mid Staffordshire NHS foundation Trust Public Inquiry: Executive Summary.* The Stationery Office: London.

Frankel, M, Chinitz, D, Salzberg, CA & Reichman, K 2013. 'Sustainable health information exchanges: The role of institutional factors.' *Israel Journal of Health Policy Research,* vol. 2, no. 1, p. 21.

Frenk, J 2006. 'Bridging the divide: Global lessons from evidence-based health policy in Mexico.' *The Lancet,* vol. 368, no. 9539, pp. 954–61.

Frenk, J, González-Pier, E, Gómez-Dantés, O, Lezana, MA & Knaul, FM 2006. 'Comprehensive reform to improve health system performance in Mexico.' *The Lancet,* vol. 368, pp. 1525–34.

Frølich, A, Talavera, JA, Broadhead, P & Dudley, RA 2007. 'A behavioral model of clinician responses to incentives to improve quality.' *Health Policy,* vol. 80, no. 1, pp. 179–93.

Fuchs, VR 2009. 'Health care reform—Why so much talk and so little action?' *New England Journal of Medicine,* vol. 360, no. 3, pp. 208–9.

Funck, E 2009. 'Ordination balanced scorecard' [doctoral thesis]. Växjö University Press: Växjö.

Fundación Mexicana para la Salud 1994. *Encuesta Nacional de Satisfacción con los Servicios de Salud.* Fundación Mexicana para la Salud: Mexico City.

Fung, CH, Lim, YW, Mattke, S, Damberg, C & Shekelle, PG 2008. 'Systematic review: The evidence that publishing patient care performance data improves quality of care.' *Annals of Internal Medicine*, vol. 148, no. 2, pp. 111–23.

Gallagher, MP & Krumholz, HM 2011. 'Public reporting of hospital outcomes: A challenging road ahead.' *The Medical Journal of Australia*, vol. 194, no. 12, pp. 658–60.

Ganguly, SS, Al-Shafaee, MA, Al-Lawati, JA, Dutta, PK & Duttagupta, KK 2009. 'Epidemiological transition of some diseases in Oman: A situational analysis.' *Eastern Mediterranean Health Journal*, vol. 15, no. 1, pp. 209–18.

Gargiulo, L, Iannucci L, Orsini, S, Cislaghi, C & de Belvis, AG 2011. 'Patients' satisfaction for hospital care among the Italian Regions between 1997 and 2009.' *Annali di Igiene: Medicina Preventiva e di Comunita*, Jul–Aug, vol. 23, no. 4, pp. 295–302.

Gauld, R 2009. *Revolving Doors: New Zealand's Health Reforms—The Continuing Saga*. 2nd edn. Institute of Policy Studies and the Health Services Research Centre: Wellington.

Gemeinsamer Bundesausschuss 2014. *Qualitätssicherung. Risikomanagement- und Fehlermeldesysteme zur Verbesserung der Patientensicherheit in Klinik und Praxis* [media release]. Gemeinsamer Bundesausschuss: Berlin, January 23.

Gerdtham, UG, Löthgren, M, Tambour, M & Rehnberg, C 1999. 'Internal markets and health care efficiency: A multiple-output stochastic frontier analysis.' *Health Economics*, vol. 8, no. 2, pp. 151–64.

Ghana Aids Commission 2014. *About*. Ghana Aids Commission [online]. Viewed May 23, 2014: http://ghanaids.gov.gh/gac1/about.php.

Ghana Health Nest 2014. *National Aids Control Programme*. Ghana Health Nest [online]. Viewed May 23, 2014: http://ghanahealthnest.com/tag/national-aids-control-programme/.

Ghana Health Service & Christian Health Association of Ghana 2013. *Memorandum of Understanding between The Ghana Health Service and The Christian Health Association of Ghana 2013*, December.

Ghana Health Service & Ghana Statistical Service 2008. *Ghana Demographic and Health Survey 2008*. Ghana Statistical Service, Ghana Health Service, and ICF Macro: Accra.

Ghana Health Service 2014. *About Us*. Ghana Health Service [online]. Viewed May 23, 2014: http://www.ghanahealthservice.org/aboutus.php?inf=Background.

Ghana News Agency 2012. 'Parliament goes on recess, approves 1.34 billion dollars on last day.' *Ghana News Agency* [online]. Viewed May 23, 2014: http://www.ghananewsagency.org/politics/parliament-goes-on-recess-approves-1-34-billion-dollars-on-last-day-51516.

Ghirardini, A, Cardone, R, De Feo, A, Leomporra, G, Cannizzaro, GD, Sgrò, A & Palumbo, F 2010. 'National policies for risk management in Italy.' *Transplantation Proceedings*, Jul–Aug, vol. 42, no. 6, pp. 2181–3.

Global Health Workforce Alliance & World Health Organization, GHWA Task Force on Scaling Up Education and Training for Health Workers 2006. *Country Case Study: Ghana: Implementing a National Human Resources for Health Plan.* World Health Organization & Global Health Workforce Alliance [pdf]. Viewed May 23, 2014: http://www.who.int/workforcealliance/knowledge/case_studies/CS_Ghana_web_en.pdf.

Gloede, TD, Pulm, J, Hammer, A, Ommen, O, Kowalski, C, Groß, SE & Pfaff, H 2013. 'Interorganizational relationships and hospital financial performance: A resource-based perspective.' *The Service Industries Journal,* vol. 33, no.13–14, pp. 1260–74.

Gobierno Federal Estados Unidos Mexicanos 2011. *Sistema de Protección Social en Salud: Informe de Resultados 2011.* Seguro Popular, Gobierno Federal Estados Unidos Mexicanos [pdf]. Viewed February 1, 2012: http://www.seguro-popular.gob.mx//images/Contenidos/informes/Informe_Resultados_2011.pdf.

Government of Ghana 1996. The Ghana Health Service and Teaching Hospitals Act, 1996, Act 525. Parliament of the Republic of Ghana: Accra.

Government of Papua New Guinea 2011. *National Health Services Standards for Papua New Guinea, (2011–2020).* National Department of Health, Government of Papua New Guinea: Port Moresby.

Government of the Hong Kong Special Administrative Region 2014. *Health Facts of Hong Kong.* 2014 edn. Department of Health, Surveillance & Epidemiology Branch, Centre for Health Protection, Hong Kong [pdf]. Viewed July 14, 2014: http://www.dh.gov.hk/english/statistics/statistics_hs/files/Health_Statistics_pamphlet_E.pdf.

Greenfield, D & Braithwaite, J 2008. 'Health sector accreditation research: A systematic review.' *International Journal for Quality in Health Care*, vol. 20, no. 3, pp. 172–83.

Greer, S 2008. 'Devolution and divergence in UK health policies.' *British Medical Journal*, vol. 337, p. a2616.

Greer, S 2009. *The Politics of European Union Health Policies.* Open University Press: Maidenhead.

Gregory, S, Dixon, A & Ham, C (eds) 2012. *Health Policy under the Coalition Government: A Mid-Term Assessment.* King's Fund: London.

Grol, R, Wensing, M, Eccles, M & Davis, D (eds) 2013. *Improving Patient Care: The Implementation of Change in Health Care.* John Wiley & Sons: West Sussex.

Gross, R 2006. 'How can data from consumers contribute to promoting quality of care in the health system?' *In:* Porat, A & Rosen, B (eds), *Quality Forum: Strategies for Promoting Quality of Care in Israel.* Myers-JDC-Brookdale Institute: Jerusalem, pp. 177–96.

Gulf Talent 2012. *Employment and salary trends in the Gulf 2012.* Annual Review, GulfTalent.com, April 29.

Hagemeister, J, Schneider, CA, Barabas, S, Schadt, R, Wassmer, G, Mager, G, Pfaff, H & Höpp, HW 2001. 'Hypertension guidelines and their limitations—The impact of physicians' compliance as evaluated by guideline awareness.' *Journal of Hypertension*, vol. 19, no. 11, pp. 2079–86.

Hall, E & McGarrol, S 2013. 'Progressive localism for an ethics of care: Local area co-ordination with people with learning disabilities.' *Social and Cultural Geography*, vol. 14, no. 6, pp. 689–709.

Ham, C, Heenan, D, Longley, M & Steel, D 2013. *Integrated Care in Northern Ireland, Scotland and Wales: Lessons for England*. The King's Fund: London.

Hammer, A 2012. *Zur Messung von Sicherheitskultur in deutschen Krankenhäusern*. Universität zu Köln: Köln.

Haraden, C & Leitch, J 2011. 'Scotland's successful national approach to improving patient safety in acute care.' *Health Affairs*, vol. 30, no. 4, pp. 755–63.

Harbour, R, Lowe, G & Twaddle, S 2011. 'Scottish Intercollegiate Guidelines Network: The first fifteen years (1983–2008).' *Journal of the Royal College of Physicians of Edinburgh*, vol. 41, no. 2, pp. 163–8.

Health Foundation 2011. *Learning Report: Safer Patients Initiative. Lessons from the First Major Improvement Programme Addressing Patient Safety in the UK*. The Health Foundation: London.

Health Fund Association of New Zealand 2013. *Health Insurance Numbers Down 0.5 percent*. Health Funds Association of New Zealand [media release], May 24, Wellington.

Health Quality and Safety Commission New Zealand 2013a. *Statement of Intent 2013–2016*. Health Quality and Safety Commission: Wellington.

Health Quality and Safety Commission New Zealand 2013b. *Annual Report 2012–2013*. Health Quality and Safety Commission: Wellington.

Health Systems Trust 2014. *Hospital CEOs*. Health Systems Trust [online]. Viewed June 10, 2014: http://www.hst.org.za/category/facility/hospital-ceos.

Helou, A 2003. 'Medizinische Leitlinien.' *In:* Schwartz, FW, Badura, B, Busse, R, Leidl, R, Raspe, H, Siegrist, J & Walter, U (eds), *Das Public Health Buch. Gesundheit und Gesundheitswesen*, vol. 2. Urban & Fischer: München, pp. 739–45.

Hinchcliff, R, Greenfield, D, Moldovan, M, Westbrook, J, Pawsey, M, Mumford, VN & Braithwaite, J 2013. 'Narrative synthesis of health service accreditation literature.' *BMJ Quality & Safety*, vol. 21, no. 12, pp. 979–91.

Hindle, D, Braithwaite, J, Iedema, R & Travaglia, J 2006. *Patient Safety: A Comparative Analysis of Eight Inquiries in Six Countries*. University of New South Wales: Sydney.

Hippe, JM & Trygstad, SC 2012. *Ti år etter – ledelse, ansvar og samarbeid i norske sykehus*. Report No. 2012:57. FAFO: Oslo.

Hoffman, B 2003. 'Health care reform and social movements in the United States.' *American Journal of Public Health*, vol. 93, no. 1, pp. 75–85.

Hong Kong Special Administrative Region 2003. *Public Charges–Eligible Persons*. Government of Hong Kong Special Administrative Region: Hong Kong.

Hong Kong Special Administrative Region 2008. *Serving the Community by Using the Private Sector: An Introductory Guide to Pubilc Private Partnership (PPPs)*. 2nd edn. Efficiency Unit: Hong Kong.

Hood, C & Margetts, H 2007. *The Tools of Government in the Digital Age*. Palgrave Macmillan: Basingstoke.

Hort, K, Hanevi, D & Utarini, A 2013. *Regulating the Quality of Health Care: Lessons from Hospital Accreditation in Australia and Indonesia*. Working Paper Series, Number 28. The Nossal Institute for Global Health, University of Melbourne [pdf]. Viewed May 13, 2014: http://ni.unimelb.edu.au/__data/assets/pdf_file/0006/782115/WP_28.pdf.

Hospital Authority 2014. *About Us. Clusters, Hospitals & Institutions*. Hospital Authority [online]. Viewed February 27, 2014: http://www.ha.org.hk/visitor/ha_visitor_index.asp?Content_ID=10036&Lang=ENG&Dimension=100&Parent_ID=10004&Ver=HTML.

Housden, P 2014. 'This is us: a perspective on public services in Scotland.' *Public Policy and Administration*, vol. 29, no. 1, pp. 64–74.

House of Commons Health Committee 2013. *After Francis: Making a Difference, Third Report of Session 2013–14*. House of Commons Health Committee, HC 657. The Stationery Office: London.

Human Sciences Research Council 2013. *Strategic Plan for the Prevention and Control of Non-Communicable Diseases 2013-17*. Human Sciences Research Council [pdf]. Viewed June 17, 2014: http://www.hsrc.ac.za/uploads/pageContent/3893/NCDs STRAT PLAN CONTENT 8 april proof.pdf.

Hunter, D 1982. 'Organising for health: The National Health Service in the United Kingdom.' *Journal of Public Policy*, vol. 2, no. 3, pp. 263–300.

Hutcheon, R 1999. *Bedside Manner–Hospital & Health Care in Hong Kong*. The Chinese University Press: Hong Kong.

Information and Statistics Division Scotland 2014. *Hospital Standardised Mortality Ratios: Quarterly HSMR Release*. Information and Statistics Division: Edinburgh.

Institute for Healthcare Improvement 2003. *The Breakthrough Series: IHI's Collaborative Model for Achieving Breakthrough Improvement*. Institute for Healthcare Improvement: Boston, MA.

Institute of Medicine 1999. *To Err is Human – Building a Safer Health System*. National Academy Press: Washington, DC.

Institute of Medicine 2001. *Crossing the Quality Chasm: A New Health System for the 21st Century*. National Academies Press: Washington, DC.

Institute of Medicine, Committee on Quality of Health Care in America 2001. *Crossing the Quality Chasm: A New Health System for the 21st Century*. National Academy Press: Washington, DC.

Instituto Brasileiro de Geografia e Estatística 2012. *Conta-Satélite de Saúde Brasil 2007–2009*. Instituto Brasileiro de Geografia e Estatística: Rio de Janeiro.

Integrated Performance and Incentive Framework Expert Advisory Group 2013. *Integrated Performance and Incentive Framework: Achieving the Best Health Care Performance for New Zealand* 2013. Health Quality Measures New Zealand: Wellington.

Italian Federation of Health Clinics and Hospitals 2012. *Libro bianco della buona sanità* [Whitepaper of good healthcare practices]. Iniziative sanitarie: Roma.

Jaffe, DH, Shmueli, A, Ben-Yehuda, A, Paltiel, O, Calderon, R, Cohen, AD, Matz, E, Rosenblum, JK, Wilf-Miron, R & Manor, O 2012. 'Community healthcare in Israel: quality indicators 2007–2009.' *Israel Journal of Health Policy Research*, vol. 1, no. 1, p. 3.

Janlöv, N 2010. 'Measuring efficiency in the Swedish health care sector – levels, trade-offs and determinants' [doctoral thesis]. Department of Economics, Lund University: Lund.

Japan Council for Quality Health Care 2011. *Project to Collect Medical Near-miss/Adverse Event Information 2011 Annual Report*. Division of Adverse Event Prevention, Japan Council for Quality Health Care: Tokyo.

Jiang, J, Lockee, C, Bass, K & Fraser, I 2008. 'Board engagement in quality: findings of a survey of hospital and system leaders.' *Journal of Healthcare Management*, vol. 53, no. 2, pp. 121–34.

Johnsen, J 2006. *Health Systems in Transition: Norway*. World Health Organization, Regional Office for Europe on behalf of the European Observatory on Health Systems and Policies: Copenhagen.

Johnston, M 2013. 'Doctor's fees for school-age children too high, say critics.' *New Zealand Herald*, July 29, 2013.

Jonsson, E 1994. *Har den s.k. Stockholmsmodellen genererat mer vård för pengarna?* IKE: Stockholm.

Jonsson, E 1995. *Har den s.k. Dala- respektive Örebromodellen genererat mer vård för pengarna?* Landstingsförbundet: Stockholm.

Juran, JM 1989. *Juran on Leadership for Quality, an Executive Handbook*. Free Press: New York.

Kaiser Family Foundation 2012. *Health Care Costs: A Primer*. Kaiser Family Foundation [online]. Viewed May 1, 2014: http://kff.org/health-costs/report/health-care-costs-a-primer/.

Karbach, U, Schubert, I, Hagemeister, J, Ernstmann, N, Pfaff, H & Höpp, HW 2011. 'Physicians' knowledge of and compliance with guidelines: An exploratory study in cardiovascular diseases.' *In: Deutsches Ärzteblatt International*, vol. 108, no. 5, pp. 61–9.

Kase, P & Thomason, J 2009. 'Chapter 7: Policy Making in Health.' *In:* May, RJ (ed), *Policy Making and Implementation: Studies from Papua New Guinea*. State Society and Governance in Melanesia vol. 5, Australian National University Press: Canberra, pp. 117–30.

Kase, P 2006. 'Prioritization in the Papua New Guinea health sector: Progress towards a health Medium Term Expenditure Framework.' *Papua New Guinea Medical Journal*, vol. 49, no. 3–4, pp. 76–82.

Keating, M & Midwinter, A 1983. *The Government of Scotland*. Mainstream: Edinburgh.

Kenagy, J, Berwick, D & Shore, M 1999. 'Service quality in health care.' *Journal of the American Medical Association*, vol. 281, no. 7, pp. 661–5.

Kennedy, I 2001. *Learning from Bristol: Public Inquiry into Children's Heart Surgery at the Bristol Royal Infirmary, 1984–1995*. The Stationary Office: London.

Kenney, C 2008. *The Best Practice–How the New Quality Movement is Transforming Medicine*. Public Affairs: New York.

Keogh, Sir B 2013. *Review into the Quality of Care and Treatment Provided by 14 Hospital Trusts in England: Overview Report*. National Health Service [pdf]. Viewed May 15, 2014: http://www.nhs.uk/nhsengland/bruce-keogh-review/documents/outcomes/keogh-review-final-report.pdf.

Kerguelén, C 2008. *Calidad en Salud en Colombia; los principios*. Health Reform Support Program, Ministry of Social Protection: Bogota.

Khoja, TAM, Kamel, AA & Rawaf, S (eds) 2011. *Glossary of Patient Safety*. 4th edn. Executive Board of the Health Ministers' Council for GCC States: Riyadh.

Kim, CS, Spahlinger, DA, Kin, JM & Billi, JE 2006. 'Lean health care: What can hospitals learn from a world-class automaker?' *Journal of Hospital Medicine*, vol. 1, no. 3, pp. 191–9.

King, A 2001. *The Primary Health Care Strategy*. Ministry of Health: Wellington.

Klein, R 2013. *The New Politics of the NHS*. 7th edn. Radcliffe Publishing: London.

Kolata, G 2014. 'Method of Study is Criticized in Group's Health Policy Tests.' *New York Times*, February 2 [online]. Viewed June 25, 2014: http://www.nytimes.com/2014/02/03/health/effort-to-test-health-policies-is-criticized-for-study-tactics.html?_r=0.

Kominski, G 2014. 'The Patient Protection and Affordable Care Act of 2010.' *In:* Kominski, G (ed.), *Changing the U.S. Health Care System: Key Issues in Health Services Policy and Management*. 4th edn. Jossey-Bass: San Francisco.

Kuisma, M 2013. 'Understanding welfare crises: The role of ideas.' *Public Administration*, vol. 91, no. 4, pp. 797–805.

La Puma, J & Lawlor, EF 1990. 'Quality-adjusted life-years: Ethical implications for physicians and policymakers.' *Journal of the American Medical Association*, vol. 263, no. 23, pp. 2917–21.

Lawn, JE & Kinney, M 2009. 'Health in South Africa. An executive summary for *The Lancet* series.' *The Lancet*, August 2009.

Leatherman, S & Sutherland, K 2003. *The Quest for Quality in the NHS: A Mid-Term Evaluation of the Ten-Year Quality Agenda*. Nuffield Trust: London.

Leatherman, S & Sutherland, K 2008. *The Quest for Quality: Refining the NHS Reforms*. Nuffield Trust: London.

Lejbkowicz, I, Denekamp, Y, Reis, S & Goldenberg, D 2004. 'Electronic medical record systems in Israel's public hospitals.' *Israel Medical Association Journal*, vol. 6, no. 10, pp. 583–7.

Linder-Gantz, R 2012. 'Patient satisfaction survey for hospitals: A castrated report that reveals nothing.' *The Marker* [online]. Viewed February 28, 2014: http://www.themarker.com/consumer/health/1.1649712.

Lo, W 2014. 'Operations delayed as Hong Kong hospitals struggle to cope with flu surge.' *South China Morning Post*. Hong Kong, January 21.

Lo Scalzo, A, Donatini, A, Orzella, L, Cicchetti, A, Profili, S & Maresso, A 2009. 'Italy: Health system review.' *Health Systems in Transition*, vol. 11, no. 6, pp. 1–216.

Luis Vera Benavides, L 2012. *Normas de Seguridad del Paciente y Calidad de Atención*. Departmento Calidad y Seguridad del Paciente, Ministerio de Salud [powerpoint presentation] [online]. Viewed June 11, 2014: http://www.powershow.com/view/28c0e6-ODQ4M/CALIDAD_Y_SEGURIDAD_DEL_PACIENTE_powerpoint_ppt_presentation.

Macfarlane, F, Exworthy, M, Wilmott, M & Greenhalgh, T 2011. 'Plus ça change, plus c'est la même chose: senior NHS managers' narratives of restructuring.' *Sociology of Health & Illness*, vol. 33, no. 6, pp. 914–29.

Mahama, JD 2012. *Critical Policy Actions of the John Mahama Administration: September to December 2012* [pdf]. Viewed June 10, 2014: http://www.presidency.gov.gh/sites/default/files/speeches/policy_statement_by_president_mahama.pdf.

Maja, P 2012. *Health Minister Launches Health Academy*. South Africa Government [media release] [online]. Viewed June 17, 2014: http://www.gov.za/events/view.php?sid=31946.

Mangione-Smith, R, DeCristofaro, AH, Setodji, CM, Keesey, J, Klein, DJ, Adams, JL, Schuster, MA & McGlynn, EA 2007. 'The quality of ambulatory care delivered to children in the United States.' *New England Journal of Medicine,* vol. 357, no. 15, pp. 1515–23.

Marmot, M, Friel, S, Bell, R, Houweling, TAJ & Taylor, S 2008. 'Closing the gap in a generation: Health equity through action on the social determinants of health.' *The Lancet,* vol. 372, no. 9650, pp. 1661–9.

Mascia, D, Morandi, F & Cicchetti, A 2014. 'Looking good or doing better? Patterns of decoupling in the implementation of clinical directorates.' *Health Care Management Review,* Apr-Jun, vol. 39, no. 2, pp. 111–23.

Mays, N, Cumming, J & Tenbensel, T 2007. *Health Reforms 2001 Research: Overview Report*. Health Services Research Centre: Wellington.

McGlynn, EA, Asch SM, Adams, J, Keesey, J, Hicks, J, DeCristofaro, A & Kerr, EA 2003. 'The Quality of Health Care Delivered to Adults in the United States.' *New England Journal of Medicine,* vol. 348, no. 26, pp. 2635–45.

McKay, J & Lepani, K 2010. *Revitalizing Papua New Guinea's Health System: The Need for Creative Approaches*. Policy Brief, Lowy Institute for International Policy [online]. Viewed March 18, 2014: http://www.lowyinstitute.org/files/mckay_and_lepani_revitalising_web.pdf.

McLean, J & Walsh, MK 2003. 'Lessons from the Inquiry into Obstetrics and Gynaecology Services at King Edward Memorial Hospital 1990–2000.' *Australian Health Review*, vol. 26, no. 1, pp. 12–23.

Medicaid.gov. 2014. *Children's Health Insurance Program (CHIP)*. Medicaid [online]. Viewed June 24, 2014: http://www.medicaid.gov/Medicaid-CHIP-Program-Information/By-Topics/Childrens-Health-Insurance-Program-CHIP.html.

Merriam-Webster.com n.d., *Crusade*. Merriam-Webster Dictionary [online]. Viewed March 12, 2012: http://www.merriam-webster.com/dictionary/crusade.

Midgam LTD 2011. *Satisfaction of Hospitalized Patients in the General Surgery and Medicine Departments – A Report to the Ministry of Health*. Ministry of Health Israel [pdf]. Viewed February 2, 2013: http://www.health.gov.il/PublicationsFiles/sekerALL.pdf.

Minister for Health and Aging 2008. *National Health and Hospitals Reform Commission*. February 25. National Health and Hospitals Reform Commission, Ministry of Health [media release] [pdf]. Viewed December 20, 2013: http://www.health.gov.au/internet/nhhrc/publishing.nsf/Content/AD03A7290849CE03CA25741F001482D0/$File/NatRefCommMediaRel.pdfht.

Ministerial Review Group 2009. *Meeting the Challenge: Enhancing Sustainability and the Patient and Consumer Experience within the Current Legislative Framework for Health and Disability Services in New Zealand: Report of the Ministerial Review Group*. Ministerial Review Group: Wellington.

Ministerial Task Team 2012. *District Clinical Specialist Teams in South Africa: Ministerial Task Team Report to the Honourable Minister of Health, Dr Aaron Motsoaledi*. Department of Health: Tshwane.

Ministerio de Salud 2002. *Documentos del Plan de Acceso Universal con Garantías Explícitas (AUGE)*. Ministerio de Salud [online]. Viewed March 10, 2014: http://www.emol.com/noticias/documentos/auge.asp.

Ministerio de Salud 2013. *Más Enfermedades AUGE 80: Chile avanza con todo*. Ministerio de Salud [pdf]. Viewed May 10, 2014: http://web.minsal.cl/portal/url/item/e03c41d3232c00ffe0400101640175e6.pdfht.

Ministero della Salute 2010a. *Piano sanitario nazionale 2011–2013*. Ministry of Health [pdf]. Viewed January 28, 2014: http://sanita.formez.it/sites/all/files/Schema_PSN_2011_2013.pdf.

Ministero della Salute 2010b. *Rapporto sui risultati del progetto ministeriale: 'Sviluppare strumenti idonei ad assicurare il coinvolgimento attivo dei pazienti e degli operatori e di tutti gli altri soggetti che interagiscono con il S.S.N.'* Ministry of Health [pdf]. Viewed May 25, 2010: http://www.salute.gov.it/imgs/C_17_pagineAree_1322_listaFile_itemName_0_file.pdf.

Ministry of Health & Christian Health Association of Ghana 2003. *Memorandum of Understanding and Administrative Instructions* 2003, Ministry of Health (MOH), Christian Health Association of Ghana (CHAG).

Ministry of Health and Care Services 2001. *Ot.prp. nr. 66 – Om lov om helseforetak m.m.* Ministry of Health: Oslo.

Ministry of Health and Care Services 2005. *Fra stykkevis til helt – en sammnhengende helsetjeneste*. Report No. 2005/3. Ministry of Health and Care Services: Oslo.

Ministry of Health and Care Services 2009. *The Coordination Reform. Proper treatment-at the right place and right time.* White paper no. 47. Ministry of Health: Oslo.

Ministry of Health and Care Services 2012. *God kvalitet – trygge tjenester: Kvalitet og pasientsikkerhet i helse- og omsorgstjenesten.* Whitepaper no. 10. Ministry of Health: Oslo.

Ministry of Health and Family Welfare India 2010. *The Clinical Establishments (Registration and Regulation) Act.* Government of India [online]. Viewed February 14, 2014: http://clinicalestablishments.nic.in/cms/Home.aspx.

Ministry of Health and Family Welfare India 2011. *Annual Report to the People on Health.* Government of India [pdf]. Viewed May 20, 2014: http://mohfw.nic.in/WriteReadData/l892s/6960144509Annual Report to the People on Health.pdf.

Ministry of Health Ghana 2014. *Holistic Assessment of the Health Sector Programme of Work 2013, Ghana.* Ministry of Health, Republic of Ghana: Accra.

Ministry of Health Indonesia 2013. *Hospital Report in Indonesia 2013.* Ministry of Health [online]. Viewed April 25, 2014: http://sirs.buk.depkes.go.id/rsonline/report/report_by_catrs.php.

Ministry of Health New Zealand 2008a. *A Portrait of Health. Key Results of the 2006/07 New Zealand Health Survey.* Ministry of Health: Wellington.

Ministry of Health New Zealand 2008b. *Health Targets: Moving Towards Healthier Futures.* Ministry of Health: Wellington.

Ministry of Health New Zealand 2012. *Health Expenditure Trends in New Zealand 2000–2010.* Ministry of Health: Wellington.

Ministry of Health New Zealand 2013a. *Annual Report for the Year Ended 30 June 2013: Including the Director-General of Health's Annual Report on the State of Public Health.* Ministry of Health: Wellington.

Ministry of Health New Zealand 2013b. *Elective Services.* Ministry of Health [online]. Viewed March 5, 2014: http://www.health.govt.nz/our-work/hospitals-and-specialist-care/elective-services?mega=Our work&title=Elective services.

Ministry of Health Norway 1984. *Lov om statlig tilsyn med helse- og omsorgstjenesten m.m.* Ministry of Health: Oslo.

Ministry of Health of the People's Republic of China 2004. *China Health Statistics Yearbook 2004.* Ministry of Health: Beijing.

Ministry of Health of the People's Republic of China 2012. *China Health Statistical Yearbook 2012.* Peking Union Medical College Press: Beijing.

Ministry of Health Oman 2002. *Manual on Expanded Program on Immunization.* 3rd Edn. Communicable Disease Surveillance and Control [pdf]. Viewed May 7, 2014: http://www.cdscoman.org/uploads/cdscoman/EPI_Manual.pdf.

Ministry of Health Oman 2010a, *The 8th Five-year Plan for Health Development (2011–2015): The National Strategic Plan.* Ministry of Health Oman [pdf]. Viewed April 9, 2014: http://www.nationalplanningcycles.org/sites/default/files/country_docs/Oman/five_year_plan_for_health_development_2011-2015.pdf.

Ministry of Health Oman 2010b. *Congenital Hypothyroidism Guidelines for Neonatal Screening and Management.* Department of Family and Community Health, Ministry of Health Oman [pdf]. Viewed April 10, 2014: http://www. moh.gov.om/en/mgl/Manual/CONGENITAL HYPOHYROIDISM-1.pdf.

Ministry of Health Oman 2012. *Annual Health Report.* Ministry of Health [online]. Viewed March 2, 2014: http://www.moh.gov.om/stat/2009/index.htm.

Ministry of Health Oman website n.d., [online]. Viewed January 19, 2014: http:// www.moh.gov.om/en/nv_menu.php?o=fiveyearPlan/fiveyear Plan.html&SP=1.

Ministry of Human Resources and Social Security of the People's Republic of China 2012. *Statistical Bulletin of Human Resources and Social Security Development in the Year of 2011.* Ministry of Human Resources and Social Security [online]. Viewed May 10, 2014: http://www.mohrss.gov.cn.

Ministry of Human Resources and Social Security of the People's Republic of China 2013. *Statistical Bulletin of Human Resources and Social Security Development in the Year of 2012.* Ministry of Human Resources and Social Security [online]. Viewed May 10, 2014: http://www.mohrss.gov.cn.

Missoni, E & Solimano, G 2010. *Towards Universal Health Coverage: the Chilean experience.* World Health Report 2010 background paper, no. 4. World Health Organization [pdf]. Viewed May 5, 2014: http://www.who.int/healthsystems/ topics/financing/healthreport/4Chile.pdf.

Mooney, G 2000. 'Vertical equity in health care resource allocation.' *Health Care Analysis,* vol. 8, no. 3, pp. 203–15.

Mooney, G & Jan, S 1997. 'Vertical equity: weighting outcomes? Or establishing procedures?' *Health Policy,* vol. 39, no. 1, pp. 79–87.

Mortimer, D & Segal, L 2008. 'Comparing the incomparable? A systematic review of competing techniques for converting descriptive measures of health status into QALY-weights.' *Medical Decision Making,* vol. 28, no. 1, pp. 66–89.

Musgrove, P 1996. *Public and Private Roles in Health: Theory and Financing Patterns.* Health, Nutrition, and Population Discussion Paper. World Bank: Washington, DC.

Nasjonalt folkehelseinstitutt 2009. *Gode helseregistre – bedre helse. Strategi for modernisering og samordning av sentrale helseregistre og medisinske kvalitetsregistre 2010–2020.* Folkehelseinstituttet: Oslo.

NasjonaltKunnskapssenterforHelsetjenesten2014.*Pasientsikkerhetskultur–nasjonal plan for måling og tiltak i 2014.* I trygge hender, pasientsikkerhetsprogrammet. no [online]. Viewed March 11, 2014: http://www.pasientsikkerhetsprogrammet. no/no/Ledere/Materiell/_attachment/2744?_ts=1441af1e978.

Nasjonalt Kunnskapssenter for Helsetjenesten n.d., *Veileder for tverrfaglige pasientsikkerhetsmøter.* I Trygge Hender, pasientsikkerhetsprogrammet.no [online]. Viewed March 11, 2014: http://www.pasientsikkerhetsprogrammet. no/no/Ledere/Materiell/_attachment/497?_ts=138233822ed.

National Agency for Regional Healthcare Services 2011. *I tempi di attesa nei siti web di Regioni e Aziende Sanitarie: la prospettiva del cittadino.* National

Agency for Regional Healthcare Services [online]. Viewed January 27, 2014: http://www.agenas.it.

National Audit Office 2005. *A Safer Place for Patients: Learning to Improve Patient Safety*. The Stationery Office: London.

National Board of Health 2002. *Nasjonal strategi for kvalitetsutvikling i helsetjenesten – rapport til Helsedepartementet*. Rapport fra Helsetilsynet 5/2002. Statens helsetilsyn: Oslo.

National Bureau of Statistics of China 2012. *China Statistical Yearbook 2012*. China Statistics Press: Beijing.

National Department of Health 2013. *Sector Performance Annual Review: Assessment of Sector Performance 2008–2012. National Report*. National Department of Health, Papua New Guinea [pdf]. Viewed May 13, 2014: http://www.health.gov.pg/publications/SPAR_2013.pdf.

National Department of Health South Africa 2006. *Standard Treatment Guidelines and Essential Drugs List for South Africa: Hospital Level Paediatrics*. 2nd edn. KwaZulu-Natal Department of Health [pdf]. Viewed June 17, 2014: http://www.kznhealth.gov.za/edlpaed06.pdf.

National Department of Health South Africa 2012, *Standard Treatment Guidelines and Essential Medicines List for South Africa: Hospital Level Adults*. 3rd edn. KwaZulu-Natal Department of Health [pdf]. Viewed June 17, 2014: http://www.kznhealth.gov.za/pharmacy/edladult_2012.pdf.

National Economic and Fiscal Commission 2010. *Green Shoots of Change: The 2009 Provincial Expenditure Review With Trend Analysis from 2005 to 2009*. National Economic and Fiscal Commission [online]. Viewed May 15, 2014: http://www.nefc.gov.pg.

National Expert Advisory Group on Safety and Quality in Australian Health Care 1999. *Implementing Safety and Quality Enhancement in Health Care: National Actions to Support Quality and Safety Improvement in Australian Healthcare, Australian Commission on Safety And Quality In Healthcare*. National Expert Advisory Group on Safety and Quality in Australian Health Care [pdf]. Viewed April 5, 2014: http://www.safetyandquality.gov.au/wp-content/uploads/2012/01/final_fullrep.pdfht.

National Health and Family Planning Commission, People's Republic of China 2013. *The 2012 Statistical Bulletin on Development of China Health and Family Planning Career*. Ministry of Health [online]. Viewed January 24, 2014: http://www.moh.gov.cn/mohwsbwstjxxzx/s7967/201306/fe0b764da4f74b858eb55264572eab92.shtml.

National Health and Hospitals Reform Commission 2009. *A Healthier Future for All Australians – Final Report of the National Health and Hospitals Reform Commission*. National Health and Hospitals Reform Commission [online]. Viewed April 6, 2014: http://www.health.gov.au/internet/nhhrc/publishing.nsf/Content/nhhrc-report.

National Health Committee 2013. *National Health Committee*. Ministry of Health [online]. Viewed March 5, 2014: http://nhc.health.govt.nz/ht.

National Health Performance Authority 2013. *Hospital Performance: Healthcare-associated Staphylococcus aureus bloodstream infections in 2011–12*, National Health Performance Authority [pdf]. Viewed January 2, 2014: http://nhpa. gov.au/internet/nhpa/publishing.nsf/Content/Report-Download-Healthcare-associated-Staphylococcus-aureus-bloodstream-infections-in-2011–12/$file/ HospitalPerformance_SAB_2011_12.pdf

National Institute of Population and Social Security Research 2012. *Population Projections for Japan (January 2012): 2011 to 2060*. National Institute of Population and Social Security Research [pdf]. Viewed June 10, 2014: http:// www.ipss.go.jp/site-ad/index_english/esuikei/ppfj2012.pdf.

National Research Council & Institute of Medicine 2013. *U.S. Health in International Perspective: Shorter Lives, Poorer Health*. The National Academies Press: Washington, DC.

National Rural Health Mission 2013. *NRHM in the Eleventh Five Year Plan (2007–12)*. National Health Systems Resource Centre [pdf]. Viewed June 10, 2014: file:// localhost/Staff088$/z3496845/Downloads/NRHM in 11th five year plan.pdf.

National Statistical Office 2011. *National Population and Housing Census of Papua New Guinea–Final Figures*. National Statistical Office [online]. Viewed May 13, 2014: http://www.nso.gov.pg.

Nationella Patientenkäten 2013. *National Patient Survey*. Institutet för kvalitetsindikatorer [online]. Viewed July 25, 2013: www.indikator.org/publik.

Nerland, SM 2001. 'Kurpengeordningen før 1980—den glemte finansieringsordningen.' *Tidsskr Nor Legeforen*, vol. 121, pp. 2983–5.

NHS England 2014. 'The biggest patient safety initiative in the history of the NHS–Mike Durkin.' NHS England [online]. Viewed May 12, 2014: http:// www.england.nhs.uk/2014/01/21/mike-durkin-3/.

Nirel, N, Rosen, B, Sharon, A, Samuel, H & Cohen, AD 2011. 'The impact of an integrated hospital-community medical information system on quality of care and medical service utilization in primary-care clinics.' *Informatics for Health and Social Care*, vol. 36, no. 2, pp. 63–74.

Nordentoft, M, Wahlbeck, K, Hällgren, J, Westman, J, Ösby, U, Alinaghizadeh, H, Gissler, M & Laursen, TM 2013. 'Excess mortality, causes of death and life expectancy in 270,770 patients with recent onset of mental disorders in Denmark, Finland and Sweden.' *PLoS One*, vol. 8, no. 1, p. e55176.

Noronha, J & Rosa, M 1999. 'Quality of health care–growing awareness in Brazil.' *International Journal for Quality in Health Care*, vol. 11, no. 5, pp. 437–41.

Norwegian Directorate of Health 2005. *...og bedre skal det bli! Nasjonal strategi for kvalitetsforbedring i sosial- og helsetjenesten (2005–2015)*. Social and Health Services, Norwegian Directorate of Health: Oslo.

Norwegian Medical Association 2009. *Gjennombruddsprosjekter*. Norwegian Medical Association [online]. Viewed May 10, 2014: http://www. legeforeningen.no/id/79985.

Nothacker, M, Muche-Borowski, C, Kopp, I, Selbmann, HK & Neugebauer, EAM 2013. 'Leitlinien – attraktivität, implementierung und evaluation.' *Zeitschrift für Evidenz, Fortbildung und Qualität im Gesundheitswesen*, vol. 107, no. 2, pp. 164–9.

Nuffield Trust 2010. *Funding and Performance of Healthcare Systems in the Four Countries of the UK before and after Devolution (revised version 2011)*. Nuffield Trust: London.

Nyonator, F 2005. *In:* 'Community-based Health Planning and Services (CHPS), The Operational Policy, A Ghana Health Service Policy.' Document No. 20, May 2005.

Nyonator, F 2013. 'Strengthening Health Systems through Quality Improvement Initiatives in Ghana.' ISQua [online]. Viewed May 5, 2014: http://www.isqua. org/docs/future-conferences/dr-frank-nyonator.pdf?sfvrsn=0.

Olsson, BS, Kullberg, M & Landgren, M 2010. 'Förbättrad hjärtsviktsvård med Q-svikt.' *Läkartidningen*, vol. 37, no. 107, pp. 2154–7.

Oman Observer 2013. 'Vision-2050 envisages 10,000 health centres.' *Oman Observer*, August 24 [online]. Viewed February 9, 2014: http://main. omanobserver.om/?p=9005ht.

Ommen, O, Ullrich, B, Janßen, C & Pfaff, H 2007. 'Die ambulant-stationäre schnittstelle in der medizinischen versorgung: probleme, erklärungsmodell und lösungsansätze.' *Medizinische Klinik,* vol. 102, no. 11, pp. 913–7.

Organisation for Economic Cooperation and Development 2012. *OECD Reviews of Health Care Quality: Israel 2012–Raising Standards*. OECD Publishing: Paris.

Organisation for Economic Cooperation and Development 2013a. *Health at a Glance 2013: OECD Indicators*. Organisation for Economic Cooperation and Development [online]. Viewed February 28, 2014: http://dx.doi.org/10.1787/ health_glance-2013-en.

Organisation for Economic Cooperation and Development 2013b. *Health Policies and Data* Organisation for Economic Cooperation and Development [online]. Viewed March 13, 2014: http://www.oecd.org/els/health-systems/ oecdhealthdata2013.

Organisation for Economic Cooperation and Development 2013c. *OECD Reviews of Health Care Quality: Denmark. Executive Summary, Assessment and Recommendations.* Organisation for Economic Cooperation and Development [pdf]. Viewed March 10, 2014: http://www.oecd.org/els/health-systems/ ReviewofHealthCareQualityDENMARK_ExecutiveSummary.pdf.

Organisation for Economic Cooperation and Development & World Health Organization 2012. *Health at a Glance: Asia/Pacific 2012*. Organisation for Economic Cooperation and Development [online]. Viewed May 10, 2014: http://dx.doi.org/10.1787/9789264183902-en.

Øvretveit, J 1992. *Health Service Quality*. Blackwell Scientific Press: Oxford.

Øvretveit, J 2001. *The Changing Public Private Mix in Nordic Healthcare*. The Nordic School of Public Health: Goteborg.

Øvretveit, J 2009. *Does Improving Quality Save Money. A Review of Evidence of Which Improvements to Quality Reduce Costs to Health Service Providers.* The Health Foundation: London.

Padarath, A, Chamberlain, C, McCoy, D, Ntuli, A, Rowson, M & Loewenson, R 2003. *Health Personnel in Southern Africa: Confronting Maldistribution and Brain Drain.* Discussion Paper No. 3. Regional Network for Equity in Health in Southern Africa (EQUINET), Health Systems Trust (South Africa), and MEDACT (UK).

Paganini, J 1999. 'Argentina: current activities in the field of quality in health care.' *International Journal for Quality in Health Care*, vol. 11, no. 5, pp. 435–6.

Paim, J, Travassos, C, Almeida, C & Macinko, J 2011. 'The Brazilian health system: history, advances, and challenges.' *The Lancet*, vol. 377, no. 9779, pp. 1778–97.

Pan-American Health Organization–Latin American Hospital Federation 1992. *La Garantía de Calidad, Acreditación de Hospitales para América Latina y el Caribe.* PAHO/WHO, HSD/SILOS: Washington, DC.

Paraje, G & Vásquez, F 2012. 'Health equity in an unequal country: the use of medical services in Chile.' *International Journal for Equity in Health*, vol. 11, no. 81.

Paterson, R 2005. *National Arrangements for Safety and Quality of Health Care in Australia: The Report of the Review of Future Governance Arrangements for Safety and Quality in Health Care.* Department of Health and Ageing: Canberra.

Israel 1996. Patient's Rights Act. State if Israel [online]. Viewed February 2, 2013: http://waml.haifa.ac.il/index/reference/legislation/israel/israel1.htmht.

Paton, C 2013. 'Garbage-can policy-making meets neo-liberal ideology: twenty five years of redundant reform of the English National Health Service.' *Social Policy and Administration*, Jun, vol. 48, no. 3, pp. 319–42.

Pattinson, RC 2013. *Saving Babies 2010–2011: Eighth Report on Perinatal Care in South Africa (Appendix 1).* Tshepesa Press: Pretoria.

Pawson, R & Tilley, N 1997. *Realistic Evaluation.* Sage: London.

Penoyer, DA 2010. 'Nurse staffing and patient outcomes in critical care: a concise review.' *Critical Care Medicine*, Jul, vol. 38, no. 7, pp. 1521–8.

Penter, V (ed.) 2014. *Untersuchung. Das deutsche Gesundheitssystem–Qualität und Effizienz.* KPMG [pdf]. Viewed May 10, 2014: http://www.kpmg.com/DE/de/Documents/deutsche-gesundheitssystem-qualitaet-effizienz-2014-kpmg.pdf.

Peres, LM 1974. 'The politics of industrial policy.' *In:* McCarthy, G (ed.), *Industrial Australia, 1975–2000: Preparing for Change. Proceedings of the 40th Summer School. Australian Institute of Political Science.* Australia and New Zealand Book Co.: Sydney.

Peterburg, Y 2010. *Israel's Health IT Industry: What Does the American Recovery and Reinvestment Act Mean for Israeli Collaborative Opportunities?* Milken Institute [online]. Viewed February 25, 2014: http://www.milkeninstitute.org/publications/publications.taf?function=detail&ID=38801229&cat=resrep.

Peters, BG 2011. 'Governance responses to the fiscal crisis–comparative perspectives.' *Public Money and Management*, vol. 31, no. 1, pp. 75–80.

Project Fives Alive! 2013. *Improvement Collaborative Report. November 2012–May 2013*. Project Fives Alive! [online]. Viewed May 5, 2014: http://fivesalive.org/improvement-collaborative-report-november-2012-may-2013/.

Pfaff, H, Ernstmann, N & Pritzbuer, E von 2005. 'Das Fehlerkultur-Modell—Warum gibt es im Krankenhaus keine Fehlerkultur?' *Deutsche Gesellschaft für Chirurgie–Mitteilungen,* vol. 34, no. 1, pp. 39–41.

Pharmaceutical Management Agency [PHARMAC] 2006. *Annual Report.* Pharmac: Wellington.

Pharmaceutical Management Agency [PHARMAC] 2013. *Annual Report.* Pharmac: Wellington.

Plsek, PE & Greenhalgh, T 2001. 'The challenge of complexity in health care.' *British Medical Journal,* vol. 323, no. 7313, pp. 625–8.

Powell, M 1997. *Evaluating the National Health Service.* Open University Press: Buckingham.

Powell, M, Millar, R, Mulla, A, Brown, H, Fewtrell, C, McLeod, H, Goodwin, N, Dixon, A & Naylor, C 2011. *Comparative Case Studies of Health Reform in England, Report submitted to the Department of Health Policy Research Programme (PRP).* University of Birmingham [pdf]. Viewed May 3, 2014: http://www.birmingham.ac.uk/Documents/college-social-sciences/social-policy/HSMC/news-events/health-reform-england.pdf.

Pronovost, PM, Weast, BM, Rosenstein, BM, Sexton, JBP, Holzmueller, CGB, Paine, LM, Davis, R & Rubin, HR 2005. 'Implementing and validating a comprehensive unit-based safety program.' *Journal of Patient Safety*, vol. 1, no. 1, pp. 33–40.

Propper, C & Venables, MA 2013. 'An assessment of Labour's record on health and healthcare.' *Oxford Review of Economic Policy*, vol. 29, no. 1, pp. 203–26.

Prüss-Üstün, A & Corvalán, C 2006. *Preventing Disease through Healthy Environments: Towards an Estimate of the Environmental Burden of Disease.* World Health Organization: Geneva.

QualityWatch 2013. *Is the Quality of Care in England Getting Better? QualityWatch Annual Statement 2013: Summary of Findings.* Health Foundation & Nuffield Trust: London.

Quince, A 2009. 'The Lost Reform–USA Health Reform.' *Rear Vision* [radio broadcast]. August 19, 8:30AM. ABC Radio National, Sydney.

Raleigh, V & Foot, C 2010. *Getting the Measure of Quality.* King's Fund: London.

Ranmuthugala, G, Cunningham, FC, Plumb, JJ, Long, J, Georgiou, A, Westbrook, JI & Braithwaite, J 2011. 'A realist evaluation of the role of communities of practice in changing healthcare practice.' *Implementation Science,* vol 6, pp. 49–54.

Raymont, A, Cumming, J & Gribben, B [in press]. *Evaluation of the Primary Health Care Strategy: Changes in Fees and Consultation Rates between 2001 and 2007.* Health Services Research Centre: Wellington.

Rehnberg, C, Janlöv, N, Khan, J & Lundgren, J 2010. *Uppföljning av husläkarsystemet inom Vårdval Stockholm–redovisning av de två första årens erfarenheter.* Karolinska Institutet: Stockholm.

Reinhold, T, Thierfelder, K, Müller-Riemenschneider, F & Willich, SN 2009. 'Gesundheitsökonomische auswirkungen der DRG-einführung in Deutschland–eine systematische Übersicht.' *Gesundheitswesen*, vol. 71, no. 5, pp. 306–12.

Republic of Indonesia 2009a. *The Health Law of The Republic of Indonesia No. 36/2009.* Republic of Indonesia: Jarkarta.

Republic of Indonesia 2009b. *The Hospital Law of The Republic of Indonesia No. 44/2009.* Republic of Indonesia: Jarkarta.

Republica de Chile 2008. *Ley 19.966. Projecto de ley: título I del régimen general de garantías en salud.* Ministerio de Salud [pdf]. Viewed July 14, 2014: http://webhosting.redsalud.gov.cl/minsal/archivos/guiasges/leyauge.pdf.

Retegan, C, Russell, C, Harris, D, Andrianopoulos, N & Beiles, CB 2013. 'Evaluating the value and impact of the Victorian audit of surgical mortality.' *ANZ Journal of Surgery*, vol. 83, no. 10, pp. 724–8.

Revans, RW (ed.) 1972. *Hospitals: Communication, Choice and Change.* Tavistock: London.

Review of Future Governance Arrangements for Safety and Quality in Health Care 2005. *National Arrangements for Safety and Quality of Health Care in Australia. The Report of the Review of Future Governance Arrangements for Safety and Quality in Health Care.* Australian Institute of Health and Welfare [online]. Viewed June 5, 2014: https://www.aihw.gov.au/WorkArea/DownloadAsset.aspx?id=6442472804&libID=6442472785.

Rigsrevisionen 2012. *Report to the Public Accounts Committee on the quality programmes at Danish hospitals.* Rigsrevisionen, February.

Ringard, Å, Brudvik, M, Krogstad, U & Lindahl AK 2012. 'Taxonomies of adverse events in hospitals–initial experiences of using WHO's classification system in Norway.' Poster presented at the International Society for Quality in Health Care 29th International Conference, Geneva.

Ringard, Å, Sagan, A, Saunes, IS & Lindahl, AK 2013. 'Norway: health systems review.' *Health Systems in Transition*, vol. 15, no. 8, pp. 1–164.

Rosen, B & Samuel, H 2009. 'Israel: health system review.' *Health Systems in Transition,* vol. 11, no. 2. European Observatory on Health Systems and Policies. World Health Organization, Regional Office for Europe [pdf]. Viewed February 2, 2013: http://www.euro.who.int/__data/assets/pdf_file/0007/85435/E92608.pdfht.

Rosen, B, Porath, A, Pawlson, LG, Chassin, MR & Benbassat, J 2011. 'Adherence to standards of care by health maintenance organizations in Israel and the USA.' *International Journal for Quality in Health Care*, Feb, vol. 23, no. 1, pp. 15–25.

Ruelas, E & Poblano, O 2007. *Certificación y Acreditación en los servicios de salud. Modelos, estrategias y logros en México y Latinoamérica.* 2nd edn. Instituto Nacional de Salud Pública: Morelos.

Ruelas, E & Querol, J 1994. *Calidad y eficiencia en las organizaciones de atención a la salud.* Fundación Mexicana para la Salud: Mexico City.

Ruelas, E 2006. 'Citizen's quality councils: an innovative mechanism for monitoring and providing social endorsement of healthcare providers' performance?' *Healthcare Papers*, vol. 6, no. 3, pp. 33–7.

Ruelas, E, Reyes, H, Zurita, B, Vidal, LM & Karchmer, S 1990. 'Círculos de calidad como estrategia de un programa de garantía de calidad.' *Salud Pública de México*, vol. 32, pp. 207–20.

Ryall, HT 2007. *Better, Sooner, More Convenient: Health Discussion Paper.* National Party of New Zealand: Wellington.

Ryall, T 2013. *Wellington Future Proofing Health Services in Wairoa.* Minister of Health [media release], New Zealand Government, November 22.

Ryall, T & Te Heuheu, G 2010. *Pacific PHO Begins Work on Integrated Health Centres.* Minister of Health and Minister of Pacific Island Affairs [media release], New Zealand Government, July 22.

Ryan, AM, Nallamothu, BK & Dimick, JB 2012. 'Medicare's public reporting initiative on hospital quality had modest or no impact on mortality from three key conditions.' *Health Affairs*, vol. 31, no. 3, pp. 585–92.

Sánchez Rodríguez, H & Nancuante Almonacid, U 2013. 'La judicialización no es el mayor problema de las ISAPRES: es un síntoma de un sector en crisis.' *Cuadernos Médico-Sociales (Chile)*, vol. 53, no. 1, pp. 49–60.

Sánchez Zinny, J 1979. *Acreditación hospitalaria sobre bases voluntarias. AMA Magazine*, no. III-IV, Buenos Aires.

Sandoval, G, Fernandez, O & Perez, JL 2013. 'Fonasa alerta a hospitales del país por aumento en lista de espera Auge.' *La Tercera* [online]. Viewed May 10, 2014: http://www.latercera.com/noticia/nacional/2013/08/680-539106-9-fonasa-alerta-a-hospitales-del-pais-por-aumento-en-lista-de-espera-auge.shtml.

Scally, G & Donaldson, L 1998. 'Clinical governance and the drive for quality improvement in the new NHS in England.' *British Medical Journal*, vol. 317, pp. 61–5.

Schilling, L, Dearing, JW, Staley, P, Harvey, P, Fahey, L & Kuruppu, F 2011. 'Kaiser Permanente's performance improvement system, Part 4: Creating a learning organization.' *Joint Commission Journal on Quality and Patient Safety*, vol. 37, no. 12, pp. 532–43.

Schoen, C & Osborn, R 2011. *The Commonwealth Fund 2011 International Health Policy Survey of Sicker Adults in Eleven Countries.* The Commonwealth Fund: New York.

Schön, DA 1971. *Beyond the Stable State: Public and Private Learning in a Changing Society.* Temple-Smith: London.

Schoon, M 2013. 'Impact of inter-facility transport on maternal mortality in the Free State.' *South African Medical Journal*, vol. 103, no. 8, pp. 534–7.

Schroeder, SA 2007. 'Shattuck Lecture. We can do better—improving the health of the American people.' *New England Journal of Medicine,* vol. 357, no. 12, pp. 1221–8.

Schumacher, A 2012. *Nasjonal plattform for ledelse i helseforetak.* Norwegian Ministry of Health and Care Services: Oslo.

Schwaber, MJ & Carmeli, Y 2014. 'An ongoing national intervention to contain the spread of carbapenem-resistant enterobacteriaceae.' *Clinical Infectious Diseases*, vol. 58, no. 5, pp. 697–703.

Scott, T, Mannion, R, Davies, HTO & Marshall, MN 2003. 'Implementing culture change in health care: Theory and practice.' *International Journal for Quality in Health Care*, vol. 15, no. 2, pp. 111–8.

Scott, WR 1987. 'The adolescence of institutional theory.' *Administrative Science Quarterly*, vol. 32, no. 4, pp. 493–511.

Scott, WR 2001. *Institutions and Organizations.* Sage: London.

Scottish Executive 2000. *Our National Health: A Plan for Action, a Plan for Change.* Scottish Executive: Edinburgh.

Scottish Executive 2001. *Patient Focus and Public Involvement.* Scottish Executive: Edinburgh.

Scottish Executive 2005. *Delivering for Health.* Scottish Executive: Edinburgh.

Scottish Government 2007. *Better Health, Better Care: Action Plan.* Scottish Government: Edinburgh.

Scottish Government 2010. *The Healthcare Quality Strategy for NHSScotland.* Scottish Government: Edinburgh.

Scottish Government 2011a. *The Scottish Health Survey. Topic Report: Obesity.* Scottish Government: Edinburgh.

Scottish Government 2011b. *Report on the Future Delivery of Public Services by the Commission (chaired by Dr Campbell Christie).* Scottish Government: Edinburgh.

Scottish Government 2011c. *Achieving Sustainable Quality in Scotland's Healthcare: A '20:20' Vision.* Scottish Government: Edinburgh.

Scottish Government 2012. *Charter of Patient Rights and Responsibilities.* Scottish Government: Edinburgh.

Scottish Government 2013a. *Public Bodies (Joint Working) (Scotland) Bill.* Scottish Government: Edinburgh.

Scottish Government 2013b. *NHSScotland Chief Executive's Annual report 2012/13.* Scottish Government [online]. Viewed December 30, 2013: http://www.scotland.gov.uk.

Scottish Government 2013c. *Scotland's Future: Your Guide to an Independent Scotland.* Scottish Government: Edinburgh.

Scottish Office 1989. *Working for Patients.* Scottish Office: Edinburgh.

Scottish Office 1997. *Designed to Care: Renewing the NHS in Scotland.* Scottish Office: Edinburgh.

Scottish Office 1998. *Clinical Governance. (MEL(75)1998).* Scottish Office: Edinburgh.

Scottish Public Health Observatory 2013. *Homepage.* Scottish Public Health Observatory [online]. Viewed December 30, 2013: http://www.scotpho.org.uk.

Secretaría de Salud 2001a. *Programa de Acción de la Cruzada Nacional por la Calidad de los Servicios de Salud.* Secretaría de Salud: Mexico City.

Secretaría de Salud 2001b. *Programa Nacional de Salud 2001–2006: La democratización de la salud en México: Hacia un sistema universal de salud.* Secretaría de Salud: Mexico City.

Selby, JV & Lipstein, SH 2014. 'PCORI at 3 years—Progress, lessons, and plans.' *New England Journal of Medicine*, vol. 370, no. 7, pp. 592–5.

Shaw, C, Braithwaite, J, Moldovan, M, Nicklin, W, Grgic, I, Fortune, T & Whittaker, S 2013. 'Profiling health-care accreditation organizations: an international survey.' *International Journal for Quality in Health Care*, vol. 25, no. 3, pp. 222–31.

Shekelle, PG 2013. 'Nurse-patient ratios as a patient safety strategy: a systematic review.' *Annals of Internal Medicine*, Mar 5, vol. 158, no. 5, pp. 404–9.

Shekelle, PG, Pronovost, PJ, Wachter, RM, McDonald, KM, Schoelles, K, Sydney, M, Dy, SM, Shojania, K, Reston, JT, Adams, AS, Peter, B, Angood, PB, Bates, DW, Bickman, L, Carayon, P, Donaldson, L, Duan, N, Farley, DO, Greenhalgh, T, Haughom, JL, Lake, E, Lilford, R, Lohr, KN, Meyer, GS, Miller, MR, Neuhauser, DV, Ryan, G, Saint, S, Shortell, SM, Stevens, DP & Walshe, K 2013. 'The top patient safety strategies that can be encouraged for adoption now.' *Annals of Internal Medicine,* vol. 158, no. 5, pp. 365–8.

Shields, L & Hartati, LE 2003. 'Nursing and health care in Indonesia.' *Health and Nursing Policy Issues*, vol. 44, no. 2, pp. 209–16.

Sicilani, L & Hurst, J 2004. 'Explaining waiting-time variations for elective surgery across OECD countries.' *OECD Economic Studies*, vol. 38, no. 1, pp. 96–122.

Siciliani, L & Hurst, J 2005. 'Tackling excessive waiting times for elective surgery: a comparative analysis of policies in 12 OECD countries.' *Health Policy,* vol. 72, no. 2, pp. 201–15.

Siegel-Itzkovich, J 2012. *Health Ministry Survey Rates Eleven State Hospitals.* The Jerusalem Post [online]. Viewed February 28, 2014: http://www.jpost.com/Health/Article.aspx?id=259406.

Smith, J 2009. *Critical Analysis of the Primary Health Care Strategy and Framing of Issues for the Next Phase.* Ministry of Health: Wellington.

Sodzi-Tettey, S 2012. 'Bright future for mental health in Ghana.' *Affirmatively Disruptive*, September 18 [blog]. Viewed March 15, 2014: http://www.sodzisodzi.com/?s=+mental+health+&searchsubmit.

Sodzi-Tettey, S 2014a. 'Health experts dissect President's address.' *Affirmatively Disruptive*, February 28 [blog]. Viewed March 15, 2014: http://www.sodzisodzi.com/?s=health+experts+dissect+&searchsubmit.

Sodzi-Tettey, S 2014b. *Report Guinea Worm Case for GH¢200*. GhanaWeb [online]. Viewed May 23, 2014: http://www.ghanaweb.com/GhanaHomePage/NewsArchive/artikel.php?ID=310371.

Sodzi-Tettey, S, Aikins, M, Awoonor-Williams, JK & Agyepong, IA 2012. 'Challenges in provider payment under the Ghana National Health Insurance Scheme: a case study of claims management in two districts.' *Ghana Medical Journal*, vol. 46, no. 4, pp.189–99.

Song, X 2009. 'Reflections on 60 years development of health insurance system in China: retrospect and prospect.' *Chinese Journal of Health Policy*, vol. 2, no. 10, pp. 6–13.

Soop, M, Fryksmark, U, Köster, M & Haglund, B 2009. 'The incidence of adverse events in Swedish hospitals: a retrospective medical record review study.' *International Journal for Quality in Health Care*, vol. 21, no. 4, pp. 285–91.

South African Nursing Council 2014. *Statistics of South African Nursing Council*. South African Nursing Council [online]. Viewed June 17, 2014: http://www.sanc.co.za/stats/stat2013/Distribution 2013.htm.

Spandonaro, F, Mennini, FS & Atella, V 2004. 'Criteri per l'allocazione regionale delle risorse per la sanità: riflessioni sul caso italiano.' *Politiche Sanitarie*, vol. 5, no. 1, pp. 27–32.

State Statistics Bureau & Ministry of Human Resources and Social Security 2003. *China Labour Statistical Yearbook*. State Statistics Bureau [online]. Viewed March 15, 2014: http://tongji.cnki.net/overseas/engnavi/HomePage.aspx?id=N2011010069&name=YZLDT&floor=1.

State Statistics Bureau & Ministry of Human Resources and Social Security 2010. *China Labour Statistical Yearbook*. State Statistics Bureau [online]. Viewed March 15, 2014: http://tongji.cnki.net/overseas/engnavi/HomePage.aspx?id=N2011010069&name=YZLDT&floor=1.

Statistics Norway 2014. *StatBank Norway*. Statistics Norway [online]. Viewed May 5, 2014: https://www.ssb.no/en/statistikkbanken.

Statistics South Africa 2011a. *Census 2011*. Statistics South Africa: Pretoria.

Statistics South Africa 2011b. *General Household Survey*. Statistics South Africa: Pretoria.

Statistisches Bundesamt (ed.) 2013. *Gesundheit–Personal*. Fachserie 12, Reihe 7.3.1. Statistisches Bundesamt: Wiesbaden.

Steel, D & Cylus, J 2012. 'United Kingdom (Scotland): Health System review.' *Health Systems in Transition*, vol. 14, no. 9, pp. 1–150.

Stockholms läns landsting 2013a. *Stockholm Healthcare Plan 2011–2018*. Stockholms läns landsting [online]. Viewed July 25, 2013: http://www.sll.se/sll/templates/NormalPage.aspx?id=61664ht.

Stockholms läns landsting 2013b. *Freedom to Choose*. Stockholms läns landsting [online]. Viewed July 30, 2013: http://www.vardguiden.se/Om-Vardguiden/Andra-sprak/English/Freedom-to-choose/.

342 *Healthcare Reform, Quality and Safety*

Sun, N 2012. 'Reflecting and prospecting of patient safety and medical risk early warning and monitoring system construction in China.' *Chinese Hospitals*, vol. 16, no. 10, pp. 2–6.

Sveriges Kommuner och Landsting 2009. *Swedish Health Care in Transition – Structure and Methods for Better Results.* Sveriges Kommuner och Landsting: Stockholm.

Sveriges Kommuner och Landsting 2010. Översyn av de nationella kvalitetsregistren. Guldgruvan i hälso- och sjukvården. Förslag till gemensam satsning 2011–2015. Sveriges Kommuner och Landsting: Stockholm.

Sveriges Kommuner och Landsting 2011. *Produktivitet och effektivitet i hälso- och sjukvården. Jämförelse mellan landsting.* Sveriges Kommuner och Landsting: Stockholm.

Sveriges Kommuner och Landsting 2013. *Quality and Efficiency in Swedish Health Care–Regional Comparisons.* Sveriges Kommuner och Landsting [online]. Viewed May 10, 2014: http://english.skl.se/activities/open_comparisons/compareht.

Sveriges Riksdag 2012. *Freedom of Choice throughout Sweden.* Sveriges Riksdag [online]. Viewed June 10, 2014: http://www.riksdagen.se/sv/Dokument-Lagar/Forslag/Motioner/Valfrihet-i-hela-Sverige_H002So441/.

Swedish Competition Authority 2010. *Omregleringen av apoteksmarknaden–redovisning av ett regeringsuppdrag.* Konkurrensverket: Stockholm.

Tan, J, Wen, HJ & Awad, N 2005. 'Health care and services delivery systems as complex adaptive systems.' *Communications of the ACM,* vol. 48, no. 5, pp. 36–44.

Teasdale, G 2002. 'Learning from Bristol: Report of the public inquiry into children's heart surgery at Bristol Royal Infirmary 1984–1995.' *British Journal of Neurosurgery,* vol. 16, no. 3, pp. 211–6.

The Economist 2012. 'Rethinking the welfare state: Asia's next revolution.' *The Economist,* September 8.

The Treasury 2013. *Key Facts for Taxpayers.* The Treasury [online]. Viewed March 5, 2014: http://www.treasury.govt.nz/budget/2013/taxpayersht.

Thompson, G 2009. *Health Expenditure: International Comparisons, Standard Note: SN/SG/2584.* House of Commons Library: London.

Thorlby, R & Maybin, J (eds) 2010. *A High-Performing NHS? A Review of Progress 1997–2010.* King's Fund: London.

Tilman, D, Cassman, KG, Matson, PA, Naylor, R & Polasky, S 2002. 'Agricultural sustainability and intensive production practices.' *Nature,* vol. 418, pp. 671–7.

Timmins, N 2001. *The Five Giants.* HarperCollins: London.

Timmins, N 2012. *Never Again.* Kings Fund: London.

TNS New Zealand 2013. *Assessing the Demand for Elective Surgery amongst New Zealanders.* Health Funds Association of New Zealand and New Zealand Private Surgical Hospitals Association: Wellington.

Tollman, SM 1994. 'The Pholela Health Centre—The origins of community-oriented primary health care (COPC). An appreciation of the work of Sidney and Emily Kar.' *South African Medical Journal*, vol. 84, no. 10, pp. 653–8.

Topham-Kindley, L 2013. 'They love you, they love you not: DHBs and primary care.' *New Zealand Doctor,* April 24. MIMLtd: Auckland.

Tukuitonga, C 1999. *Primary Healthcare for Pacific People in New Zealand.* National Advisory Committee on Health and Disability: Wellington.

Tuohy, CH 1999. *Accidental Logics: The Dynamics of Change in the Health Care Arena in the United States.* Oxford University Press: New York.

Unger, JP, De Paepe, P, Solimano, G & Arteaga, O 2008. 'Chile's neoliberal health reform: An assessment and a critique.' *PLoS Medicine*, vol. 5, no. 4, p. e79.

University of Health and Allied Sciences 2012. *Homepage.* University of Health and Allied Sciences [online]. Viewed May 23, 2014: http://www.uhas.edu.gh/.

US Congress 2010. The *Patient Protection* and Affordable Care Act, Mar 23. Pub. L. No. 111-148, 124 *Stat.* 119.

US Department of Health and Human Services 2014. *Healthcare Homepage.* US Department of Health and Human Services [online]. Viewed February 6, 2014: http://www.HHS.gov/HealthCare.

van der Weyden, MB 2004. 'The "Cam affair:" An isolated incident or destined to be repeated?' *The Medical Journal of Australia*, vol. 180, no. 3, pp. 100–1.

van der Weyden, MB 2005. 'The Bundaberg Hospital scandal: The need for reform in Queensland and beyond.' *The Medical Journal of Australia*, vol. 183, no. 6, pp. 284–5.

VanLare, JM & Conway, PH 2012. 'Value-based purchasing—National programs to move from volume to value.' *New England Journal of Medicine*, vol. 367, no. 4, pp. 292–5.

Vasselli, S, Filippetti, G & Spizzichino, L 2005. *Misurare la performance del sistema sanitario. Proposta di una metodologia.* Il Pensiero Scientifico Editore, p. 214.

Velasquez, MS 2012. 'Política de Acreditación de Calidad en Salud en Chile: objetivos y desafíos.' Presentation at 2° Encuentro Internacional de Salud en Chile EISACH-Expo Hospital 2012, June 29. Superintendencia de Salud, Ministerio de Salud: Santiago de Chile.

Vettore, L 2008. 'Ragionando sulla storia dell'ECM'. *Dialogo sui farmaci,* vol. 1, pp. 20–22.

Vincent, C, Burnett, S & Carthey, J 2013. *The Measurement and Monitoring of Safety.* Health Foundation: London.

Waddington, CJ & Enyimayew, KA 1989. 'A price to pay: The impact of user charges in Ashanti-Akim district, Ghana.' *International Journal of Health Planning and Management*, vol. 4, pp. 17–47.

Walley, J, Lawn, JE, Tinker, A, de Francisco, A, Chopra, M, Rudan, I, Bhutta, ZA & Black, RE 2008. 'Primary health care: Making Alma-Ata a reality.' *The Lancet,* vol. 372, no. 9642, pp. 1001–7.

Walshe, K 2009. 'Pseudoinnovation: The development and spread of healthcare quality improvement methodologies.' *International Journal for Quality in Health Care,* vol. 21, no. 3, pp. 153–9.

Wendt, C 2014. 'Changing healthcare system types.' *Social Policy and Administration* [online]. Viewed June 10, 2014: http://dx.doi.org/10.1111/ spol.12061.

Wikipedia 2013. *Healthcare in Sweden.* Wikipedia [online]. Viewed June 10, 2014: http://en.wikipedia.org/wiki/Healthcare_in_Sweden.

Wilsford, D 1994. 'Path dependency, or why history makes it difficult but not impossible to reform health care systems in a big way.' *Journal of Public Policy,* vol. 14, no. 3, pp. 251–83.

Wilson, RM, Runciman, WB, Gibberd, RW, Harrison, BT, Newby, L & Hamilton, JD 1995. 'The Quality in Australian Health Care Study.' *Medical Journal of Australia*, vol. 163, no. 9, pp. 458–71.

Winblad, U & Andersson, C 2010. *The Medical Profession and Waiting Times for Patients.* Report from an expert group ESO. Finansdepartementet: Stockholm.

Winful, EA 2010. *Speech Delivered by GMA President at the 52nd Annual General Conference, Ghana Medical Association.* News, Modern Ghana [online]. Viewed June 5, 2014: http://www.modernghana.com/news/303609/1/use-oil-revenue-to-support-nhis.html.

Worldatlas n.d. *Planet Earth.* Worldatlas [online]. Viewed June 10, 2014: http:// www.worldatlas.com/aatlas/infopage/earth.htmht.

World Bank 2011. *PNG Health Workforce Crisis: A Call to Action.* World Bank [online]. Viewed March 18, 2014: http://www.worldbank.org/en/news/ feature/2013/04/26/papua-new-guinea-health-workforce-crisis-a-call-to-action.

World Bank 2014a. *Data, Land Area (sq. km).* World Bank Group [online]. Viewed May 13, 2014: http://data.worldbank.org/indicator/AG.LND.TOTL.K2.

World Bank 2014b. *GDP (Current US$).* World Bank Group [online]. Viewed May 13, 2014: http://data.worldbank.org/indicator/NY.GDP.MKTP.CD/ countries?order=wbapi_data_value_2012 wbapi_data_value wbapi_data_ value-last&sort=desc&display=default.

World Bank 2014c. *Gross National Income per Capita 2012, Atlas Method and PPP.* World Development Indicators database, World Bank Group [pdf]. Viewed May 7, 2014: http://databank.worldbank.org/data/download/GNIPC. pdf.

World Health Organization 2000. *Health Systems: Improving Performance.* The World Health Report 2000. WHO: Geneva.

World Health Organization 2002. *Quality of Care: Patient Safety.* Report by the Secretariat to the Fifty-Fifth World Health Assembly, A55/13, March 23. World Health Organization: Geneva.

World Health Organization 2007. *Patient Safety Solutions.* World Health Organization [online]. Viewed May 1, 2014: http://www.who.int/mediacentre/ news/releases/2007/pr22/en/.

World Health Organization 2008. *WHO Country Cooperation Strategy 2007–2011—Indonesia*. WHO Regional Office for South East Asia: New Delhi.

World Health Organization 2011a. *Global Status Report on Noncommunicable Diseases 2010*. World Health Organization [online]. Viewed June 10, 2014: http://whqlibdoc.who.int/publications/2011/9789240686458_eng.pdf?ua=1.

World Health Organization 2011b. *mHealth: New Horizons for Health through Mobile Technologies: Based on the Findings of the Second Global Survey on eHealth*. Global Observatory for eHealth Series, vol. 3. World Health Organization: Geneva.

World Health Organization 2012. *Global Tuberculosis Report 2012*. World Health Organization: Geneva.

World Health Organization 2013a. *World Health Statistics 2013*. World Health Organization: Geneva.

World Health Organization 2013b. *Country Summaries: Papua New Guinea Key Indicators*. World Health Organization [online]. Viewed May 13, 2014: http://apps.who.int/gho/data/node.cco.

World Health Organization 2014a. *Countries*. World Health Organization [online]. Viewed May 13, 2014: http://www.who.int/countries/en/.

World Health Organization 2014b. *Global Health Expenditure Database*. World Health Organization [online]. Viewed June 17, 2014: http://apps.who.int/nha/database/ViewData/Indicators/en.

World Population Review 2014. *China Population 2014*. World Population Review [online]. Viewed June 19, 2014: http://worldpopulationreview.com/countries/china-population/.

Zimlichman, E & Bates, DW 2012. 'National patient safety initiatives: Moving beyond what is necessary.' *Israel Journal of Health Policy Research*, vol. 1, no. 1, p. 20.

Zimlichman, E, Rozenblum, R & Millenson, ML 2013. 'The road to patient experience of care measurement: Lessons from the United States.' *Israel Journal of Health Policy Research*, vol. 2, no. 1, p. 35.

Zohar, D, Livne, Y, Orly, T, Admi, H & Donchin, Y 2007. 'Healthcare climate: A framework for measuring and improving patient safety.' *Critical Care Medicine*, vol. 35, no. 5, pp. 1312–7.

Zohar, D & Luria, G 2005. 'A multilevel model of safety climate: Cross-level relationships between organization and group-level climates.' *Journal of Applied Psychology*, vol. 90, no. 4, pp. 616–28.

Index